Palpation and Assessment Skills

Please retu.

For Churchill Livingstone:

Editorial Director: Mary Law
Project Development Manager: Katrina Mather
Project Manager: Wendy Gardiner
Design: Judith Wright
Illustrations Manager: Bruce Hogarth

Palpation and Assessment Skills

Assessment Through Touch

with accompanying CD-ROM

Leon Chaitow ND DO
Osteopathic Practitioner and Senior Lecturer, University of Westminster, London, UK

Foreword by

Viola M Frymann DO FAAO FCA MBBS MFHOM
Osteopathic Center for Children,
San Diego, California, USA

Illustrated by

Graeme Chambers BA (Hons)
Medical Artist

SECOND EDITION

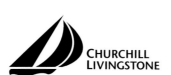

CHURCHILL
LIVINGSTONE

EDINBURGH LONDON NEW YORK OXFORD PHILADELPHIA ST LOUIS SYDNEY TORONTO 2003

CHURCHILL LIVINGSTONE
An imprint of Elsevier Limited

First edition 1997
Second edition 2003
    Reprinted 2004, 2006, 2007 (twice)

ISBN 978 0 443 07218 5

British Library Cataloguing in Publication Data
A catalogue record for this book is available from the British Library

Library of Congress Cataloguing in Publication Data
A catalogue record for this book is available from the Library of Congress

Note
Medical knowledge is constantly changing. Standard safety precautions must be followed, but as new research and clinical experience broaden our knowledge, changes in treatment and drug therapy may become necessary or appropriate. Readers are advised to check the most current product information provided by the manufacturer of each drug to be administered to verify the recommended dose, the method and duration of administration, and contraindications. It is the responsibility of the practitioner, relying on experience and knowledge of the patient, to determine dosages and the best treatment for each individual patient. Neither the Publisher nor the author assumes any liability for any injury and/or damage to persons or property arising from this publication.

Contents

The CD-ROM accompanying this text includes video sequences of all the techniques indicated by the ⊚ icon. To look at the video for a given technique, click on the relevant icon on the CD-ROM. The CD-ROM is designed to be used in conjunction with the text and not as a stand-alone product.

Foreword

The encroachment of technology into diagnosis and treatment threatens to erode the long-established field of touch. But every mother knows the comforting healing impulse of her hand on her troubled child and many proxy grandmothers are being recruited into the neonatal nurseries to hold, and tenderly touch, abandoned babies, comfort and reassure them and enhance their weight gain and development. Intuition is the teacher of these mothers and grandmothers. May the intuitive dimension never depart from the physician and therapists regardless of technology. Perish the day when a robot arm will be 'less expensive', 'more available' and 'more enduring' than the compassionate ministrations of a nurse's or physician's hands.

A. T. Still abandoned the practice of medicine after three members of his immediate family died of spinal meningitis despite the best care that his profession had to offer. Before that his distress began in finding himself helpless before the ravages of acute illness which decimated his soldiers during the Civil War. But he reasoned that if God had permitted such diseases, he had also provided answers to them. So his research began. A diligent detailed study of human anatomy led him to the recognition that structure governs function, and efficient healthy function is dependent upon precisely integrated structure. Furthermore, the patient is a total being, a dynamic unit of function. Thus life and matter can be united but that union cannot continue with any hindrance to free and absolute motion. Thus motion is the fundamental function of the living body. As a result the inevitable conclusion must be that diseases are only effects. These are the central conclusions of A. T. Still as osteopathy came into being.

Structural integrity and its potential for physiologic motion inspired William Garner Sutherland in his studies of the cranial mechanism following the incredible thought given to him about the sphenosquamous articulation – 'beveled like the gills of a fish for respiratory motion of an articular mechanism.' As with his original teacher Dr Still, Sutherland embarked on an intensive study of cranial anatomy – bone, membrane, fluid and nervous system and their extensions through the spinal mechanism to the sacrum.

Eventually, came the recognition of the continuity of intracranial and intraspinal membranes with the fascial system of the body, the recognition of the relationship between cerebrospinal fluid and the lymphatic system thus returning to the dynamic unity of the whole patient.

Motion is the measure between health and dysfunction, between vitality and fatigue, between joy and despair, and ultimately between life and death. Motion may be external, visible, voluntarily initiated, limited by pathology or enhanced by diligent training. Its dimension provides a valuable record of the state of the musculoskeletal system today and the progress manifested in response to the therapeutic modality.

The far greater field of motion of vital significance to the health and well-being of our patients, however, is inherent, invisible, subtle in its dimensions and continuous whether awake or asleep as long as life persists. Food that enters the mouth is digested, assimilated, selectively absorbed or eliminated as it passes down the extensive digestive system. Blood is pumped from the heart to be oxygenated by the lungs and thence dynamically distributed to every cell in the body from the scalp to the toe. The reproductive system has its own inherent rhythmic motion from its preparatory monthly cycle until such time as the intense inherent motility of the sperm fertilises the ovum at the exact right time and a rapid motile developmental panorama of events is set in motion until such time as a fully developed newborn is propelled by a powerful rhythmic cycle of activity out into the external world. The water system is efficiently maintained by the inherent rhythmic activity of the renal system. Each of these internal, invisible, involuntary systems functions quietly and effectively so long as there is no disturbance, diversion or interruption in its remarkable involuntary rhythmic motion.

But the respiratory system has some unique characteristics. It has an inherent, involuntary rhythm highly sensitive to the gaseous composition of the atmospheric air, and to fluctuating oxygen demands of the inner physiology. It may be interrupted voluntarily for a period of time, the duration of which is ultimately determined by another inherent rhythm, which will never be interrupted as long as life persists, and which is beyond the will to control for it is the primary respiratory mechanism (PRM) (see p. 51).

Becker (p 201–207) provides vivid directions for palpating these inherent rhythms, the diagnostic touch whereby he searches for what the patient's body wants to tell him. The potency within the patient and the fulcrum established by the operator need to be understood if Becker is to be fully appreciated. But what are we palpating? (p. 202)

Inherent slow rhythmic motion of the central nervous system has been known for generations and was in fact first described by Magendie in 1845. However, Sutherland also recognised the motion of the cerebrospinal fluid, a slow rhythmic fluctuating motion. His initial inspired thought concerning respiratory motion of an articular mechanism prompted an intensive study of all the bones of the cranium and the dural membranes which bind them together and reciprocally integrate their motion. The palpation of cranial motion has been reported in patients of all ages. This rhythmic motion of the cranial bones was recorded in 1971 (VF). Skull bone motion may be considered as very small comparative changes of the position of bones at their sutures: the mobility of skull bones is in fact localised in sutures. Rhythmic periodicity of skull bone motion of 6–15 cycles/minutes has been clearly demonstrated (Chaitow 1999; Moskalenko 2000).

Understanding the PRM underlying these bone motions requires a recognition of the nature of the inherent forces, namely fluctuation of vascular tone and the replacement of cerebrospinal fluid inside the cranial cavity and between the cranial and spinal cavities. Still declared that 'the rule of the artery is supreme but the cerebrospinal fluid is in command.' Transcranial Dopplerography integrated with Bioelectrical Impedance have substantiated this, but have also demonstrated conclusively that skilfully applied therapeutic touch can enhance the CV and CSF motility. Following from this fundamental basis of the PRM its activity can be described by the complex of objective parameters as well as from the results of spectrum analysis which is the most adequate method for the analysis of slow fluctuations with changeable frequency and amplitude (Moskalenko 2001). It is the relation of these control links with different time constants that support brain metabolic supply and water balance of brain tissue. They are responsible for motion of the brain tissue and skull bone motion. As Still stated long ago, the brain is the dynamo.

Functional palpation, the evaluation of this primary respiratory mechanism is the essential sequel to structural palpation. It provides a vital measure of the level of wellness of this person, the potential for positive change in the inherent physiology. It may reveal underlying etiologies and the appropriate strategy for addressing them. Structural palpation with the precise recognition described in this text will provide a picture of the traumatic forces and their consequences which have caused the problems presented by the patient. Functional palpation, through the inherent motility of the PRM, provides wisdom concerning the therapeutic potential, the inherent therapeutic potency of the physician within this patient. Develop those 'thinking, feeling, seeing, knowing fingers' and then 'be up and touching' (Sutherland).

San Diego, CA, USA   Viola M. Frymann

REFERENCES

Chaitow L 1999 Cranial manipulation: theory and practice. Churchill Livingstone, Edinburgh
Moskalenko Y 2000 Physiologic of mechanism of slow fluctuations inside the cranium. Part 2. Osteo 51: 4–11
Moskalenko Y, Weinstein GB 2001 Development of current concepts of physiology of cerebral circulation: a comparative analysis. Journal of Evolution Biochemistry and Physiology 37: 492–605

Preface

How can the practitioner/therapist, using manual methods of treatment, best learn to evaluate accurately the status of the tissues being palpated or assessed? How are the best skills acquired to achieve effective extraction of knowledge and information from living tissue, via touch?

The answer to these two questions is simple: by application (and repetition) of hundreds of carefully designed exercises that are capable of refining palpation skills to an astonishing degree of sensitivity. As Frymann (1963) has said: 'Palpation cannot be learned by reading or listening; it can only be learned by palpation.' This learning process is not just about hard dedicated labour; it should be fun and it should be exciting. The thrills to be experienced when taking this journey of exploration of the tissues of the human body is hopefully contagious; as an example see Ida Rolf's words in chapter 1.

Leaving aside non-specific, 'wellness' massage, and similar approaches that are designed to have an overall constitutional, relaxing or stimulating influence, it is safe to say that manual treatment, if it is to have a therapeutic effect, should ideally relate to the particular perceived needs of the tissues, region or person concerned. Haphazard, unstructured, manual approaches are unlikely to achieve optimal results.

So, determination of the *needs* of the tissues, and of the person, are paramount. Whether the objective is mobilisation of a joint; restoration of joint play or range of motion; release of tense, shortened structures; enhanced circulation to, or drainage of, needy tissues; toning of weak or inhibited musculature; deactivation of trigger points, or other pain modulating initiative, or any of a range of other 'bodywork' approaches, it is axiomatic that there should be in place an adequate degree of awareness of the nature and current level of dysfunction, as well as an ability to compare this current state with whatever is conceived of as 'normal', before treatment commences. The decisions made as to what form and degree of treatment to offer will always depend on the training and belief system of the practitioner/therapist, responding to information gathered through history-taking, palpation, observation and assessment.

Whatever the system of treatment, any local findings (muscle, joint, etc.), naturally enough, need to be related to the needs and status of the person as a whole, before treatment starts. In Chapter 9 examples are given of assessment methods by means of which the current ability of the individual to respond favourably or unfavourably to treatment can be assessed, based on criteria relating to the degree of adaptive compensation/decompensation evident in the tissues. In some therapeutic systems – take as an example cranial osteopathy (and/or craniosacral, sacro-occipital therapies – see Chapter 6) or neuromuscular therapy (see Chapter 5) – assessment and treatment are virtually synchronous, with responses to what is being palpated determining the immediate therapeutic input.

Whether palpation and assessment is used to build a clinical picture from which treatment flows, or whether assessment/palpation and treatment are simultaneous, what is evaluated offers the basis for the intervention, a yardstick by means of which to measure progress, a documentable, ideally measurable, foundational (to the therapeutic endeavour) record of the current state of the target tissues.

The ability of a skilled practitioner to switch from palpation/assessment to treatment and back again, seamlessly, marks out the truly skilled individual. As discussed in the Preface to the first edition of this book, in 1997, this ability is often spoken of as an *intuitive* approach. Intuition in this sense is not a vague esoteric phenomenon, but rather a demonstration of 'knowing in action' (Schon 1984) in which apparently spontaneous therapeutic skills emerge from a background of deep understanding and refined actions, acquired by diligent practice.

Clearly much such evaluation can now be performed using technology. Patients can be photographed, video'd, scanned, X-rayed and in a multitude of other ways investigated as to the current state of their structures, functions and dysfunctions. Biotechnology is advancing by leaps and bounds, and tools and equipment, previously only available in hospital and major clinic settings, are increasingly available to the individual practitioner and therapist, to assist in the clinical application of such methods.

So is the ancient art of palpation becoming redundant? Are assessments involving subjective judgement, old-fashioned and inaccurate?

In recent years the value of palpation has been challenged, with research studies suggesting that reproducible results cannot always be demonstrated when the accuracy of palpation is tested. The reliability of palpation performed by individuals, as well as the degree of agreement between experts palpating the same patient, or tissues, is increasingly questioned. These issues, as well as the suggested remedies for individuals as well as for teaching and training organisations, are explored in Chapter 2.

The truth is that as with the acquisition of any skill there are a number of variables that can determine whether the outcome is a skilled individual or not. These variables include:

- the quality of the teaching of the skill, particularly the tactics and methods used in hands-on practice;
- the degree of application and practice (amount of time, number of repetitions, as well as the degree of focus and thought, given to particular tasks and methods, etc.) that the person brings to skill acquisition; and
- the underlying depth of knowledge of anatomy, physiology and patho-physiology to which the findings can be applied, and from which deductions and conclusions can be drawn.

This book contains a distillation of the methods and thoughts of hundreds of wonderfully skilled individuals, from diverse therapeutic backgrounds. The commonality that emerges is that despite the doubts expressed as to the value of palpation (see Chapter 2), there is no equivalent in technology to replace what can be gleaned from truly skilful hands-on touch and assessment methods.

You are recommended to work through the book, chapter by chapter, exercise by exercise (more than once), recording your findings and refining your skills. This is as relevant to the student as to the person currently in active practice, for we should never cease striving for even better subtlety of palpatory literacy.

REFERENCES

Frymann V 1963 Palpation: its study in the workshop. Academy of Applied Osteopathy Yearbook, pp. 16–30
Schon D 1984 In: Christensen C, Hansen A (eds) Teaching by the case method. Harvard Business School, Boston, MA.

London 2003   LC

Dedication

This book and the tradition it represents is dedicated with profound and sincere thanks to the pioneers – osteopaths, chiropractors, physiotherapists, massage therapists, doctors of physical medicine, researchers into the field of human health – past and present, who inspired it and from whom I have drawn so much in its writing; in particular to: Beryl Arbuckle, Myron Beal, Alan Becker, Rollin Becker, CA Bowles, Boris Chaitow, Frank Chapman, Bertrand DeJarnette, Elizabeth Dicke, Jiri and Vaclav Dvorak, Clyde Ford, Viola Frymann, George Goodheart, Philip Greenman, Gregory Grieve, Laurie Hartman, Marshall Hoag, HV Hoover, Vladimir Janda, William Johnstone, Lawrence Jones, Brugh Joy, Deane Juhan, Dolores Krieger, Freddie Kaltenborn, Irvin Korr, Philip Latey, Karel Lewit, Stanley Lief, Harold Magoun, Carl McConnell, Fred Mitchell Jr., Raymond Nimmo, Charles Owen, Marion Rosen, Ida Rolf, David Simons, Fritz Smith, Edward Stiles, WG Sutherland, Andrew Taylor Still, R McFarlane Tilley, Janet Travell, John Upledger, Paul Van Allen, Dewananchand Varma, William Walton – and to those many others I have not listed, whose work has been credited in the text.

Glossary

AC	acromioclavicular
AMT	adverse mechanical tension
AP	anteroposterior
ASIS	anterior superior iliac spine
CNS	central nervous system
CSF	cerebrospinal fluid
CTM	connective tissue massage
F-AB-ER-E	flexion-abduction-external rotation-extension
FMS	fibromyalgia syndrome
GAS	general adaptation syndrome
HSZ	hyperalgesic skin zone
HVS	hyperventilation syndrome
LAS	local adaptation syndrome
MET	muscle energy technique
MI	mechanical interface
NMT	neuromuscular technique
PKB	prone knee bending
PNF	passive neck flexion
PSIS	posterior superior iliac spine
PPP	periosteal pain point
SI	sacroiliac
SLR	straight leg raising
SOT	sacrooccipital technique
TCC	thermal conducting coefficient
TCM	Traditional Chinese Medicine
TFL	tensor fascia lata
TMJ	temporomandibular joint
TP	trigger point
TR	thermoreceptor
ULTT	upper limb tension test

SPECIAL TOPIC 1
Using appropriate pressure (and the MPI)

When palpating lightly, advice varies as to how to learn to achieve appropriate levels of contact pressure. Upledger (Upledger & Vredevoogd 1983) speaks of 5 grams of pressure, which is very light indeed. Many experts advise discovering how hard you can press on your own (closed) eyeball before discomfort starts, as a means of learning just how lightly to press. Other advice includes keeping an eye on the degree of blanching of the nailbed, to ensure uniformity of pressure.

In truth, the art of palpation, and of using applied pressure, requires sensitivity, involving awareness of when tissue tension/resistance is being 'met' and when overcome. This is particularly important in the evaluation mode of neuromuscular technique (see Chapter 5).

When we palpate more deeply or apply digital pressure to a tender point in order to ascertain its status ('Does it hurt?', 'Does it refer?', etc.), it is important to have some way of knowing that the pressure being applied is uniform. For example, when assessing people with the symptoms of fibromyalgia, the criteria for a diagnosis depend upon 11 of 18 designated sites testing as positive (i.e. hurting severely), on application of 4 kilograms of pressure (American College of Rheumatologists 1990). If it takes more than 4 kg of pressure to produce pain, the point does not count in the tally.

The question then is, how does a person learn to apply 4 kg of pressure, and no more? It has been shown that, using a simple technology (such as bathroom scales), physical therapy students could be taught to accurately produce specific degrees of pressure on request. Students were tested applying posteroanterior pressure force to lumbar tissues. After training, using bathroom scales to evaluate pressure levels, the students showed significantly reduced error, both immediately after training as well as a month later (Keating et al 1993).

The term 'pressure threshold' is used to describe the least amount of pressure required to produce a report of pain and/or referred symptoms when a trigger point is compressed (Hong et al 1996). It is obviously useful to know how much pressure is required to produce pain and/or referred symptoms and whether this degree of pressure is different before and after treatment or at a subsequent clinical encounter (see Pain Index discussion below). Without a measuring device such as an algometer there would be no accurate means of achieving, or measuring, a standardised degree of pressure application. An algometer is a hand-held, spring-loaded, rubber-tipped, pressure-measuring device, which offers a means of achieving standardised pressure application. Using an algometer, sufficient pressure to produce pain is applied to palpated or preselected points, at a precise 90° angle to the skin. The measurement is taken when pain is reported.

Baldry (referring to research by Fischer) discusses algometer use (he calls it a 'pressure threshold meter') and suggests it should be employed to measure the degree of pressure required to produce symptoms, 'before and after deactivation of a trigger point, for when this is successful, the pressure threshold over the trigger point increases by about 4 kg' (Baldry 1993, Fischer 1988).

Valuable as it is in research and in training pressure sensitivity, use of an algometer is not really practical in everyday clinical work. It is, however, an important tool in research, as an objective measurement of a change in the degree of pressure required to produce symptoms. It also helps a practitioner to train themselves to apply a standardised degree of pressure when treating and to 'know' how hard they are pressing.

MPI

One use of an algometer is in order to identify a 'myofascial pain index' (MPI). This is an objective base which is calculated from the patient's subjective pain reports, when pressure is applied to test points. The calculation of the MPI determines the average degree of pressure required to evoke pain in a trigger or tender point.

Using an algometer, pressure is applied to each of the points being tested (which could be the 18 fibromyalgia test points) or, more logically, a selection of active trigger points identified by standard palpation. Pressure is applied, using the algometer, at a precise 90° angle to the skin, sufficient to produce pain, with the pressure measurement being taken when this is reported. The values are recorded and then averaged, producing a number which is the MPI. This allows comparison at a later stage to see whether the trigger point requires greater pressure to produce pain, indicating that it is less active, or the same or less pressure, indicating that it has not changed or is more sensitive.

REFERENCES

American College of Rheumatologists 1990 Criteria for the classification of fibromyalgia. Arthritis and Rheumatism 33:160–172

Baldry P 1993 Acupuncture trigger points and musculoskeletal pain. Churchill Livingstone, Edinburgh

Fischer A 1988 Documentation of muscle pain and soft tissue pathology. In: Kraus H (ed) Diagnosis and treatment of muscle pain. Quintessence, Chicago

Hong C-Z, Chen Y-N, Twehouse D, Hong D 1996 Pressure threshold for referred pain by compression on trigger point and adjacent area. Journal of Musculoskeletal Pain 4(3):61–79

Keating J, Matuyas T, Bach T 1993 The effect of training on physical therapist's ability to apply specified forces of palpation. Physical Therapy 73(1):38–46

Upledger J, Vredevoogd J 1983 Craniosacral Therapy. Eastland Press, Seattle

1

Objective – palpatory literacy

It is axiomatic that practitioners who use their hands to manipulate soft or bony structures should be able, accurately and relatively swiftly, to feel, assess and judge the state of a wide range of physiological and pathological conditions and parameters, relating not only to the tissues with which they are in touch but others associated with these, perhaps lying at greater depth. The information a practitioner needs to gather will vary according to the therapeutic approach; it might be the range of motion and the feel of joint play, the relative weakness or tightness in muscles, the amount of induration, oedema or fibrosis in soft tissues, identification of regions in which reflex activity is operating or even differences in the quality of perceived 'energy' variations in regions of the body.

Karel Lewit (1999) sums up a major problem in learning to palpate:

Palpation is the basis of our diagnostic techniques [and yet] it is extremely difficult to describe exactly, in words, the information palpation provides.

We will try, nevertheless, to do just this, with the help of numerous experts from a variety of disciplines, all the while keeping in mind the words of Viola Frymann (1963):

Palpation cannot be learned by reading or listening; it can only be learned by palpation.

Much of this book comprises descriptions of various forms of palpation, highlighting different ways in which this may be best achieved, along with numerous examples of exercises which can help in the development of perceptive exploratory skills. Of course, what we make of the information we derive from palpation will depend upon how it fits into a larger diagnostic picture, which needs to be built up from case history taking and other forms of assessment. Such interpretation is naturally essential in order for treatment to have any direction; palpation is anything but an end in itself. However, interpretation of the information derived from palpation is not a major purpose of this text; the main purpose is learning to palpate. (This concentration on the process of learning to palpate is not because interpretation of information is regarded as being of only secondary importance – for it is not – but because to have ventured too far into that realm would have expanded the text to an unmanageable size.)

For example, in Chapter 3, which deals with the assessment of skin tone elasticity, we will discover how to make an accurate assessment of local or general areas in which there is a relative loss of the skin's ability to stretch due to reflex activity. The section therefore deals with the art of palpation of these particular tissues in terms of this particular characteristic (elasticity, adherence). What the finding of local skin 'tightness' may actually mean in terms of pathological or physiological responses, and what to do about it, will also be touched on in terms of the opinion of various experts, but it is not possible to give a comprehensive survey of all possible opinions on the topic.

In other words, the individual practitioner will have to fit the acquired information into their own belief system and use it in accordance with their own therapeutic methodology. The aim of the book is to help in identifying what is under our hands.

We can equate palpation with learning to make sense of some other form of information, say that relating to music. It is possible to learn to read music, to understand its structure, the theory of harmony, tones and chords and even something of the application of such knowledge to different forms of composition. However, this would not enable us to play an instrument. The instrument that therapists play is the human body and the development of palpatory literacy allows us to 'read' that body.

One of osteopathy's major figures, Frederick Mitchell Jr (1976), makes a different comparison when he equates the learning of palpatory literacy with that of visual literacy.

> Visual literacy is developed in visual experiences, and the exercise of visual perceptions in making judgments. Visual judgments and perceptions may be qualitative, or quantitative, or both. Although the objectives in training the diagnostic senses do not include aesthetic considerations, aesthetic experiences probably are developmental in terms of visual literacy. In making aesthetic value judgments one must be able to discriminate between straight lines and crooked lines, perfect circles and distorted circles . . . To evaluate the level of sensory literacy, one may (also) test for specific sensory skills in a testing situation.

In later chapters I will suggest ways in which this can be done.

Assumptions and paradoxes

The assumption is made that the reader has at least a basic knowledge of anatomy and physiology, and, ideally, of pathology. It is necessary to emphasise that we must distinguish between what we are palpating, what we actually sense, and the way we interpret the information thus gained. It is all too easy for practitioners (even those with wide experience) to feel what they 'want' to feel or what they expect to feel. A relative degree of detachment from the process of assessment is therefore helpful, if not essential.

An open mind is also vital to the task of learning palpatory literacy; those practitioners with the greatest degree of 'rigidity' in terms of their training and the system of therapy they follow often have the hardest time in allowing themselves to sense new feelings and become aware of new sensations. Those with the most open, eclectic approaches (massage therapists are a prime example) usually find it easiest to 'trust' their senses and feelings.

The other side of the coin is the fact that many (though by no means all) such 'open' therapists also have the poorest knowledge of anatomy/physiology and pathology against which to relate their palpatory evaluations. This paradox can only be resolved by highly trained professionals becoming more intuitive and open, trusting that they really are sensing very subtle sensations as they open themselves to developing the delicate skills necessary for many palpatory methods. At the same time, many less 'well-trained' professionals may need to accept the necessity of adding layers of knowledge to their intuitive and nurturing talents.

Unless a practitioner is able to 'read' with the hands the information which abounds in all soft tissues and is also able to relate this to the problems of the patient (as well as to a good deal of other diagnostic information) much potentially vital data will be missed.

No one in the osteopathic field has done more to stress the importance of sound palpatory skills than Viola Frymann and we will be learning from a number of her observations as we progress through the text. She summed up the focusing of these skills, and the importance of making sense of them, when she said (Frymann 1963):

> The first step in the process of palpation is detection, the second step is amplification, and the third step must therefore be interpretation. The interpretation of the observations made by palpation is the key which makes the study of the structure and function of tissues meaningful. Nevertheless it is like the first visit to a foreign country. Numerous strange and unfamiliar sights are to be seen, but without some knowledge of the language with which to ask questions, or a guide to interpret those observations in the life and history of the country, they have little meaning to us. The third step in our study then is to be able to translate palpatory observations into meaningful anatomic, physiologic or pathologic states.

Palpation objectives

Philip Greenman, in his superb analysis *Principles of manual medicine* (Greenman 1989), summarises the five objectives of palpation. You, the practitioner/therapist, should be able to:

1. detect abnormal tissue texture
2. evaluate symmetry in the position of structures, both physically and visually
3. detect and assess variations in range and quality of movement during the range, as well as the quality of the end of the range of any movement
4. sense the position in space of yourself and the person being palpated
5. detect and evaluate change in the palpated findings, whether these are improving or worsening as time passes.

As will become clear, others have added more subtle but still palpable factors, such as energy variations, 'tissue memory' and emotional residues, to these basic requirements of what can (and should) be palpated and assessed. The elements described by Greenman are, however, our major objectives in obtaining palpatory literacy. Karel Lewit (1999), the brilliant Czech physician who has eclectically combined so much of osteopathic, chiropractic, physical therapy and orthopaedic knowledge, states his objective in palpating the patient as follows:

> Palpation of tissue structures seeks to determine the texture, resilience, warmth, humidity and the possibility of moving, stretching or compressing these structures. Concentrating on the tissues palpated, and pushing aside one layer after another, we distinguish skin, subcutaneous tissue, muscle and bone, we recognise the transition to the tendon, and finally the insertion. Palpating bone, we recognise tuberosities (and possible changes) and locate joints. Reflex changes due to pain affect all these tissues, and can be assessed by palpation; one of the most significant factors is increased tension.

We will examine Lewit's methods of ascertaining the presence of tense, tight tissues in some detail in later chapters.

Regarding the learning process, Gerald Cooper (1977) says:

> To begin to learn palpatory skill one must learn to practise to palpate bone or muscle or viscera. Gradually one learns to distinguish between a healthy muscle, a spastic muscle, and a flaccid one, and gradually one learns there is a difference in feel between a hard malignant tumour and a firm benign tumour. *Palpation cannot be learned by reading or listening, it can only be learned by palpation.*
>
> [My italics]

This message is basic and vital and many experts repeat it. Read, understand and then practise, practise and practise some more. It is the only way to become literate in palpation.

George Webster (1947) said:

We should feel with our brain as well as with our fingers, that is to say, into our touch should go our concentrated attention and all the correlated knowledge that we can bring to bear upon the case before us . . . The principle employed by Dr Still [founder of osteopathy] in so carefully educating his tactile sense as he did with his Indian skeletons and living subjects, together with the knowledge to properly interpret the findings, accounted for his success over such a wide field. He had a way of letting his fingers sink slowly into the tissues, feeling his way from the superficial to the deep structures, that gave him a comprehensive picture of local as well as general pathology.

On the learning of palpatory skills, Frederick Mitchell Jr (1976) states:

Although visual sensing of objects is done through an intervening medium (the atmosphere or other transparent material), students are rather uncomfortable with the notion that palpation is also performed through an intervening medium. The necessity for projecting one's tactile senses to varying distances through an intervening medium* must seem mystical and esoteric to many beginning students. Yet even when one is palpating surface textures the information reaches one's nervous system through one's own intervening integument. Students are often troubled by the challenge of palpating an internal organ through overlying skin, subcutaneous fascia and fat, muscle, deep fascia, subserous fascia and peritoneum.

Palpate by 'feeling', not thinking

It is just that 'troubled' feeling towards such challenges which the exercises and advice in the text will hopefully overcome, for along with the assertion of so many experts that palpation can only be learned by palpating, there is another common theme; there must be a trusting of what is being felt, a suspension of critical judgement while the process is being carried out.

Later on, critical judgement becomes essential when interpreting what was felt but the process of 'feeling' needs to be carried out with that faculty silenced. No one has better expressed this need than John Upledger (1987), the developer of craniosacral therapy. He states:

Most of you have spent years studying the sciences and have learned to rely heavily upon your rational, reasoning mind. You probably have been convinced that the information which your hands can give you is unreliable. You may consider facts to be reliable only when they are printed on a computer sheet, projected on a screen or read from the indicator of an electrical device. In order to use your hands and to begin to develop them as reliable instruments for diagnosis and treatment, you must learn to trust them and the information they can give you.

Learning to trust your hands is not an easy task. You must learn to shut off your conscious, critical mind while you palpate for subtle changes in the body you are examining. You must adopt an empirical attitude so that you may temporarily accept without question those perceptions which come into your brain from your hands. Although this attitude is unpalatable to most scientists it is recommended that you give it a trial. After you have developed your palpatory skill, you can criticise what you have felt with your hands. If you criticise before you learn to palpate, you will never learn to palpate, you will never learn to use your hands effectively as the highly sensitive diagnostic and therapeutic instruments which, in fact, they are.

---

* Becker (1974), whose work is discussed in later chapters, suggested we palpate *through* our fingers, not with them.

'Accept what you sense as real' is Upledger's plea. This is a valid motto for the exploration of palpatory skills only if the palpation is accurately performed. As will be discussed in the next chapter (and with periodic references in later chapters), the accuracy of palpatory findings is frequently questioned by researchers (Panzer 1992, Van Duersen et al 1990, Vincent Smith & Gibbons 1999).

The ability of an individual practitioner to regularly and accurately locate and identify somatic landmarks, and changes in function, lies at the very heart of palpatory reliability. Upledger's injunction to 'trust what you feel' is only valid if what you think you feel really is what you intended to feel, that the vertebra or rib being assessed is actually the one you meant to investigate!

WG Sutherland (1948), the primary osteopathic researcher into cranial motion, gave his uncompromising instruction as follows.

> It is necessary to develop fingers with brain cells in their tips, fingers capable of feeling, thinking, seeing. Therefore first instruct the fingers how to feel, how to think, how to see, and then let them touch.

Palpation variations

As though the fears outlined by Mitchell were insufficient, or Upledger's and Sutherland's directions not difficult enough, there are also those therapists who make an assessment a short distance from the skin, although it should be clear that what they are 'palpating' is rather different from the tissues that Mitchell's students were palpating.

This approach is far less indefensible than might be assumed, following the publication of the results of double blind studies into the use of 'therapeutic touch' methods, in which no contact with the (physical) body is made at all. This will be discussed further in Chapters 6 and 11 where an array of methods aimed at increasing sensitivity to subtle energy patterns will be detailed.

Other forms of assessment involving very light skin contact, either with the palpating hand(s)/digit(s) stationary or moving in a variety of ways, will also be explored at length. Palpation of this sort often employs, as Lewit (1999) mentions, awareness of variations in skin tone, temperature, feel and elasticity (which may reflect or be associated with altered electrical resistance) or other changes.

Some methods, such as the German system of *bindegewebsmassage* (connective tissue massage), employ a sequential examination of the relative adherence of different layers of tissue to each other, either at an interface (say, between muscle and connective tissue) or above it (skin over muscle, muscle over bone and so on) (Bischof & Elmiger 1960). Lewit too has shown the relevance of identifying changes in skin adherence over reflexogenic areas which are active (trigger points, for example) (Lewit 1999).

Recent developments, as well as the reintroduction of older concepts, have led to methods of assessment of visceral structures, in terms of both position and 'motion', and some of the methods involved will be outlined – specifically those which involve evaluation of drag, or tension, on mesenteric attachments (Kuchera 1997). Craniosacral and 'zero-balancing' methods (among others) involve the sensing of inherent rhythms, felt on the surface, to make assessments of relative physiological or pathological states or even of 'tissue memory' relating to trauma, either physical or emotional. Variations on these methods will be examined and described together with exercises which can assist in developing appropriate degrees of sensitivity for their effective use.

Deeper palpation of the soft tissues, involving stretching, probing, compressing and the use of various movements and positions, is commonly employed to seek out information relating to local and reflex activity; these approaches will also be examined and explained. Such methods are frequently combined with the use of sequential assessment of the relative degree of tension (shortness), or strength, of associated muscles and such a sequence will be described in detail.

Examination of some of the ways in which joint status can be judged, from its 'end-feel', when range of motion and motion palpation are used for this purpose, add a further dimension to the art of palpation and will be presented with appropriate exercises.

What the various palpation findings may actually mean will be surveyed, both in relation to obvious biomechanical changes as well as possible reflex and psychological implications. This latter element is something we should always be aware of, as there are few chronic states of dysfunction which are not overlaid (or often caused) by psychosomatic interactions. Indeed, research by German connective tissue massage therapists has clearly demonstrated specific, palpable, soft tissue changes which relate to particular emotional or psychological states.

Osteopathy, chiropractic, physiotherapy, massage therapy and a host of other systems associated with bodywork have all developed individualised diagnostic methods, some of which have become universally applied and valued by other systems. In order not to upset professional sensitivities, credit will be given to the system which first developed particular palpatory methods, wherever this is known.

Poetry of palpation

Ida Rolf, the developer of structural integration through the system known as Rolfing, gave an idea of just how exciting an experience palpation can be. She suggests (Rolf 1977) that the beginner in the art of palpation should feel their own thigh (as an example). Initially, she says, this will feel 'undifferentiated', either overly dense or soft, lacking in tone or as though large lumps were held together under the skin. These 'extremes in the spectrum of spatial, material and chemical disorganisation' make recognition of the ideally well-organised elements of the structures difficult. However, after appropriate normalisation of such tissues the 'feel' is quite different:

> You can feel the energy and tone flow into and through the myofascial unit . . . dissolving the 'glue' that, in holding the fascial envelopes together, has given the feeling of bunched and undifferentiated flesh.
> As fascial tone improves, individual muscles glide over one another, and the flesh – no longer 'too, too solid' – reminds the searching fingers of layers of silk that glide on one another with a suggestion of opulence.

Rolf's excitement is not feigned. Palpation of the body should change with practice from being a purely mechanical act into a truly touching and moving experience, in all senses of those words. Inspired by having studied with Rolf, Tom Myers (2001) has developed a model which demonstrates concrete fascial continuities or networks. These 'trains', or connective tissue meridians, link all parts of the body in functional ways and awareness of the particular connections can change the way we see the musculoskeletal system and its problems. Some of Myers' lines will be discussed and illustrated in later chapters.

Paul Van Allen (1964) pinpointed the need for concentrated application to the task of heightening one's perceptive (and therapeutic) skills.

> Let us lay down a few principles to guide us in the development of manual skills . . . It is commonplace to accept the need for basic principles and for practice, in developing manual skill to strike a golf ball, or a baseball, to roll a bowling ball, to

strike a piano key or to draw a bow across strings, but we seldom, if ever any more, think of manual skills in osteopathic practice in this way. Is it possible that osteopathic manipulation began to lose its effectiveness and to fall into disrepute even among our own people, when students no longer practised to see through how many pages of *Gray's Anatomy* they could feel a hair?

Note that this was written at a traumatic time for osteopathy in the United States, when 2000 Californian osteopaths gave up their DO status and accepted MD status in return for the turning of an osteopathic college into an allopathic medical school. A resurgence of basic osteopathic teaching and skills has since reversed that catastrophe.

Describing what we feel

All therapists who use their hands can ask themselves whether they spend enough time refining and heightening their degree of palpatory sensitivity. The answer in many cases will be 'no' and hopefully this text will encourage a return to exercises such as this useful application of *Gray's Anatomy* (a telephone directory was used for this purpose in the author's training; it is equally effective).

Moving beyond his despair at the loss of interest in palpatory skills, Van Allen makes another useful contribution.

We will understand better what we feel if we attempt to describe it. In describing what is experienced through palpation we try to classify the characteristics of tissue states, thus not only clarifying our own observations but broadening our collective experience by affording a better means of communication between us and discussing [osteopathic] theory and method. We are accustomed to describing crude differences in what we feel by touch, the roughness of the bark of a tree or of a tweed coat, the smoothness of a glass or silk. We must now develop a language of nuances and I shall suggest only a few words from many to apply to palpable tissue states in an effort to describe them accurately.

Van Allen then launches into detailed descriptions of the meanings, as he sees them, of words such as 'density', 'turgidity', 'compressibility', 'tensile state' (or response to stretch) and 'elasticity'. His choice of words may not suit everyone but the idea is sound. We need to unleash a torrent of descriptive words for what we feel when we palpate and the chapters covering various approaches to this most vital of procedures will hopefully inspire the reader to follow Van Allen's advice, to obtain a thesaurus and to look up as many words as possible in order to describe accurately the subtle variations in what is being palpated.

Viola Frymann reminds us that Dr Sutherland used the analogy of a bird alighting on a twig and then taking hold of it, when he tried to teach his students how to palpate the cranium. Some of the exercises in this book are derived from Frymann's work and in many of these she echoes Van Allen's idea that the student of palpation should also practise the art of describing what she is feeling, either verbally or in writing. Dr Frymann's words (Frymann 1963) may serve as a guide throughout this text.

It is one thing to understand intellectually that physiological functions operate, and what may happen if they become disorganised. It is quite another thing, however, to be able to place the hands on a patient and analyse the nature and the extent of the disorganisation and know what can be done to restore it to normal, unimpeded, rhythmic physiology. This then is the task before us; to know what has happened and is happening to the tissues under our hands, and then to know what can be done about it and be able to carry it through . . . [however] . . . palpation alone is virtually worthless without the rest of the patient evaluation. The value comes from the entire package – history, examination [including palpation], special tests, and response to treatment.

Current views

A modern British osteopathic view is offered by Stone (1999) who describes palpation as the 'fifth dimension'.

> Palpation allows us to interpret tissue function. Different histological make-up brings differing amounts of inherent pliability and elasticity; because of this a muscle feels completely different from a ligament, a bone and an organ, for example. Thus there is a 'normal' feel to healthy tissues that is different for each tissue. This has to be learned through repeated exploration of 'normal' and the practitioner builds his/her own vocabulary of what 'normal' is. Once someone is trained to use palpation efficiently, then finer and finer differences between tissues can be felt. This is vital, as one must be able to differentiate when something has changed from being 'normal' to being 'too normal'.

Touching on the palpatory qualities of tissues in relation to emotional states (see also Chapter 12), Stone continues:

> Each practitioner must build up their own subjective description of what the tissue states mean to them clinically, whether this is to do with the degree of actual injury or some sort of emotional problem. Experience and careful reflection on the nature of the tissue reactions and responses to manipulations are an important part of maturing as a professional, and by their very nature are descriptive terms unique to the individual practitioner.

A challenging physiotherapy perspective is offered by Maitland (2001), one of the giants of that profession.

> In the vertebral column, it is palpation that is the most important and the most difficult skill to learn. To achieve this skill it is necessary to be able to feel, by palpation, the difference in the spinal segments – normal to abnormal; old or new; hypomobile or hypermobile – and then be able to relate the response, site, depth and relevance to a patient's symptoms (structure, source and causes). This requires an honest, self-critical attitude, and also applies to the testing of functional movements and combined physiological test movements. It takes at least 10 years for any clinician (even one who has an inborn ability) to learn the relationship between her hands, the pain responses, and her mind.

Chiropractic examination depends a great deal on direct palpation, both static and active. Murphy (2000) describes that profession's modern perspective.

> Palpation encompasses static palpation, such as for skin temperature and texture, masses, myofascial trigger points, or soft tissue changes; motion palpation for assessing joint function; and muscle length tests for assessing muscle function. So it is used in the detection of red flags for serious disease, the primary pain generator(s), and the key dysfunctions and dysfunctional changes. There is no substitute for good palpation skills in examining patients . . . The two most important tools that are used in the process of examination are those of sight and touch (in addition to hearing) . . . palpation in particular, is a skill that is invaluable in the assessment of locomotor system function.

American osteopathic medicine training places great emphasis on palpation skills. Kappler (1997) explains:

> The art of palpation requires discipline, time, patience and practice. To be most effective and productive, palpatory findings must be correlated with a knowledge of functional anatomy, physiology and pathophysiology. It is much easier to identify frank pathological states, a tumor for example, than to describe signs, symptoms, and palpatory findings that lead to or identify pathological mechanisms . . . Palpation with fingers and hands provides sensory information that the brain interprets as: temperature, texture, surface humidity, elasticity, turgor, tissue tension, thickness, shape, irritability, motion. To accomplish this task, it is necessary to teach the fingers to feel, think, see, and know. One feels through

the palpating fingers on the patient; one sees the structures under the palpating fingers through a visual image based on knowledge of anatomy; one thinks what is normal and abnormal, and one knows with confidence acquired with practice that what is felt is real and accurate.

By heeding the words of the experts, quoted throughout this book, and by evaluating and reflecting on some of the insights to be found in the special topic areas between chapters, as well as by assiduously practising the exercises given in all subsequent chapters and some of the special topic areas, palpation skills can be refined to an extraordinary degree, bringing both satisfaction and benefit to practitioner and patient alike. The acquisition of greater skills will also reduce the frequency with which researchers find unreliability to be common. These issues are discussed in the next chapter.

REFERENCES

Bischof I, Elmiger G 1960 Connective tissue massage. In: Licht E (ed) Massage, manipulation and traction. New Haven, Connecticut

Cooper G 1977 Clinical considerations of fascia in diagnosis and treatment. Academy of Applied Osteopathy Yearbook, Newark, OH

Frymann V 1963 Palpation – its study in the workshop. Academy of Applied Osteopathy Yearbook, Newark, OH, pp 16–30

Greenman P 1989 Principles of manual medicine. Williams and Wilkins, Baltimore

Kappler R 1997 Palpatory skills. In: Ward R (ed) Foundations for osteopathic medicine. Williams and Wilkins, Baltimore

Kuchera W 1997 Lumbar and abdominal region. In: Ward R (ed) Foundations for osteopathic medicine. Williams and Wilkins, Baltimore

Lewit K 1999 Manipulation in rehabilitation of the motor system, 3rd edn. Butterworths, London

Maitland G 2001 Maitland's vertebral manipulation, 6th edn. Butterworth Heinemann, Oxford

Mitchell F Jr 1976 Training and measuring sensory literacy. Yearbook of the American Academy of Osteopathy, Newark, OH, pp 120–127

Murphy D 2000 Conservative management of cervical spine syndromes. McGraw-Hill, New York

Myers T 2001 Anatomy trains. Churchill Livingstone, Edinburgh

Panzer DM 1992 The reliability of lumbar motion palpation. Journal of Manipulative and Physiological Therapeutics 15(8): 518–524

Rolf I 1977 Rolfing: the integration of human structures. Harper and Row, New York

Stone C 1999 Science in the art of osteopathy. Stanley Thornes, Cheltenham

Sutherland WG 1948 The cranial bowl. Mankato, Minnesota

Upledger J 1987 Craniosacral therapy. Eastland Press, Seattle

Van Allen P 1964 Improving our skills. Academy of Applied Osteopathy Yearbook, pp 147–152

Van Duersen L, Patijn J, Ockhuysen A, Vortman B 1990 The value of some clinical tests of the sacroiliac joint. Manual Medicine 5: 96–99

Vincent Smith B, Gibbons P 1999 Inter-examiner and intra-examiner reliability of palpatory findings for the standing flexion test. Manual Therapy 4(2): 87–93

Webster G 1947 Feel of the tissues. Yearbook of the American Academy of Osteopathy, pp 32–35

2

SPECIAL TOPIC 2
Structure and function: are they inseparable?

One of the oldest maxims in osteopathic medicine highlights the total interdependence of structure and function; structure determines function and vice versa. Anything which causes a change to occur in structure will cause function to modify and any functional change will result in structural change (for example, fibrosis of muscle, alteration in length of any soft tissue, change in joint surface smoothness).

There is no way that a shortened or fibrosed muscle can function normally; there will always be a degree of adaptation, a modification from normal patterns of use, some degree of malcoordination or imbalance in the way it works.

Similarly, all changes in the way any part of the body is used (breathing function, for example) or the way the whole body is used (posture, for example), which vary from the way it was designed to work, will produce alterations in structure. If posture is poor or habitual use is incorrect (sitting cross-legged and writing with the head tilted to one side are common examples) structural changes will develop in response to, or in order to support and cement, these functional changes.

We can summarise factors which produce functional and subsequently structural change as involving overuse, misuse, abuse and disuse, which in turn can be reduced to one word: stress. Conversely, if we palpate structure and find alterations from the expected norm, we should be able to confirm related functional changes. For example, if we palpate shortened or fibrosed soft tissues it should be possible to register that the area does not function optimally (for example, a shortened hamstring is palpable and the leg will be restricted during a straight-leg raising test as well as when normal functional demands are made of that muscle).

It is worth considering, however, that just because something is other than the way it 'should' be, this does not mean that it needs to be modified by treatment or rehabilitation exercises. Take, for example, the same short hamstring muscle mentioned above. There may be times when this is actually serving a useful purpose; for example, if there is a dysfunctional, unstable, sacroiliac joint, a tight hamstring, placing additional load on the sacrotuberous ligament, might be acting as a stabilising influence (see Chapter 9). In such a situation stretching the tight hamstring group might make these more 'normal' but could produce instability in the SI joint (Vleeming et al 1997). Similar consideration should be given to the presence of active trigger points, which may be serving some stabilising function because they produce heightened tone in the muscles in which they exist, as well as in the muscles to which they refer (Chaitow & DeLany 2000).

When we observe functional change we should readily be able to identify structural alterations which relate to this. Thus when posture or breathing function is not as it should be, we should target the tissues which are most likely to carry evidence of associated structural change.

On a more local scale, when skin elasticity (a function dependent on normal structure) is reduced, we know that underlying reflex change (function) is involved (see Chapter 4). Palpation and observation are as inseparable as structure and function and this should be kept in mind both during our exploration of palpatory methods which experience both structure and function and also as we observe the physical manifestation of these two concepts – what the body looks and feels like and what its working looks and feels like.

When we palpate we are feeling structure, the physical manifestation of functional tissues and units, and we are also sensing the changes which take place as a result of the functioning of the body or part.

When we observe we are seeing these same things.

Ida Rolf (1977) suggests that we have an ever-enquiring mind focused on what we are feeling and that we should ask ourselves:

> What is structure? What does it look like? What am I looking for when I look for structure, and how do I recognise it? Structure in general, structure in human bodies in particular – what is its function? What is its mechanism? To what extent can it be modified in humans? If you modify the physical structure of a body, what have you modified, and what can you hope to influence?

REFERENCES

Chaitow L, DeLany J 2000 Clinical applications of neuromuscular techniques: volume 1 (upper body). Churchill Livingstone, Edinburgh
Rolf I 1977 Rolfing: the integration of human structures. Harper and Row, New York
Vleeming A, Mooney V, Dorman T, Snijders C, Stoeckart R (eds) 1997 Movement, stability and low back pain. Churchill Livingstone, Edinburgh

Palpatory accuracy – mirage or reality?

Many research studies suggest a relatively poor degree of accuracy in standard assessment and palpation tests. This should be cause for concern amongst responsible practitioners and educators and yet apart from the regular appearance of ever more reports questioning the value of individual manual assessment and palpation procedures, the methods in question continue to be widely used and taught as the basis for the development of subsequent treatment protocols.

Lord & Bogduk (1996) state:

> There have been many claims regarding the accuracy of manual diagnosis, but few data. Only one study (Jull et al 1988) compared manual diagnosis to the criterion standard of local anaesthetic blocks. The authors found the sensitivity and specificity of the manual examination technique to be 100%, the manual therapist having correctly identified in all patients with proven joint pain, the symptomatic and asymptomatic segments. The ability of other manual examiners to replicate these results has not been tested.

It seems extraordinary that this one study, involving one physical therapist, which displayed 100% accuracy, is the single most widely quoted example of a perfect palpation result, whereas hundreds of studies have shown inadequate clinical results (see discussion of this in the responses, below).

When research is carried out on intra- and interrater reliability the results are frequently poor and often bad. Results can be divided into those that evaluate:

- the individual practitioner's degree of consistency in performance of palpation assessment methods (intrarater reliability)
- the degree of agreement of findings between different practitioners performing the same palpation assessment (interrater reliability).

The key questions which emerge from the many studies which show poor inter- and intraexaminer reliability relate to whether the problems lie in palpation as a method of assessment or in the way palpation is taught and therefore practised. In this chapter these questions will be analysed, as will possible solutions to the problems which are identified. This book as a whole, if used appropriately, is hopefully part of that solution.

Not only palpation!

Before listing a selection of some of the negative evidence regarding palpation results, it is worth reflecting that other forms of assessment, such as radiography, can also demonstrate relative inaccuracy. In one example, Christensen et al (2001) conducted a study to evaluate the accuracy of radiographic interpretation of a posterolateral spinal fusion mass. They noted that, in general, the literature describing the classification criteria used for radiographic interpretation of spinal posterolateral fusion has serious deficiencies. The study they designed involved four experienced observers who each evaluated radiographs of posterolateral fusion masses. The mean interobserver agreement was 86% (kappa 0.53), while the mean intraobserver agreement was 93% (kappa 0.78) (see Box 2.1 for summary of kappa meanings). All mean kappa values were classified as 'fair' or 'good' and yet the conclusion was that it is 'extremely difficult' to interpret radiographic images of lumbar posterolateral fusion.

Box 2.1 Kappa values (Fleiss 1981)

Kappa greater than 0.75 = excellent
Kappa between 0.4 and 0.75 = good reproducibility
Kappa less than 0.4 = poor reproducibility

Comeaux et al (2001) comment on this study that:

> the interpretation of x-rays . . . in the Christensen article, demonstrated actual kappa scores of .53 and .78 which is in the same range as in some of the palpation studies which are questioned as to accuracy.

Professor Comeaux further observed:

> Any clinician who reads the radiologists' report of imaging procedures recognizes the interpretation challenge and variation of interpretation with the same films. Why should palpation be expected to be any less of an art? (personal communication, June 2001)

It seems therefore that the questionable palpation results (as detailed below) are no worse than the sort of accuracy we might expect on the reading of some (albeit 'difficult') X-ray plates. Should we be satisfied with this or appalled?

Is palpation an art? Or are there good scientific and clinical reasons for using the subjective evidence of palpation in making therapeutic decisions? And if so, what are we to make of the negative research studies, such as those listed below?

Examples of apparently poor palpation results

1. Standing flexion test for sacroiliac dysfunction (see Figure 9.1, Chapter 9). A study by Vincent Smith & Gibbons (1999) showed that 'the reliability of the standing flexion test as an indicator of SIJ dysfunction still remains questionable'. Interexaminer reliability showed 'a mean percentage agreement of 42% and a κ [kappa] coefficient of 0.052 demonstrating statistically insignificant reliability'. Intraexaminer reliability data demonstrated a mean percentage agreement of 68% and a kappa coefficient of 0.46, indicating moderate reliability.

2. Slipman et al (1998) investigated the predictive value of SI joint 'provocation' tests, as compared with what they describe as the medical 'gold standard' approach of a joint block injection. Fifty patients were selected to be tested by joint block if they tested positive using at least three manual methods. The manual provocation tests always included Patrick's F-AB-ER-E test (Fig. 2.1), as well as direct palpation for pain in the ipsilateral sacral sulcus, plus one other from the wide range of choices available, such as pain provocation by means of the transverse anterior distraction compression test, transverse posterior distraction test or Gaenslen's test.

The working hypothesis was that if the joint block injections (performed using fluoroscopically guided needling) effectively eliminated SI pain, the manual assessment had been accurate. The results showed that 30 of the 50 patients were relieved of symptoms by 80% or more, by means of joint block, whereas 20

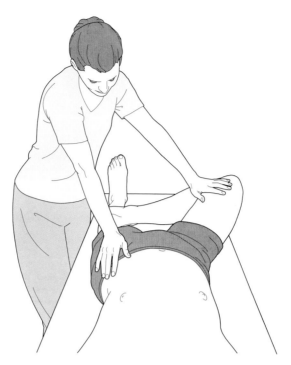

Fig. 2.1 Patrick's F-AB-ER-E test (adapted from Vleeming et al 1997).

achieved less than 80% relief. A 60% degree of accuracy in identifying SI joint syndrome was therefore noted using manual testing, in this study. Conclusion: 'Our results do not support the use of provocative SIJ manoeuvres to confirm SIJ syndrome diagnosis'.

3. Static palpation was performed for the location of three standard landmarks used in assessment of the SI joint – posterior superior iliac spine (PSIS), sacral sulcus (SS), sacral inferior lateral angle (SILA) – on 10 asymptomatic individuals, by 10 senior osteopathic students. Intraexaminer agreement results were: for SILA less than chance; for PSIS and SS slight to moderate. Interexaminer results were 'slight'. Conclusion: 'The poor reliability of clinical tests involving palpation may be partially explained by error in landmark location' (O'Haire & Gibbons 2000). Clearly, if the practitioner, or student, cannot locate the landmark, the test will be meaningless.

4. Fourteen physiotherapists were tested for intertherapist reliability to see whether they could accurately identify specific spinal levels (which had been pre-marked with ultraviolet ink) by palpation of five normal subjects, while for intratherapist reliability three therapists palpated five normal subjects. There was only fair agreement between physiotherapists ($\kappa=0.28$) but intratherapist agreement ranged from substantial to almost perfect ($\kappa=0.61, 0.70, 0.90$). 'The lack of intertherapist reliability suggests that further research into reliability of spinal palpation is required, if it is to remain an important component of spinal therapy' (McKenzie & Taylor 1997).

It is obviously important that an individual therapist is able to consistently locate a spinal landmark. However, different therapists should also be able to agree that the same location represents the spinal landmark in question.

5. Gillet's test (Fig. 2.2), which assesses sacroiliac mobility, is widely used, albeit with variations in manual contacts (including L5 spinous process, different aspects of the PSIS, sacral spinous processes, etc.) as the patient removes weight from and raises one leg or the other. A study was conducted in which some 40 symptomatic and asymptomatic subjects were evaluated, using variations on the test. The conclusion was that 'The Gillet test – as performed in this study – does

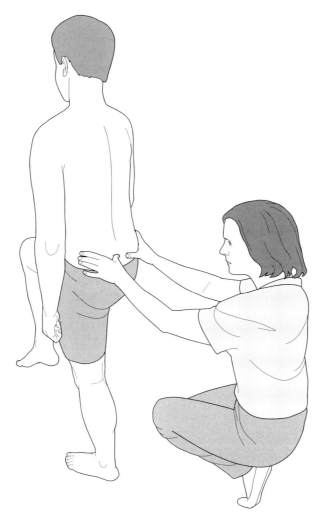

Fig. 2.2 Ipsilateral posterior rotation test (Gillet). Note the inferomedial displacement of the PSIS.

not appear to be reliable' (Meijne et al 1999). Since the Gillet (stork) test is widely used, this study offers a cautionary warning that a single assessment result should not be taken as diagnostic of dysfunction (this caution is discussed later in the chapter). Gillet's test is described in Chapter 9.

6. A complex study involved chiropractic assessment of possible lumbopelvic dysfunction – low back pain (LBP) – in 83 pairs of twins. The study evaluated use of a variety of different tests, each of which has the option of a 'yes', a 'no' or a 'don't know' answer to the question of 'is there dysfunction?'. Some of the tests used were observational: stork test, non-reversal of lordosis, antalgic posture, gearbox movement on flexion. Additional tests assessed pain on movement, including flexion, extension, left and right side bending and rotation. Pain-provoking tests were also evaluated, such as forced extension and percussion of spinous processes. The tests were evaluated to see if they met the following criteria: (1) logical pattern in relation to low back pain status; (2) high sensitivity; (3) high specificity; (4) high positive and (5) high negative predictive values.

The researchers' results were: 'None of the single tests fulfilled all five of the criteria. However, the variable of at least one painful movement did fulfil all of the criteria. Each of the individual lumbar movements (except left rotation) fulfilled all the criteria but one (high sensitivity). The gearbox test was only present in one person, who was correctly classified as "LBP today". Conclusion: Although no individual test was accurate, the diagnostic discrimination on the basis of these tests was satisfactory' (Lebouef-Yde & Kyvik 2000).

Again we see that while single tests are vulnerable to misinterpretation, a combination of results seems to point to an accurate assessment.

A need to compound evidence

This final study reported above suggests that clinically no single test should be used diagnostically but that a picture should be built up based on the compounding of evidence. Accuracy may then be sufficient for the purpose of devising subsequent treatment protocols.

Lee (1999) seems to agree with Bogduk (1997) that ideally a 'biomechanical diagnosis requires biomechanical criteria' and that 'pain on movement is not that criteria'. A subtext for debate seems to be emerging as to whether or not pain on movement should be used as part of clinical evaluation, an idea supported by chiropractic researchers (see Lebouef-Yde & Kyvik 2000) but not by physiotherapy (as per Lee's opinion, given above).

The fact that there is relatively poor interexaminer reliability when applying tests does not necessarily negate their value, merely the efficiency with which they are applied, according to Lee, who continues:

> The tests for spinal and sacroiliac function (i.e. mobility/stability, not pain) continue to be developed, and hopefully will be able to withstand the scrutiny and rigor of scientific research and take their place in a clinical evaluation which follows a biomechanical, and not a pain, model.

Discussing the value of tests, she notes that while individually, in isolation, some may fail evaluation as to their reliability and validity, when such tests are combined into a sequence involving a number of evaluation strategies, and especially when 'a clinical reasoning process is applied to their findings', they offer a logical biomechanical diagnosis and 'without apology, they continue to be defended'.

The palpation reliability debate – the experts respond

In order to establish the attitudes of different experts, working in different professions within 'bodywork', the *Journal of Bodywork and Movement Therapies* invited leading figures in manual medicine, physiotherapy, chiropractic, osteopathy and massage therapy to answer a series of questions and to discuss the issues raised by the negative research results reported on above (Editorial: JBMT 2001; 5(4): 223–226).

The questions were as follows.

1. Does the poor interobserver reliability of palpation methods make you question the validity and usefulness of an examination based upon this skill? If not, why not?

2. How do you think palpation and clinical assessment should be taught/ studied so that its validity and clinical potential can be best demonstrated?

3. Should we depend less on palpation and assessment methods in clinical settings, since their reliability seems to be so poor?

4. What other tests do you use so that your clinical examination's reliability can be bolstered?

5. If treatment based on possibly unreliable assessment and palpation methods is apparently effective, what does this say about the value of the methods being used? (For example, is apparently successful treatment, based on apparently unreliable assessment methods, valuable mainly for its placebo effects?)

6. Should palpatory diagnostic findings be accepted as having a subjective/interpretative value similar to interpretation of radiographic findings or other laboratory data and therefore be capable of being integrated into a treatment plan by a skilled therapist?

The responses (JBMT 6(2) 2002) are both encouraging and positive. It seems that there are solutions to the problems which result from research showing inadequate palpation results and many suggestions as to how these solutions might be achieved are outlined. There are also some quite depressing messages – that standards of teaching and practice are not what they could be. The overall understanding, which emerged from many of the responses, emphasises the need for the foundational level of palpation and assessment skills, on which all manual treatment ultimately rests, to be well taught, well learned and well practised.

This is not a surprising message and is certainly timely. Therapists already in practice need to ensure that they do not just coast along, employing assessment and palpation methods in habitual ways. They may need to review, reflect and polish palpation skills, so ensuring the likelihood of extracting the most reliable information possible from patient encounters.

If treatment choices depend on data derived from palpation sources, all practitioners owe it to themselves and their patients to achieve palpatory excellence, consistency and reliability, as evidence is gathered. The implications of current palpation skill levels, for both educators and students, are equally profound and urgent.

What's to be done?

David Simons MD, in his response to the palpation questions (see below), notes that one-to-one tuition is best. In establishing that the student actually palpates what is supposed to be palpated (trigger points in his example), Simons offers his own tissues for evaluation. This is an exceptional approach to teaching, which is not reproducible to any widespread degree in teaching settings. However, Simons makes suggestions for educators which are practical, as do a number of the other experts. It is to be hoped that teachers and institutions will take note of the need for the repetition of closely monitored exercises in palpation skill enhancement.

Additionally, it seems there exists, in many institutions (and some professions), a need to broaden the knowledge and skill base incorporated into palpation training so that a greater understanding of anatomy and physiology and pathophysiology is available on which to build palpation skills.

The response to such suggestions from educators is often that courses are already overloaded and that there is just no time, or space, for more topics or for more detailed study of practical skills. These statements may be valid but simply represent logistical conundrums in search of solutions. The need for better palpation training is far greater than the scheduling problems raised and cannot be dismissed as being too difficult to solve.

The professions and individuals represented in the palpation debate were:

- chiropractic – Craig Liebenson DC and Don Murphy DC
- massage therapy – Shannon Goossen LMT
- medicine – Karel Lewit MD and David Simons MD
- osteopathy – Peter Gibbons DO and Philip Tehan DO
- physiotherapy – Joanne Bullock-Saxton PT and Dianne Lee PT.

The responses are given below, in alphabetical order (Gibbons and Teahy, as well as Liebenson and Lewit, chose to offer jointly composed answers). Some of the experts elected to answer the individual questions as posed, whereas others presented 'position statements' which reflected their overall response to the questions.

Responses

Dr Joanne Bullock-Saxton PhD, MAppPhty St (Manips), BPhty (Hons)

Q1. Does the poor interobserver reliability of palpation methods make you question the validity and usefulness of an examination based upon this skill? If not, why not?

A1. When reviewing the literature in this area, it is very important to keep in mind the quality of the research question asked, whether the protocol was sufficiently well designed to answer this question and thirdly, whether the conclusions drawn by the authors are confined to the limits of the study. Much research has been published that throws a negative light on clinical practice because of poor inception or design. This has resulted in ramifications that go far beyond clinical practice to stakeholders in the health-care system whose agenda may be to prove or disprove the efficacy of practice on the basis of any literature (regardless of its quality). It is also important to remember that conclusions drawn about reliability of an assessment method for one joint cannot be extrapolated to reflect on reliability of assessment for other joints. The sacroiliac joint (SIJ), for instance, is a joint that has minuscule movement and in many cases, assessment of the degree of any movement that does exist in it may be inherently unreliable, particularly if dysfunction is associated with changes in muscle tone. Study designs that attempt to determine reliability between examiners of dysfunctional SIJ joints may be inherently confounded by the fact that the assessment movements may also be treatment movements, and accordingly, variables may differ between examiners due to 'treatment effect'. Evaluations of reliability of palpation of joints such as the SIJ need to be considered in parallel with studies reporting the repeatability of movements of the SIJ, to be able to determine the source of any error in measurement. Unfortunately, many studies fail to do this and the total error is sometimes inappropriately attributed fully to 'between rater' error.

An example of a simple, well-designed study that attempted to avoid potential confounding variables has been quoted in the prelude to these questions. Jull et al (1988) asked the straightforward and answerable question, can a skilled manual therapist identify correctly the zygapophyseal joint responsible for neck pain? The researchers did not attempt to answer any question about the degree of hypo- or hypermobility existing in the dysfunctional cervical spine joints. This is highly relevant to clinical practice, for it is my perception that many skilled clinicians seeking a diagnosis do not base their findings on the results of a single assessment parameter.

Therefore, the answer that I provide to this question is this. Questions of validity and usefulness of any assessment procedure need to be asked and researched wisely by our professions. Researchers need to be careful that their design is not doomed to failure before starting due to the potential of incorporating other confounding variables that if not revealed, will produce results that reflect poorly on the profession as a whole. It takes time to develop manual palpation skills and novices of palpation should not be included in a research design, unless the protocol is specifically interested in a question about skill acquisition. I am not yet convinced that there is sufficient evidence in the current literature to condemn the use of some commonly taught palpation techniques. One must always keep an open mind and discriminate each contribution to the literature for its capacity to reveal the truth of the issue.

Q2. How do you think palpation and clinical assessment should be taught/studied so that its validity and clinical potential can be best demonstrated?

A2. In answering this question, I would like to make it clear that in my judgement, palpation is a component part of the physical examination of a patient. In making a diagnosis, palpation alone is insufficient and the information it provides must be considered in context with the subjective information from the subject, as well as related to other findings associated with appropriate assessment of the articular, neural and muscular systems.

An approach to education related to assessment of musculoskeletal disorders, applied at the University of Queensland, Australia, is an adult-based learning model directed at developing a student's clinical reasoning skills. Initially, a hypothetical deductive model is taught where, at all levels of the patient examination, students must generate a number of hypotheses regarding diagnosis. These hypotheses must be tested throughout the examination and intervention phases. The patterns of subjective or physical patient responses both to directed tests and in response to specific treatment must be used to confirm or reject evolving hypotheses regarding diagnosis. This is a slow and cognitively demanding process. However, it is valuable in establishing the essential questioning and confirmation approach that should be applied throughout patient assessment and management.

Essential elements to develop clinical reasoning skills in students are the following.

- Knowledge that is discipline specific, well understood, easy to recall and commonly applied.
- Cognitive skills of analysis, synthesis and data evaluation practised.
- Context specific, that is, that presenting conditions or events are associated with the development or maintenance of the presenting problem.

Conversely, experts in clinical practice tend to use a pattern recognition/ inductive reasoning model, that has superseded the hypothetical deductive approach. With the development of expertise, large meaningful patterns of information are interpreted quickly for problem solving. These individuals demonstrate a highly developed short- and long-term memory regarding the above three essential elements, as well as a deeper understanding of the problem that is inclusive of the patient's perspective. While this model of diagnosis is rapid, if employed too early there is a chance that the pattern recognition model may be responsible for the clinician's making assumptions without clarification, failing to collect sufficient information and demonstrating confirmation bias. The final outcome is that all presentations may be placed into a single diagnostic box. Clearly, there is a chance that without sufficient groundwork in establishing the questioning and confirming model of clinical reasoning, and applying only pattern recognition processes, a student may suffer some of these pitfalls. Again, when reviewing literature in the area of reliability or efficacy of clinical diagnosis and management, and judging the value of reported findings, it is important for the reader to establish the type of clinical reasoning model that has been employed by participants and to look for evidence of their skill and capacity to utilise either model effectively. Strategies taught to enhance a student's clinical reasoning should ensure a high level of knowledge and organisation of that knowledge; the development of a capacity to accurately perform technical and manual skills (taught in a tutor/student practical class format emphasising feedback of performance) and encouragement of the student to understand any problem at a deeper level.

Q3. Should we depend less on palpation and assessment methods in clinical settings, since their reliability seems to be so poor?

A3. For reasons stated in the answers to the initial two questions, I believe that palpation forms one component of a large range of potential assessment procedures to assess components of the muscular, articular and neural systems. Following a thorough subjective examination, decisions are made by the clinician regarding the appropriate musculoskeletal structures to assess. Responses to various assessments provide the necessary information to assist clinicians in generating a hypothesis about the nature of the problem and the most likely dysfunctional structure to manage. During the examination of the patient, a suite of positive tests will be identified and the nature of the responses recorded to provide baseline data prior to application of an intervention.

Once a decision is made about diagnosis and the form of management, treatment may commence, followed by reevaluation of the positive tests in order to ascertain the influence of treatment. Such review of management confirms the clinician's assumptions based on the suite of tests and ultimately improves the efficacy of patient management.

Q4. What other tests do you use so that your clinical examination's reliability can be bolstered?

A4. The principal issue is the development of assessment and treatment methods that have specificity and efficacy. The reassessment model described in answer 3 allows the development of such an approach. I would ensure that I had considered the total system in terms of potential causes of the presenting signs and symptoms, select the most appropriate assessments for those presenting signs, intervene and then reassess the outcome. Each treatment therefore involves outcome appraisal of decisions that are based on the range of assessments selected. The muscular system can be assessed in a number of ways for strength, fatigue, hypertrophy, atrophy, alteration in coordination and recruitment of motor units, resting length and underlying tone. The articular system can be assessed, for example, for hypomobility, hypermobility, instability, deformity, compensatory movement and biomechanics of motion. The neural system can be assessed for conductivity and sensitivity. The number of procedures that can be employed to investigate any one of these potential systems is large. From a clinical perspective, however, positive findings in any structure should alter with appropriate treatment if the clinical diagnosis is correct. If there is no change over a reasonable timeframe, then the clinician must ask the questions 'have I made the correct diagnosis?', 'is my treatment appropriate?' or 'is the problem untreatable by a musculoskeletal approach?'.

Q5. If treatment based on possibly unreliable assessment and palpation methods is apparently effective, what does this say about the value of the methods being used? (For example, is apparently successful treatment, based on apparently unreliable assessment methods, valuable mainly for its placebo effects?)

A5. For reasons stated in the answer to question 1, I believe there may still be value in assessment and palpation methods for diagnosis. I am also convinced that the issue of placebo is a very important one and is often associated with a perceived relationship between the clinician and the patient. Strong evidence exists for striking positive physical effects associated with placebo. Although a side issue to the question asked here, placebo is an effect that is understudied and needs to be embraced in the medical literature, as it suggests a high potential for patients to 'cure' themselves.

Q6. Should palpatory diagnostic findings be accepted as having subjective/interpretive value similar to interpretation of radiographic findings or other laboratory data and therefore be capable of being integrated into a treatment plan by a skilled therapist?

A6. Yes, any findings should be interpreted in relation to other findings and signs and symptoms. However, they are not all subjective and many have an objectivity that allows for intratreatment assessment.

Peter Gibbons MB, BS, DO, DM-SMed and Philip Tehan DipPhysio, DO, MMPAA

Position statement relative to the questions posed

The ability to diagnose and treat a patient rests upon a bodyworker's clinical skills, in particular the ability to take a thorough history and to undertake a comprehensive physical examination of the patient. A manual medicine practitioner uses palpation to identify somatic problems, to treat the problems found and to assess the result of treatment (Basmajian & Nyberg 1993, DiGiovanna & Schiowitz 1991, Dvorak & Dvorak 1990, Greenman 1989, Ward 1996). Despite reliance upon palpation as a diagnostic tool, the reliability of palpation as a form of physical assessment that has scientific validity remains to be proven. However, for many bodyworkers the ability to generate a treatment plan is predicated upon the use of highly refined palpatory skills.

Johnston et al (1982a,b) demonstrated that osteopaths could achieve reasonable levels of interexaminer agreement for passive gross motion testing on selected subjects with consistent findings of regional motion asymmetry. One osteopathic study demonstrated low agreement of findings for patients with acute spinal complaints, when practitioners used their own diagnostic procedures (McConnell et al 1980), but the level of agreement was improved by negotiating and selecting specific tests for detecting patient improvement (Beal et al 1980). These studies support the view that standardisation of testing procedures can improve interexaminer reliability.

It is apparent from the literature that interobserver reliability for palpatory motion testing, without pain provocation, is poor (Gonnella et al 1982, Harvey & Byfield 1991, Jull et al 1988, 1997, Laslett & Williams 1995, Lewit & Leibenson 1993, Love & Brodeur 1987, Matyas & Bach 1985, Nyberg 1993, Panzer 1992, Van Duersen et al 1990, Vincent Smith & Gibbons 1999).

Palpation as a diagnostic tool can demonstrate high levels of sensitivity and specificity in detecting symptomatic intervertebral segments (Jull et al 1988, 1997). Jull et al (1988) were able to successfully identify symptomatic upper cervical zygapophyseal joints by palpation; these findings were confirmed by the use of diagnostic blocks. For positive identification as symptomatic, the intervertebral zygapophyseal joints had to fulfil three specific criteria: abnormal end-feel, abnormal quality of resistance to motion, and reproduction of local or referred pain when passive accessory movements were tested.

Manual therapy texts advise that diagnosis should be based upon collections of clinical findings (Basmajian & Nyberg 1993, Bourdillon et al 1995, DiGiovanna & Schiowitz 1991, Dvorak & Dvorak 1990, Greenman 1989, Ward 1996). Diagnosis is not usually predicated upon a single palpatory test but upon multiple palpatory findings. Cibulka et al (1988) investigated the reliability of a combination of four palpation tests for the detection of SIJ dysfunction. They reported high levels of reliability (kappa = 0.88) for such tests. This study supports the concept of using multiple test regimes or multiple palpatory findings, in assessing for dysfunction.

There are many components of the clinical examination leading to a final diagnosis. Poor interobserver reliability of palpatory findings should not be considered as necessarily devaluing the use of palpation as a diagnostic tool. Different practitioners respond in different ways to different palpatory cues, formulating their own manipulative prescription based upon individual experience. We believe that reliability of palpatory diagnosis could be improved by:

1. standardisation of palpatory assessment procedures
2. utilisation of multiple tests
3. increased focus upon linking palpation with pain provocation.

Despite extensive research involving numerous different palpation procedures, the reliability and validity of many of these procedures remain questionable. Poor research design, use of inappropriate statistical methods and unsubstantiated conclusions have prevented musculoskeletal medicine from drawing substantive or definitive conclusions concerning the reliability of palpation as a diagnostic procedure. One might argue that the jury is still out.

Research to date has largely focused upon the reliability of palpation in diagnosis but has not adequately explored the relationship between palpatory skills and the delivery and monitoring of manipulative techniques. Even where diagnosis is not predicated upon the use of palpatory cues, palpation is still critical to the safe and effective application of 'hands-on techniques'.

While there is obviously a need to continue research and improve our abilities within the area of palpatory diagnosis, we believe the debate should also address another area where the skills of palpation make a significant impact. This is in the delivery of 'hands-on technique' in a pain-free, safe and effective manner. Proficiency in the delivery of manipulative technique takes training, practice and development of palpatory and psychomotor skills (Gibbons & Tehan 2000). The authors would contend that highly refined palpatory skills are essential for the development of the psychomotor skills necessary to perform manual therapy techniques. It has been our experience, in teaching high-velocity, low-amplitude (HVLA) thrust techniques for over 20 years, that the development of palpatory proficiency is necessary for both the intial development and the subsequent refinement of the psychomotor skills necessary for the effective delivery of HVLA thrust techniques.

The importance of palpation in the application of technique should not be underestimated and needs to be researched.

Shannon Goossen BA, LMT, CMTPT

Q1. Does the poor interobserver reliability of palpation methods make you question the validity and usefulness of an examination based upon this skill? If not why not?

A1. Before the days of MRIs, CAT scans, diagnostic spinal injections, needle EMGs and sEMG, the skilled practitioner relied upon listening to a history, observation skills and the ability to perform an examination with all of their senses. From this, practitioners formed a provisional diagnosis to explain their patient's complaints and/or suffering. New diagnostic tests came to us in the 1980s with big hopes for the definitive answers to pain and suffering. This was followed in the 1990s by the landmark study (Boden et al 1990) which showed that a portion of the population happily walks about the planet, pain free, even after an MRI has demonstrated that they have a herniated disc in the lumbar spine. Yet would anyone actually question the validity of a MRI demonstrating a L5–S1 disc herniation in a patient suffering desperately from leg pain? Well, they might, if the leg pain is on the right and the MRI report is a herniation on the left. Should we therefore discount the value of MRIs? Obviously not, they are tremendously valuable when combined with a properly focused examination. The appropriately trained manual therapist, skilled in identifying myofascial pain syndromes, should, using palpation skills, be able to differentiate an active myofascial trigger point in the gluteus minimus from a pinched L5 or S1 nerve root, both of which refer pain in similar trajectories, with subtle but clear differences.

Mense & Simons (2001) make the point that the studies performed in the early 1990s demonstrated poor interrater reliability, due to experienced examiners that were untrained in an agreed upon technique or due to examiners that were trained in a specific technique, but inexperienced.

In a more recent study, Gerwin et al (1997) demonstrated much greater interrater reliability in examiners that were both experienced and trained before the study commenced (mean kappa up to 0.74). What is demonstrated here is that even amongst experienced examiners, interrater reliability for the sake of a study is best served by standardised training for the examiners, which must in itself be tested for interrater reliability. It should be kept in mind that experienced radiologists reporting their findings on MRIs of the lumbar spine did not report annular tears until they were trained to recognise the significance of the high-intensity zone (Aprill & Bogduk 1992). It seems that studies suggest that poor interrater reliability is indicative of poor palpatory skills, poor training or poor study design.

Q2. How do you think palpation and clinical assessment should be taught/studied so that its validity and clinical potential can be best demonstrated?

A2. It is my impression that many therapists have been taught a method of evaluation as if it is 'the only way' to determine dysfunction and the aetiology of a patient's complaint. It has been said that 'You never think about the things you never think about' (Aprill 2000). This captures the essence of the challenge. A typical orthopaedic examination might focus on looking for problems with the bones or joints. A neurologist seeks for sensory and motor dysfunction in the nervous system. A chiropractor looks for spinal joint dysfunction and sub-luxation. A physical therapist evaluates for decreased strength, ROM, poor balance and gait problems. A psychiatrist might look for chemical imbalances and how to augment mood. An acupuncturist evaluates dysfunction in the meridians. And the list goes on, with the exception that there is not a specialist for muscles. There are no muscle doctors.

While we do not need to be experts in all these fields, we should know what they evaluate the patient for and why. This leads to critical, investigative thinking. Next, therapists should be exposed to the understanding that all of these fields, at one time or another, have varying degrees of reliability in their assessment techniques. If we each stay in our respective 'boxes' of thinking and evaluation, then we can only envision the patient's problem to be coming from what we evaluate and treat. Students need to see, hear and learn multiple perspectives. Then they need to learn the limitations of each. If a patient presents with muscle weakness, a PT may decide it just needs to be strengthened, a neurologist may order a EMG study to find a damaged nerve causing weakness and the myofascial trigger point therapist may stretch the muscle, because shortened muscles may test weak from taut bands and trigger points. Whereas in fact the patient may actually be showing early signs of undiagnosed MS.

In order to really be proficient in palpation one needs hundreds of hours of training and feedback. Structural evaluation also takes hundreds of hours to learn. It has been said that 'there is no technique worth knowing outside of context' (Rockwell 1998). Therapists need more training in the context of what they are evaluating and palpating. This needs to be done with a multi-disciplinary training team, where they are asked the difficult questions of 'How do you know that?', 'Are you sure that you are where you think you are, and can you prove it?'. If no one asks these questions, it may be easy to assume knowledge which is in fact absent. Surgeons may be the only ones that are regularly subjected to such scrutiny and even then, only as a result of poor outcomes.

Q3. Should we depend less on palpation and assessment methods in clinical settings, since their reliability seems to be so poor?

A3. Absolutely not. How many doctors would treat a patient based solely on what their MRI or X-rays showed and not bother to do an examination? There are no muscle doctors or specific scans/tests to objectify muscle pain and dysfunction, with the exception of surface EMG. Our most valuable tool is the ability to palpate soft tissue and assess for dysfunction. It is also true that some therapists are better than others at palpation and assessment techniques. Everyone has varying degrees of training and different levels of proficiency. Myofascial trigger point therapists, massage therapists, bodyworkers, movement therapists, chiropractors, physicians, etc. are no different than any other health-care discipline in this regard. I also take this position because of the credibility of some of the studies which form the basis for this question being asked.

Q4. What other tests do you use so that your clinical examination's reliability can be bolstered?

A4. In a general clinical examination, following recording of the patient's life and medical history, structural disparities are evaluated (feet, ankles, knees, hips, pelvis, spine, thorax, shoulders, neck and head). This is checked standing, sitting and lying down, which systematically removes muscle's functional response to gravity and loading. Are the feet only flat and pronated when standing? Is the pelvis elevated on one side while standing, but then depressed or level when sitting? Active range of motion of muscles, as well as hyper- and hypomobility of joints, are then assessed, as is passive range of motion of all major joints. The patient's gait and movement patterns are also observed. If suspicious of an underlying joint or structural problem, X-rays are requested and/or an appropriate referral. Active and latent trigger points are then palpated for, based on the patient's pain diagram, as well as assessment for restricted ROM in muscles, and performance of a structural exam.

All of this allows for a practitioner to form an impression regarding what may be the main problem. If the patient has minor trigger point involvement and global pain of unknown aetiology is a primary complaint, a focused fibromyalgia evaluation is performed including palpation for tender points. Other tests might include checking for nystagmus and screening for vestibular injuries that can result in balance and sleep disturbances.

Additionally a motor sensory exam might be performed with muscle testing and the checking of deep tendon reflexes. If there is a complaint of leg pain with physical activity, distal pulses are checked for vascular insufficiency, with appropriate referrals if findings suggest problems which lie outside of my scope of practice. Chinese pulse diagnosis for meridian disturbances and blocks may also be used.

Janet Travell MD taught that 'the magic will never fail you'. If someone has a primary myofascial pain problem, they will improve very quickly under the myofascial trigger point therapy protocol. When they don't improve, it means something else is wrong. It is the patients that I have seen and treated that didn't steadily improve that taught me that I needed to be able to do a more focused evaluation.

Q5. If treatment based on possibly unreliable assessment and palpation methods is apparently effective, what does this say about the value of the methods being used?

A5. The study by Gerwin et al (1997) seems to indicate that previous poor study design may have contributed to poor interrater reliability when palpation is involved. Bogduk has said (1999, personal communication) that he didn't really believe in so-called trigger points as a primary pain generator because, to date, few were able to reliably locate them. Bogduk (1997) may have formed this opinion from the outcome of interrater reliability studies, which he cites. Poor study design, as well as the levels of experience and training of those involved, may have contributed to those results. Physicians and therapists adequately experienced and trained to locate and treat myofascial trigger points do not question their existence.

Additionally, it would be interesting to see a study comparing sham bodywork (involving inexperienced, untrained therapists) with focused bodywork (involving experienced and trained therapists), to see if it is 'just placebo'. We need to acknowledge that what we do in a therapeutic setting may work in spite of science asking for justification. However, when it doesn't work we need to ask 'why?' and 'might something be wrong that I don't have knowledge of, or for which there is a lack of understanding?'.

Q6. Should palpatory diagnostic findings be accepted as having a subjective/interpretative value similar to interpretation of radiographic findings or other laboratory data and therefore be capable of being integrated into a treatment plan by a skilled therapist?

A6. Palpation is no more subjective than the motor sensory examination carried out by a neurologist or determining the usefulness of an X-ray or MRI. To be meaningful in developing a treatment plan, these methods all require subjective information from the patient and then subjective interpretation on the part of the examiner. Such interpretation is clearly influenced by the level of experience and training of the particular practitioner. There are not many findings in medicine which are purely objective, where findings are consistently reproducible between different qualified observers, in which cooperation is not required on the part of the patient. As the Boden study (1990) pointed out, an objective finding on an MRI does not predict a patient's complaint of pain, as there may be none. Many (possibly most) examinations rely on the information which patients provide, as well as the observations and interpretations of evidence by the practitioner. It therefore seems reasonable to integrate the findings of experienced and skilled manual therapists, including those derived from palpation and manual assessment, into the evidence used to compose a comprehensive treatment plan.

Diane Lee MCPA

Q1. Does the poor interobserver reliability of palpation methods make you question the validity and usefulness of an examination based upon this skill? If not, why not?

A1. The use of palpation for assessment and treatment of musculoskeletal conditions is a long-standing practice of many different practitioners. Confidence in these techniques grows as experience is gained, I would not want to be without them in the clinic. The research quoted pertains to joints with small amplitude of motion (vertebral zygapophyseal and sacroiliac joints) which poses a greater reliability challenge than the larger peripheral joints.

I believe that we have not been able to show inter- nor intratester reliability when motion (either active or passive) of these joints is assessed because we have not paid attention to the dynamic and changing nature of the individual being tested. To investigate, determine and then compare findings such as articular range of motion implies that the tester 'knows' what the range of motion for that joint should be. In addition, we have assumed that the range of motion will be constant from moment to moment for that individual. Recent research (Richardson et al 2000, Van Wingerden et al 2001) in the pelvic girdle has shown that the stiffness value (directly related to range of motion; Buyruk et al 1995a,b) of the sacroiliac joint is related to compression within the pelvis. In these two studies, compression was increased by activation of transversus abdominis, multifidus, erector spinae, gluteus maximus and/or biceps femoris. Whenever these muscles were activated (in isolation or combination), the stiffness value (measured with oscillations and the Echodoppler as per the method originally proposed by Buyruk et al 1995a,b) of the SIJ increased (and thus the range of motion decreased). Unless the specific muscle activation pattern is noted during whatever range of motion test (active or passive) is being evaluated for reliability, there is no way of knowing what amount of compression the SIJ is under (at that moment) and therefore what the available range of motion should be. Lee (2002) reports that Hungerford (2000, unpublished research) has shown that normal individuals performing a one-leg standing hip flexion test vary their motor control strategy each time they perform the test, implying that different muscles can be used to perform the same osteokinematic motion. This will vary the amount of compression each time they lift the leg and thus vary the range of motion. Unless trials are repeated and motions averaged, reliability is impossible – not because the tester can't feel what's happening but because the subject keeps changing from moment to moment.

Q2. How do you think palpation and clinical assessment should be taught/studied so that its validity and clinical potential can be best demonstrated?

A2. I think the teaching methods for translatoric and angular motion analysis in the spine and pelvis are fine. What we need to consider is how we are interpreting the findings from these assessments. Just because a joint has decreased amplitude of motion does not mean that the joint is stiff or hypomobile. Excessive activation of the deep stabilisers for that joint will increase compression and restrict the available range. We need to apply a clinical reasoning process from a number of different tests to reach a mobility diagnosis of hypomobility, hypermobility or instability. This cannot be reached from one test alone and yet too often we are being asked (in research) to make statements regarding range of motion based on one test.

To demonstrate validity for the test procedures I believe we need to really look at the inclusion criteria of the subjects and include subjects on the basis of a biomechanical assessment regardless of location and behaviour of pain. Pain has no relevance on motion. Exquisitely painful joints can have full range of motion whereas non-painful joints can be totally blocked in all directions.

Q3. Should we depend less on palpation and assessment methods in clinical settings, since their reliability seems to be so poor?

A3. Absolutely not – we need to continue to refine the research methods. For me, good research 'rings true' to clinical findings. An experienced clinician will already be aware of what the research 'reveals' or discovers; after all, the clinician is 'researching' every day in their practice.

Q4. What other tests do you use so that your clinical examination's reliability can be bolstered?

A4. A clinical correlation between the subjective examination and objective examination (Lee & Vleeming 1998) which includes tests for:

1. form closure (structure and anatomical restraints to motion) – stability and ligamentous stress and motion tests
2. force closure (myofascial activation and relaxation tests)
3. motor control (sequencing or timing of muscle activation)
4. influence of the emotional state on resting muscle tone.

Q5. If treatment based on possibly unreliable assessment and palpation methods is apparently effective, what does this say about the value of the methods being used? (For example, is apparently successful treatment, based on apparently unreliable assessment methods, valuable mainly for its placebo effects?)

A5. It implies that the treatment methods are valuable and effective and the research is flawed.

Q6. Should palpatory diagnostic findings be accepted as having a subjective/interpretative value similar to interpretation of radiographic findings or other laboratory data and therefore be capable of being integrated into a treatment plan by a skilled therapist?

A6. Yes – the more we understand the dynamic nature of the human body, the less structural and concrete our interpretations of the findings will be. As we gain a clearer understanding of how joints respond to compression and what can increase or decrease compression across them, the confusion will clear and many controversies will be explained. In the meantime, palpation should remain a primary tool for manual therapists in any discipline.

Craig Liebenson DC and Karel Lewit MD

Palpation's reliability: a question of science versus art

Palpation is not very reliable. Yet mankind has always relied on palpation as is borne out by language (not only English): if you have understood something you have grasped it and if you have solved a problem you have worked it out (with your hands). In a field where even the best assessment tools can provide a specific diagnosis only 15% of the time, to lobby for the exclusion of a safe, inexpensive assessment tool believed to be valuable by experts in manual medicine is highly illogical (Bigos et al 1994, Waddell et al 1996). Our entire array of evaluative procedures has low predictive validity. For example, we still lack the ability to identify subgroups of low back pain patients who would respond to specific therapeutic interventions. From this we can only conclude that our science is in its infancy. The question about palpation's reliability should not be turned against palpation but should be turned towards asking how to develop reliable, responsive and valid instruments.

The difficulty of establishing motion palpation's reliability may, in fact, point to the conclusion that our ability to measure the parameters involved in motion palpation is insufficient. The Nobel prize-winning microbiologist Rene Dubos said 'the measurable drives out the useful'. To abandon a tool because it is hard to measure does not make much sense when we are in a field where over 85% of our patients are labelled as having a 'non-specific disorder' (Bigos et al 1994, Erhard & Deritto 1994). If we were able to identify, specifically, what was wrong with most back pain patients with non-palpation tools and thereby determine the most appropriate treatment, then it would be foolish to hold onto techniques with questionable reliability and validity. However, in our field, we're just beginning to crawl. While we strive to establish proof as our goal for creating a 'best practice' scenario, we are a long way from being able to reasonably justify throwing away such a safe, low-cost, although admittedly difficult to measure technique as palpation of joint, muscle or soft tissue motion and stiffness.

The state of palpation art

The skill with which patients are diagnosed and treated in the field of manual medicine requires both science and art. Western medicine has led the way in the development of hands-off, high-tech medicine. Gordon Waddell helped us to see clearly the grave shortcomings of this approach when considering the diagnosis and treatment of spine disorders (Waddell 1998). The problems of motion palpation's reliability have been considered in a paper by Lewit (1993) which acknowledged that 'motion palpation of intersegmental movement in the spinal column has been shown repeatedly to have poor reliability'. However, four important exceptions were noted (Jull et al 1988, 1997, Leboeuf & Gardner 1989, Leboeuf et al 1989). Palpation of trigger points has also proven to be controversial. While most studies have not shown it to be reliable a recent study by Sciotti demonstrated promising results (Sciotti et al 2001). In particular, when palpating the trapezius muscle, the presence of a taut band, nodule and spot tenderness were found to be reliable while the findings of a jump sign and local twitch responses were not.

Palpation of muscles and joints is certainly controversial. However, palpation clearly has clinical utility. A full literature summary shows that it has not been convincingly proven to be unreliable and, as Lewit (1999) points out, it presents many inherent difficulties in demonstrating reliability because of the sophistication and high level of skill required for performing the technique. Is palpation a science? Or does it reflect an aspect of the artful practice of clinical manual medicine?

The craft of palpation has the merit that it encourages the development of 'palpatory literacy' (Chaitow 1997) since one at least attempts to feel restricted mobility and end-feel. In fact, although palpation is too complex to measure with a gold standard instrument, like seeing with photography or hearing with tape recorders, this does not make palpation useless. Palpation is much more than just pressure (algometry); it involves proprioception, motion and tension. The fact that it cannot be copied is no reason to abandon it.

Manipulative techniques are best performed after first sensing with the hands such things as resistance and tension. One's level of technique depends on the capacity to feel (i.e. the palpatory skill), as well as to interpret what is felt. In fact, it could be argued that without the ability to palpate, good manipulative technique is unimaginable. It is precisely the wealth of information, i.e. its sophistication including feedback with the patient, which makes it less reliable or, more precisely, less reproducible.

Clinically, palpation is a highly valued method because it tells the experienced examiner where the patient feels pain. Increased tension, especially myofascial trigger points, is a signpost for the clinician.

A promising direction

One of the reasons why motion palpation is not reliable is that the range of active movement constantly changes (Wolff 2000). Another is that individual techniques have not been properly analysed. Finally, there is no science of 'palpatorics' as there is of optics or of hearing.

If we examine the motion palpation literature regarding the sacroiliac (SI) joints, an interesting picture emerges. Erhard & Delitto (1994) reported that individual motion palpation tests (with good interobserver reliability) were not valid for classifying patients with SI syndrome. However, when a battery of SI tests are used together, valid classification of the patient can be made if the majority of the tests are found to be positive (Erhard & Delitto 1994). Many successful palpation studies benefited by having the examiners practise together. Sciotti's study on trigger point assessment utilised four 3-hour training/practice sessions (Sciotti et al 2001). Gerwin also showed modest interobserver reliability, but only after a 3-hour training session was included (Gerwin et al 1997). Similarly, in the subtle evaluation of movement coordination, practice sessions have been demonstrated to be essential to interobserver reliability (Van Dillen et al 1998). Strender also found that practice together was essential to good reliability in the physical examination of low back function (Strender et al 1997).

Since functional disturbances are so variable, our patient populations are likely very heterogeneous. Therefore, it should be expected that no single palpatory test will have high validity. Perhaps, instead of abandoning the palpation of our patients, we should perform a thorough physical examination using a battery of tests so that the heterogeneity of our patient population will not lead us to falsely conclude that there is nothing mechanically wrong.

Erhard & Delitto concluded that:

- a collection of palpation tests was more valid than any one test by itself
- classification by a combination of palpation findings and other physical examination tests has predictive validity for assigning patients into different meaningful conservative care treatment groups
- non-specific back pain patients represent a heterogeneous group.

Erhard & Delitto's work demonstrates a situation where palpation, in conjunction with other test procedures, led to the adjudication of a subclassification of non-specific back pain patients. This classification enhances the ability to assign patients to treatment groups where favourable outcomes are more likely.

Where do we go?

Harrison & Troyanovich (1998) have recommended that motion palpation be abandoned by the chiropractic profession. They come to this conclusion because, in their opinion, it is unreliable, invalid and perceived by most chiropractors as scientific. That it is unreliable and invalid is controversial. That chiropractors perceive it to be scientific is a 'straw horse' easily assailed and of little value in discrediting the technique. While we laud an effort to make a profession more critical of their assessment of analytic and therapeutic tools, it is important not to misinterpret the scientific literature regarding specific techniques (DIHTA 1999, Lewit 1999). Literature reviews in manual medicine typically are based on a small number of studies. Their conclusions are not based on health technology assessment which, in addition to a systematic literature review, includes ethical issues, health-care organisation and structure and economic analysis (DIHTA 1999, Manniche & Jordan 2001).

Palpation presents many problems to be solved. A full literature summary shows that it has not been convincingly proven to be unreliable and as Lewit (1999) points out, it presents many inherent difficulties in demonstrating its reliability because of its sophistication and the high level of skill required.

Conclusion

If palpation were to be abandoned, what is to fill the void? The field of manual medicine has a long way to go scientifically, but abandoning palpation for a 'more sophisticated' analysis would be a memorable error. Manual medicine specialists do need to realise the quicksand they are in and learn to utilise tests of greater reliability, responsiveness and validity (Bolton 1994, Yeomans & Liebenson 1997). We should learn about palpation's limitations and focus on incorporating sturdier assessment tools. However, manual medicine practitioners should not abandon palpation of joints, muscles and soft tissues any more than an internist should abandon palpating the abdomen or a cardiologist abandon auscultating the chest. The direction of combining several techniques to accurately classify and therefore accurately treat patients seems to show great promise at this point.

Donald R Murphy DC, DACAN

Preliminary remarks

It is important for us as clinicians to be guided by the scientific literature while avoiding being a slave to it. This is a fine art, that must be developed in the absence of the ego-temptation to try to mould the scientific literature to fit our preconceived beliefs – applying science in areas in which it supports our belief system and ignoring it when this support is not provided. At the same time, our scientific methods are not even close to allowing us to rely on the scientific literature to answer many of the questions that we have about how best to treat our patients. This leads to the often great dichotomy between what the scientific literature seems to suggest and what our clinical experience seems to suggest.

This having been said, I would not agree with the idea of 'poor interobserver reliability of palpation methods'. A great deal of research has been done in this area (indeed, this research is still in its infancy) and there are several conclusions that can be drawn from this research. One is that there are several problems with the reliability studies that have been done thus far in the area of joint palpation that dramatically decrease the reliability of the studies themselves. These are as follows.

In most of the studies that have assessed reliability, movement restriction only was analysed, not the combination of loss of joint play and pain provocation on palpation (Bergstrom & Courtis 1986, Carmichael 1987, DeBoer et al 1985, Haas et al 1995, Keating et al 1990, Love & Brodeur 1987, Meijne et al 1999, Mootz et al 1989, Nansel et al 1989). It is doubtful that the average experienced clinician uses movement restriction alone as the sole criterion for making the diagnosis of joint dysfunction.

In most of the studies of motion palpation of joints, a substantial percentage, and in some cases all, of the subjects were asymptomatic, rendering the studies irrelevant to the clinical setting (Bergstrom & Courtis 1986, Boline et al 1988, Carmichael 1987, DeBoer et al 1985, Love & Brodeur 1987, Meijne et al 1999, Mootz et al 1989, Nansel et al 1989). Reliability has been shown to be greater in symptomatic than asymptomatic populations (Fjellner et al 1999). Some patients, due to the thickness of the overlying tissues, general stiffness or other factors, are more difficult to palpate than others. This is a reality in clinical practice as well as in research. In a study in which such patients are included in the subject population, this can negatively affect the group kappa values but does not mean that the procedure is necessarily unreliable in all patients.

Some individuals are better able to discriminate levels of resistance to palpation than are others, as was demonstrated by Nicholson et al (1997) who found that there was a wide variability in the ability of different practitioners to detect stiffness. If a particular study includes examiners who are 'good' at assessing stiffness and others that are not, 'reliability' will likely be 'poor'.

Particularly in studies in which multiple examiners are used, changes are likely to occur in the patient with repeated palpation, i.e. it is likely that irritation to the joints and soft tissues from the palpation itself will produce restriction of motion and texture changes that are detected by subsequent examiners and that alter their findings.

The literature suggests there are some methods and criteria of palpation that can be carried out more reliably than others.

Another conclusion that can be drawn is that, if performed properly, particularly using the criteria of both movement restriction and pain provocation, motion palpation for joint dysfunction is reliable (Jull et al 1997, Marcus et al 1999, Strender et al 1997) and valid (Hides et al 1994, Jull 1985, Jull et al 1988, Lord et al 1994, Sandmark & Nisell 1995).

Finally, motion palpation for joint dysfunction in the sacroiliac joints has been found to be both reliable (Albert et al 2000, Broadhurst & Bond 1998, Cibulka et al 1988, Laslett & Williams 1994) and valid (Broadhurst & Bond 1998, Cibulka & Koldehoff 1999, Slipman et al 1998). Muscle palpation has also been demonstrated to be reliable (Gerwin et al 1997, Marcus et al 1999, Tunks et al 1995).

So, once again, I do not think that we can, based on clinical experience and a comprehensive look at the scientific literature, state flat out that palpation is not a reliable examination procedure.

Q1. Does the poor interobserver reliability of palpation methods make you question the validity and usefulness of an examination based upon this skill? If not, why not?

A1. If used appropriately, applying the most effective means and the most clinically appropriate criteria, palpation methods can be an excellent tool in patient examination. It must be noted, however, that the patient examination has many aspects, starting with history taking, through neurologic and general physical examination, to pain provocation and functional examination. It is from the entire clinical exam that we draw conclusions as to diagnosis, and thus management strategy, not from any one assessment tool.

Q2. How do you think palpation and clinical assessment should be taught/studied so that its validity and clinical potential can be best demonstrated?

A2. First, I think that students should be taught to palpate for both joint restriction and pain provocation when palpating joints (DeFranca 2000), as this is the only method that has been shown to be reliable, and should be taught tissue texture changes during joint and myofascial palpation of other tissues. When I was in school (some time ago!), there was no systematic method applied to teaching students the art of palpation. One was just told to palpate as many patients as possible and eventually one would 'get the hang of it'. It would be much more effective to teach the art of palpation and to develop the sensitivity to detect differences in texture, movement and muscle activity, in a stepwise fashion, starting with simple tasks and gradually progressing to more difficult tasks. There is some recent evidence that suggests that starting with non-biologic materials may be an effective starting point for students to be able to detect levels of stiffness in isolation from the other nuances of biological tissue (Nicholson et al 1997).

Q3. Should we depend less on palpation and assessment methods in clinical settings, since their reliability seems to be so poor?

A3. Again, I do not agree that the reliability is as poor as some would think, so I do not believe that palpation should be abandoned, but instead improved. The primary improvement should be teaching students the most reliable criteria for joint and myofascial palpation and more meticulously helping them to hone their skills in the teaching setting.

But we should also recognise that, in the clinical setting, things are not always 'black and white' and that there are patients and clinical situations in which we will apply the best methods of examination and will still not be sure of the diagnosis. It is important that we become comfortable with this and accept that this will sometimes be the case. This is where intuition and trial and error come into play. And this is where we apply the most reliable and valid diagnostic tool – a trial of treatment. That is, we first form the best diagnostic hypothesis we can of what has gone wrong with the patient that is producing the current pain syndrome, based on all of our knowledge, skills, training and intuition. We then test that hypothesis by applying the most effective treatment approaches that we know for that disorder and monitoring the result. If we see some improvement within a reasonable amount of time, we can be confident that our hypothesised diagnosis was correct and we continue in that direction. If we see no or only partial improvement, we reconsider the hypothesis in light of whatever new information we have gained in the treatment trial and form a new hypothesis to be tested. In this way, we are taking a scientific, systematic approach to blending diagnosis and treatment approaches in order to, as expeditiously as possible, uncover the key areas of the patient's problem.

Q4. What other tests do you use so that your clinical examination's reliability can be bolstered?

A4. The purpose of the clinical examination is to answer what I call the Three Essential Questions of Diagnosis (Murphy 2000).

1. Does this patient have a potentially serious or life-threatening condition?
2. What tissue(s) is(are) the primary source(s) of the patient's symptoms?
3. What has gone wrong with the patient as a whole that these symptoms would have developed and persisted?

We then set out to answer these questions with the process of examination. As I stated earlier, the patient examination is a multilevel process, that begins when the practitioner first lays eyes on the patient and continues through history taking, neurologic and general physical examination, examination for pain provocation, and examination for key dysfunctional chains and localised dysfunction. In this process, there are a variety of individual clinical tests that are available to us, some of which have been demonstrated to be reliable and valid, some of which have been demonstrated to have relatively poor reliability and validity and most of which have not yet been evaluated for reliability and validity. By being aware of the literature in the area of reliability and validity, we may then apply a 'levels of evidence' approach to the examination. That is, we can go through the examination process and arrive at a working diagnosis, the 'diagnostic hypothesis' to which I referred earlier. Those aspects of the hypothesis that are based on tests that are known to be reliable and valid will be given greater emphasis and the level of evidence for these will be high. Those aspects that are based on tests of questionable reliability and validity will be given less emphasis due to a lower level of evidence. From this we will come up with our greatest suspicion of what is the most likely diagnosis and, as I stated earlier, will test our hypothesis with treatment.

So I think that taking a systematic approach is what will lead us to the best clinical outcome for our patients, by incorporating the most reliable test whenever possible and combining this with clinical experience, intuition and trials of treatment.

Q5. If treatment based on possibly unreliable assessment and palpation methods is apparently effective, what does this say about the value of the methods being used? (For example, is apparently successful treatment, based on apparently unreliable assessment methods, valuable mainly for its placebo effects?)

A5. We should try to base our diagnostic hypotheses on the best level of evidence possible, with the use of the most reliable diagnostic tests available. So there should not be those clinical situations in which treatment is based purely on unreliable assessment and palpation methods – we should be using those methods that have been shown to be reliable if at all possible. But in reality, things will not always be as exact as we would like. There will be times in which our diagnostic hypothesis will be based on relatively weak evidence. So what if we undergo a trial of treatment and the patient improves? Does this mean that the result was 'merely' placebo?

Even if a certain examination method has poor reliability this does not mean that every time the method is used, the finding is wrong. In other words, we do not know the reliability of motion palpation for loss of joint play in the mortise joint. So if a patient is seen by a clinician for ankle pain and the clinician, based on motion palpation, makes the diagnosis of joint dysfunction in the mortise joint, treats this and the patient gets better, the lack of reliability does not mean that the diagnosis was necessarily wrong and thus the positive clinical result was necessarily placebo. It simply means that the clinician cannot prove to an outsider that the diagnosis was correct and that the positive clinical result was directly due to the treatment, a fact that, in the common clinical setting, would hardly matter to the clinician or the patient. Only the result matters to those directly involved. This, of course, does not rule out the possibility that the apparently positive clinical result may have been produced by the placebo effect but, to me, if we are not using the placebo effect in our clinical approaches, then we are likely not being very successful with our management strategies. Proper patient management inevitably will involve the placebo effect to a certain extent although, in my opinion, only the most gifted among us can solely rely on this effect.

It is for this reason, then, that we continue to assess our examination procedures for reliability and validity and continue to strive to use those that have been shown to be most reliable and valid, so that we can maximise our clinical outcomes by having greater confidence in our diagnoses. This greater confidence allows us to apply those methods that have the greatest likelihood of resolving the specific pain generators and dysfunctions that we have detected on examination as well as maximising our use of placebo by bolstering confidence on the part of the patient.

Q6. Should palpatory diagnostic findings be accepted as having a subjective/interpretative value similar to interpretation of radiographic findings or other laboratory data and therefore be capable of being integrated into a treatment plan by a skilled therapist?

A6. In theory at least, this is exactly how they should be used. One can ask the question 'what is the reliability of the interpretation of intravenous pyelogram in the detection of pyelonephritis?'. Before answering this question, one must ask 'who is doing the interpretation?'. If experienced radiologists are interpreting the study, the reliability will likely be quite a bit better than if I and several fellow non-radiologist chiropractic physicians are making this interpretation. So it should be that the experienced manual practitioner be seen as that person that possesses the skills required to make the diagnosis of locomotor system dysfunction, just as the palpation skill of the experienced neurologist can be relied upon to make the diagnosis of cogwheeling rigidity in a patient with Parkinson's disease. In this case, the neurologist cannot 'prove' the presence of rigidity because, as with joint dysfunction or myofascial trigger points, there are no common objective tests to demonstrate this finding. So we rely on the expertise of the practitioner. Whether experienced manual practitioners have the common level of skill to attain this status remains to be determined. It is my feeling that many have the skill level to fit the bill, but many do not.

Another problem with palpation findings in locomotor system pain and dysfunction in making the comparison with these other fields of medicine is that there are so many theories as to those factors that contribute to disorders in this area. This, to me, is the reason why a patient may go to five manual practitioners and walk away with five different diagnoses. It is not so much the lack of reliability of palpation methods as the difference in the theoretical constructs from which each practitioner is operating.

David G Simons MD

Q1. Does the poor interobserver reliability of palpation methods make you question the validity and usefulness of an examination based upon this skill? If not, why not?

A1. It serves as a warning flag that some examiners use different criteria than others or have a significant difference in skill level. If no study can demonstrate satisfactory interobserver reliability by palpation, then that diagnostic method is seriously suspect.

In the case of myofascial trigger points (MTrPs), five well-designed studies used raters that were either experienced or trained but not both. All five studies reported reliability ratings that were unsatisfactory. One other reliability study by four physicians who were recognised for their expertise in MTrPs started out making the same mistake and assumed that because of their individual expertise, they would have high interobserver reliability. They did poorly on their first study so, before repeating the study, they spent 3 hours comparing their examination techniques on a human subject and came to agreement regarding details as to what constituted each specific diagnostic finding. This time the study resulted in good to excellent agreement (Gerwin et al 1997).

My conclusion is that reliable diagnosis of MTrPs takes more training and skill than most teachers or investigators realise.

Q2. How do you think palpation and clinical assessment should be taught/studied so that its validity and clinical potential can be best demonstrated?

A2. Taught: in my experience of teaching physical therapists, the most effective way to teach palpation of MTrPs is one-on-one training. Have the student first study (and learn) that muscle's attachments, structure and function, then understand what they are looking for in their examination and finally realise the pathophysiological basis for the MTrP's clinical characteristics. At that point, I have the student examine one of my muscles (the SCM for pincer palpation and the third finger extensor for flat palpation for starters). First, I check the muscle myself to make sure I know what is there and then see what they can find. If they are having trouble finding it, it is easy for me to see why based on what I see them doing and what their palpation of that muscle feels like compared to what it felt like when I palpated myself. This process can be applied to most of the muscles in the body.

Another approach that is less demanding of teaching time is to have the students work in teams of three and have them take turns being paired examiners of the subject. Each examiner examines the muscle with the other examiner blinded and fills out a worksheet listing individual examination findings and what MTrPs were found. After the second examiner fills out a similar worksheet, they then compare results and, with the help of an instructor, see how they could have examined the muscle so they would have agreed as to their findings. The person who served as subject then similarly examines one of the previous examiners.

Studies: when conducting a research project that involves the identification of MTrPs, there is one simple way to establish credibility of the palpation-based diagnosis. Have all examinations of subjects be performed by two blinded examiners and then do an interrater reliability evaluation of their findings for all subjects in that study. If the ratings are unsatisfactory then the examiners must practise as described above until they develop the skill necessary to achieve good interrater reliability. If they cannot achieve this level of skill, it may be because one (or both) of them does not have the native talent for palpation that is needed to become effective at finding MTrPs. When the examiners have learned how to agree on examination techniques sufficiently to get high ratings, the readers of the published paper must conclude that those two blinded examiners knew how to identify whatever it was that they called MTrPs by using the criteria and techniques that they described fully in the paper. This confirms that for the purposes of that paper there was a credible entity MTrP which was reliably identifiable by palpation. It also helps the examiners to hone their own examination skills.

Q3. Should we depend less on palpation and assessment methods in clinical settings, since their reliability seems to be so poor?

A3. No. We should learn how to improve our palpation skills and concentrate on a better understanding of what it is that we are palpating.

Q4. What other tests do you use so that your clinical examination's reliability can be bolstered?

A4. Take a thorough history and consider the circumstances associated with the onset.

What muscles were likely overloaded or were held in the shortened position for a long time?

Ask the patient precisely what movements or positions increase their pain or relieve it.

Sleeping position problems can be very revealing as to which muscles are likely involved.

Carefully make a drawing of the patient's pain pattern and use that as a guide for further testing.

Examine the suspected muscles for painfully restricted stretch range of motion. Look for skeletal and muscular perpetuating factors such as pronated feet, a short lower extremity, an asymmetrical pelvis, short upper arms, forward head posture, paradoxical breathing, gait or movement patterns that indicate muscle imbalances, mild to moderate muscle weakness (reflex inhibition from TrPs in the same or functionally related muscles), etc.

Now you are ready to start palpating the muscles for the MTrPs that are very likely the cause of the patient's pain. Finding what you expected to find at this point greatly bolsters your confidence in the validity of your palpation findings. Not finding it presents a serious diagnostic challenge.

Q5. If treatment based on possibly unreliable assessment and palpation methods is apparently effective, what does this say about the value of the methods being used? (For example, is apparently successful treatment, based on apparently unreliable assessment methods, valuable mainly for its placebo effects?)

A5. Sometimes. There is no doubt that the placebo effect is one of our most valuable therapeutic tools. Even cancer is favourably affected by a positive psychological outlook and imaging. Only, we must be careful not to delude ourselves by attributing favourable clinical results to treatment that is ineffective for that cause of the patient's pain, when in reality the results were placebo effect. It is important to identify and treat the cause of the pain, too.

A more important factor is the common practice of doing the right thing for the wrong reason. Since MTrPs are so commonly undiagnosed, the patient is treated (often less effectively) for another diagnosis that may be related. When a vertebral joint is mobilised because of restricted joint mobility by a muscle energy technique, what is done to the patient is almost indistinguishable from performing contract–relax for releasing the rotatores or multifidus muscles that have taut bands and the TrPs which are responsible for the restricted joint movement and the pain complaint. It is important to identify and treat the cause of the patient's pain.

Q6. Should palpatory diagnostic findings be accepted as having a subjective/interpretative value similar to interpretation of radiographic findings or other laboratory data and therefore be capable of being integrated into a treatment plan by a skilled therapist?

A6. The question assumes an adequately skilled radiologist who underwent years of training and practice specifically to gain that skill and was taught by experts who really were skilful themselves. The radiologist was then critically tested and evaluated to ensure that he or she, in fact, had developed adequate skill before being certified as qualified. The same applies to the 'skilled therapist'. In my experience, when it comes to MTrPs, that is a rare bird. With regard to MTrPs the problem is lack of adequate training and practice.

Conclusion

The main thoughts and recommendations which emerge from this debate seem to be as follows.

1. Individual palpation-based assessments and tests have limited value, but when combined with other indicators and tests, along with the patient's history and presenting symptoms, are invaluable.

2. The apparent inadequacies in palpation results, exposed by research, are not very different from other assessment methods which depend on subjective interpretation of evidence (e.g. radiographic interpretation) and can be remedied by appropriate training and precise application of agreed methodology.

3. Training in palpation skills demands a sound knowledge of the terrain, as well as diligent practising of assessment techniques, in a standardised manner, until results are routinely reproducible by the individual and between individual practitioners.

REFERENCES

Albert H, Godskesen M, Westergaard J 2000 Evaluation of clinical tests used in classification procedures in pregnancy-related pelvic joint pain. European Spine Journal 9:161–166

Aprill C 2000 Sacro-iliac joint dysfunction: evaluation and treatment. Focus on Pain Conference, Mesa, AZ

Aprill C, Bogduk N 1992 High-intensity zone: a diagnostic sign of painful lumbar disc on magnetic resonance imaging. British Journal of Radiology 66 (773):361–369

Basmajian J, Nyberg R 1993 Rational manual therapies. Williams and Wilkins, Baltimore

Beal M, Goodridge J, Johnston W, McConnell D 1980 Inter examiner agreement on patient improvement after negotiated selection of tests. Journal of the American Osteopathic Association 79(7):45–53

Bergstrom E, Courtis G 1986 An inter- and intra-examiner reliability study of motion palpation of the lumbar spine in lateral flexion in the seated position. European Journal of Chiropractic 34:121–141

Bigos S, Bowyer O, Braen G 1994 Acute low back problems in adults. Clinical practice guideline. US Department of Health and Human Services, Public Health Service, Agency for Health Care Policy and Research, Rockville, MD

Boden S, Davis D, Dina T, Pastroras N, Wiesel S 1990 Abnormal magnetic resonance scans of the lumbar spin in asymptomatic subjects. Journal of Bone and Joint Surgery 72A(3):403–408

Bogduk N 1997 Clinical anatomy of the lumbar spine and sacrum, 3rd edn. Churchill Livingstone, Edinburgh, pp 195–196

Boline P, Keating J, Brist J, Denver G 1988 Inter examiner reliability of palpatory evaluations of the lumbar spine. American Journal of Chiropractic Medicine 1(1):5–11

Bolton JE 1994 Evaluation of treatment of back pain patients: clinical outcome measures. European Journal of Chiropractic 42:29–40

Bourdillon J, Day E, Boohhout M 1995 Spinal manipulation, 5th edn. Bath Press, Avon

Broadhurst NA, Bond MJ 1998 Pain provocation tests for the assessment of sacroiliac joint dysfunction. Journal of Spinal Disorders 11(4):341–345

Buyruk HM, Stam HJ, Snijders CJ, Vleeming A, Lamris JS, Holland WPJ 1995a The use of colour Doppler imaging for the assessment of sacroiliac joint stiffness: a study on embalmed human pelvises. European Journal of Radiology 21:112–116

Buyruk HM, Snijders CJ, Vleeming A, Lamris JS, Holland WPJ, Stam HJ 1995b The measurements of sacroiliac joint stiffness with colour Doppler imaging: a study on healthy subjects. European Journal of Radiology 21:117–121

Carmichael JP 1987 Inter- and intra-examiner reliability of palpation for sacroiliac joint dysfunction. Journal of Manipulative and Physiological Therapeutics 10(4):164–171

Chaitow L 1997 Palpation skills. Churchill Livingstone, Edinburgh

Christensen FB, Laursen M, Gelineck J, Eiskjaer SP, Thomsen K, Bunger CE 2001 Interobserver and intraobserver agreement of radiograph interpretation with and without pedicle screw implants: the need for a detailed classification system in posterolateral spinal fusion. Spine 26(5):538–543; discussion 543–544

Cibulka MT, Koldehoff R 1999 Clinical usefulness of a cluster of sacroiliac joint tests in patients with and without low back pain. Journal of Orthopedic and Sports Physical Therapy 29(2):83–92

Cibulka MT, DeLitto A, Koldejoff RM 1988 Changes in innominate tilt after manipulation of the sacroiliac joint in patients with low back pain: an experimental study. Physical Therapy 68(9):1359–1363

Comeaux Z, Eland D, Chila A, Pheley A, Tate M 2001 Measurement challenges in physical diagnosis: refining inter-rater palpation, perception and communication. Journal of Bodywork and Movement Therapies 5(4):245–253

Danish Health Technology Assessment (DIHTA) 1999 Low back pain: Frequency management and prevention from an HAD Perspective.

DeBoer KF, Harmon R, Tuttle CD, Wallace H 1985 Reliability of detection of somatic dysfunctions in the cervical spine. Journal of Manipulative Physiological Therapeutics 8(1):9–16

Defranca GG 2000 Evaluation of joint dysfunction in the cervical spine. In: Murphy DR (ed) Conservative management of cervical spine syndromes. McGraw-Hill, New York, pp 267–306

DiGiovanna E, Schiowitz S (eds) 1991 An osteopathic approach to diagnosis and treatment. JB Lippincott, Philadelphia

Dvorak J, Dvorak V 1990 Manual medicine diagnostics, 2nd edn. Thieme Medical Publishers, New York

Erhard RE, Delitto A 1994 Relative effectiveness of an extension program and a combined program of manipulation and flexion and extension exercises in patients with acute low back syndrome. Physical Therapy 74:1093–1100

Fjellner A, Bexander C, Falei R, Strender LE 1999 Inter examiner reliability in physical examination of the cervical spine. Journal of Manipulative and Physiological Therapeutics 22(8):511–516

Fleiss J 1981 Statistical methods for rates and proportions. Wiley, New York

Gerwin RD, Shannon S, Hong CZ, et al 1997 Inter-rater reliability in myofascial trigger point examination. Pain 69(1,2):65–73

Gonnella C, Paris S, Kutner M 1982 Reliability in evaluating passive intervertebral motion. Physical Therapy 62:436–444

Gibbons P, Tehan P 2000 Manipulation of the spine, thorax and pelvis: an osteopathic perspective. Churchill Livingstone, Edinburgh

Greenman PE 1989 Principles of manual medicine. Williams and Wilkins, Baltimore

Haas M, Raphael R, Panzer D, Peterson D 1995 Reliability of manual end-play palpation of the thoracic spine. Chiropractic Technique 7(4):120–124

Harrison D, Troyanovich S 1998 Commentary: motion palpation: it's time to accept the evidence. Journal of Manipulative and Physiological Therapeutics 21:568–571

Harvey D, Byfield D 1991 Preliminary studies with a mechanical model for the evaluation of spinal motion palpation. Clinical Biomechanics 6:79–82

Hides JA, Stokes MJ, Saide M, Jull GA, Cooper DH 1994 Evidence of lumbar multifidus muscle wasting ipsilateral to symptoms in patients with acute/subacute low back pain. Spine 19(2):165–172

Johnston W, Elkiss M, Marino R, Blum G 1982a Passive gross motion testing: Part 11. A study of inter examiner agreement. Journal of the American Osteopathic Association 81(5):65–69

Johnston W, Beal M, Blum G, Hendra J, Neff D, Rosen M 1982b Passive gross motion testing: Part 111. Examiner agreement on selected subjects. Journal of the American Osteopathic Association 81(5):70–74

Jull G 1985 Manual diagnosis of C2–3 headache. Cephalalgia 5(suppl):308–309

Jull G, Bogduk N, Marsland A 1988 The accuracy of manual diagnosis for cervical zygapophyseal joint pain syndromes. Medical Journal of Australia 148:233–236

Jull G, Zito G, Trott P et al 1997 Inter-examiner reliability to detect painful upper cervical joint dysfunction. Australian Physiotherapy 43:125–129

Keating JC, Bergmann TF, Jacobs GE, Finer BA, Larson K 1990 Inter examiner reliability of eight evaluative dimensions of lumbar segmental abnormality. Journal of Manipulative and Physiological Therapeutics 13(8):463–470

Laslett M, Williams M 1994 The reliability of selected pain provocation tests for sacroiliac joint pathology. Spine 19(11):1243–1249

Laslett M, Williams M 1995 The reliability of selected pain provocation tests for sacroiliac joint pathology. In: Leeming A, Mooney V, Dorman T, Snijders J (eds) The integrated function of the lumbar spine and sacroiliac joint. San Diego

Leboeuf C, Gardner V 1989 Chronic low back pain: orthopaedic and chiropractic test results. Journal of Australian Chiropractic Association 19:1–16

Leboeuf C, Gardner V, Carter AL, Scott TA 1989 Chiropractic examination procedures: a reliability and consistency study. Journal of Australian Chiropractic Association 19:101–104

Lebouef-Yde C, Kyvik K 2000 Is it possible to differentiate people with or without low-back pain on the basis of tests of lumbo-pelvic dysfunction? Journal of Manipulative and Physiological Therapeutics 23(3):160–167

Lee D 1999 The pelvic girdle. Churchill Livingstone, Edinburgh

Lee D 2002 How accurate is palpation? Journal of Bodywork and Movement Therapies 6(1):26–27

Lee D, Vleeming A 1998 Impaired load transfer through the pelvic girdle – a new model of altered neutral zone function. 3rd Interdisciplinary World Congress on Low Back and Pelvic Pain. November 19–21, Vienna, Austria, p 76

Lewit K 1999 Letter to the editor. Journal of Manipulative and Physiological Therapeutics 22:260–261

Lewit K, Liebenson C 1993 Palpation – problems and implications. Journal of Manipulative and Physiological Therapeutics 16(9):586–590

Lord S, Bogduk N 1996 Cervical synovial joints as sources of post-traumatic headache. In: Allen M (ed) Musculoskeletal pain emanating from head and neck. Haworth Medical Press, New York

Lord S, Barnsley L, Wallis BJ, Bogduk N 1994 Third occipital nerve headache: a prevalence study. Journal of Neurology, Neurosurgery and Psychiatry 57:1187–1190

Love RM, Brodeur RR 1987 Inter- and intra-examiner reliability of motion palpation for the thoracolumbar spine. Journal of Manipulative and Physiological Therapeutics 10(1):1–4

Manniche C, Jordan A 2001 Letter to the editor. Spine 26:843

Marcus DA, Scharff L, Mercer S, Turk DC 1999 Musculoskeletal abnormalities in chronic headache: a controlled comparison of headache diagnostic groups. Headache 39:21–27

Matyas T, Bach T 1985 The reliability of selected techniques in clinical arthrokinematics. Australian Journal of Physiotherapy 31(5):175–195

McConnell D, Beal M, Dinnar U et al 1980 Low agreement of findings in neuromusculoskeletal examinations by a group of osteopathic physicians using their own procedures. Journal of the American Osteopathic Association 79(7):59–68

McKenzie C, Taylor N 1997 Can physiotherapists locate lumbar spinal levels by palpation? Physiotherapy 83(5):235–239

Meijne W, Van Neerbos K, Aufdenkampe G, Van Der Wurff P 1999 Intraexaminer and interexaminer reliability of the Gillet test. Journal of Manipulative and Physiological Therapeutics 22(1):4–9

Mense S, Simons D 2001 Muscle pain: understanding its nature, diagnosis, and treatment. Lippincott Williams and Wilkins, Baltimore, pp 223–226

Mootz RD, Keating JC, Kontz HP, Milus TB, Jacobs GE 1989 Intra- and interobserver reliability of passive motion palpation of the lumbar spine. Journal of Manipulative and Physiological Therapeutics 12(6):440–445

Murphy DR 2000 History and examination. In: Murphy DR (ed.) Conservative management of cervical spine syndromes. McGraw-Hill, New York, pp 387–419

Nansel DD, Peneff AL, Jansen RD, Cooperstein R 1989 Inter examiner concordance in detecting joint-play asymmetries in the cervical spines of otherwise asymptomatic subjects. Journal of Manipulative and Physiological Therapeutics 12(6):428–433

Nicholson L, Adams R, Maher C 1997 The reliability of a discrimination measure for judgments of non-biological stiffness. Manual Therapy 2:150–156

Nyberg R 1993 Rational manual therapies. Williams and Wilkins, Baltimore

O'Haire F, Gibbons P 2000 Inter-examiner and intra-examiner agreement for assessing sacroiliac anatomical landmarks using palpation and observation: pilot study. Manual Therapy 5(1):13–20

Panzer DM 1992 The reliability of lumbar motion palpation. Journal of Manipulative and Physiological Therapeutics 15(8):518–524

Richardson CA, Snijders CJ, Hides JA, Damen L, Pas MS, Storm J 2000 The relationship between the transversely oriented abdominal muscles, sacroiliac joint mechanics and low back pain. Proceedings of the 7th Scientific Conference of IFOMT, Perth, Australia, November

Rockwell J 1998 Myofascial therapy: a massage therapist's perspective (Seminar). Jacksonville, FL

Sandmark H, Nisell R 1995 Validity of five manual neck pain provocation tests. Scandinavian Journal of Rehabilitation Medicine 27:131–136

Sciotti V, Mittaka V, DiMarcoa L et al 2001 Clinical precision of myofascial trigger points location in the trapezius muscle. Pain 93(3):259–266

Slipman CW, Sterenfeld EB, Chou LB et al 1998 The predictive value of provocative sacroiliac joint stress maneuvers in the diagnosis of sacroiliac joint syndrome. Archives of Physical Medicine and Rehabilitation 79:288–292

Strender LE, Sjoblom A, Sundell K et al 1997 Inter examiner reliability in physical examination of patients with low back pain. Spine 22(7):814–820

Tunks E, McCain GA, Hart LE et al 1995 The reliability of examination for tenderness in patients with myofascial pain, chronic fibromyalgia and controls. Journal of Rheumatology 22(5):944–952

Van Dillen LR, Sahrmann SA, Norton BJ 1998 Reliability of physical examination items used for classification of patients with low back pain. Journal of Orthopedic and Sports Physical Therapy 78(9):979–988

Van Duersen L, Patijn J, Ockhuysen A, Vortman B 1990 The value of some clinical tests of the sacroiliac joint. Manual Medicine 5:96–99

Van Wingerden JP, Vleeming A, Buyruk HM, Raissadat K 2001 Stabilization of the SIJ in vivo: verification of muscular contribution to force closure of the pelvis.

Vincent Smith B, Gibbons P 1999 Inter-examiner and intra-examiner reliability of palpatory findings for the standing flexion test. Manual Therapy 4(2):87–93

Waddell G 1998 The back pain revolution. Churchill Livingstone, Edinburgh

Waddell G, Feder G, McIntosh A, Lewis M, Hutchinson A 1996 Low back pain: evidence review. RCGP, London

Ward R (ed) 1996 Foundations for osteopathic medicine. Williams and Wilkins, Baltimore

Wolff HD 2000 Manuelle Medizin 38:284–288

Yeomans S, Leibenson C 1997 Applying outcomes to clinical practice. Journal of Neuromuscular Systems 5(1):14

SPECIAL TOPIC 3
Visual assessment, the dominant eye, and other issues

Many osteopathic and chiropractic texts advise that, before starting to palpate, you should identify your dominant eye. Almost all of us have one eye which dominates and the reasoning is that during the application of assessment procedures you should position yourself in relation to the patient, or body part, so that the dominant eye has the clearest possible view of what is being observed.

Clearly this is of little importance when palpating with the eyes closed (a common recommendation). There will, however, be many instances when visual impressions need to be combined with palpation, for example in use of the 'red reaction' (see Special Topic 6 for example, and the assessment of ASIS levels in Chapter 9).

Assessing the dominant eye

Make a circle with your first finger and thumb and, holding the arm out in front of your face, observe an object across the room, through that circle, with both eyes open.

Close one eye. If the object is still in the circle, you now have your dominant eye open. If, however, the image shifts out of the circle when only one eye is open, open the closed eye and close the open eye and the image should shift back into clear view, inside the circle.

The one eye which sees the same view as you saw when both eyes were open is the one to use in close observation of the body.

If the patient is on an examination couch, you should approach the couch from the side which will allow your dominant eye to be closest to the centre of the couch.

Using peripheral vision

In some instances, when symmetrical motion is being observed, such as when rib function is being assessed, it is a mistake to closely observe one side and then the other. You should instead rely on the sensitive discrimination which peripheral vision offers.

Focus on a point between your two moving fingers which rest on the ribs and allow your peripheral vision to judge variations in range of motion as the patient breathes.

The use of the dominant eye will be referred to in various exercises when it is appropriate.

By the way, if you are right-handed with a dominant left eye or left-handed with a dominant right eye – both of which are unusual combinations – you would probably make an excellent batsman in cricket or hitter in baseball!

Body position and the eyes

Vladimir Janda (1988) points to the existence of oculopelvic and pelviocular reflexes which indicate that any change in pelvic orientation alters the position of the eyes, and vice versa, and to the fact that eye position modifies muscle tone, particularly the suboccipital muscles (look up and extensors tighten, look down and flexors prepare for activity, etc.).

The implications of modified eye position due to altered pelvic and head positions therefore add yet another set of factors to be considered as we try to ensure that our observational and palpatory efficiency is optimal (Komendatov 1945).

'Sensory literacy'

Frederick Mitchell Jr (Mitchell 1976), writing on the topic of training and measurement of sensory literacy, discussed the various 'parts' of vision. Visual assessment is very important for making effective and reliable assessments and clinical judgements. As Mitchell puts it:

> Does the patient have good or poor posture and how poor is the patient's posture?
> Is a laceration 2.5 cm or 3 cm in length?
> Are the iliac crests equal in height?
> Is the patient's head tilted and by how many degrees?
> Is one knee larger than the other?
> Is dermatosis violaceous or merely pink?

In order to make such judgements, Mitchell lists the need to be able to:

1. identify and discriminate colour hues and saturations
2. quantify 'rectilinear length measurements, angular measurements, curvilinear and arcuate shapes, and their radius of curvature'
3. sense horizontal and vertical frames of reference in which to make quantitative judgements
4. appreciate motion, absolute motion or subjective awareness of motion in relation to himself or relative motion of one thing to another thing
5. demonstrate depth perception and the ability to estimate length and proportion.

All sighted individuals have these skills but the degree of keenness is variable and Mitchell suggests ways of measuring and of enhancing 'visual literacy' by means of training devices which, for example, simulate an extremity's range of motion or leg length differences in a supine patient or levels of iliac crest height in a standing patient.

When such tools are utilised in classroom settings, the student remains unaware of the true angle or length or height until having made an estimation. There then needs to be an immediate feedback of information because, as Mitchell explains:

> Success builds confidence. Failure destroys confidence. It is not unlikely that self-confidence may be an essential ingredient of reliability in accuracy of visual judgment. As accuracy and reliability in making visual judgments increases the student learns to avoid parallax errors and to deal with the possibilities of optical illusion.

Eye dominance appears to be a significant element in the accuracy of visual judgement and becoming aware of backgrounds; lighting is also a part of the training process and is important in eliminating optical illusions as a source of error.

Visual assessment in a physical examination

Dinnar et al (1982) provide the following summary of the questions you might ask yourself during the visual component – observation – of a physical examination, in which screening occurs from three viewpoints: posterior, lateral and anterior.

You might assess your ability to make these observations now, before you start to work your way through the many exercises in this book, and perhaps some time later when you have applied the exercises and hopefully enhanced those skills.

SPECIAL TOPIC EXERCISE 3.1: POSTURAL SCREENING

Time suggested: 15 minutes

This visual screening is designed to give an initial impression, it is not diagnostic.

The patient is standing.

1. Posterior view
   — Are shoulders and scapulae asymmetrical (unequal)?
   — Is there a lateral curvature of the midspinal line?
   — Is the head held to one side?
   — Is the pelvic position asymmetrical (are crests level)?
   — Is there obvious flatness or fullness of the paravertebral muscle mass?
   — Are the feet placed symmetrically or not?
   — Are the positions of the knees symmetrical?
   — Is the body rotated as a whole?
   — Are the Achilles tendons deviated or symmetrical?
   — Are the positions of the malleoli symmetrical in relation to the heels?
   — Are arm positions symmetrical?
   — Are the fat folds (creases) at the waist symmetrical?
   — Is there any obvious morphological asymmetry of the posterior skin surface such as scars, bruises?
2. Lateral view
   — Are the knees relaxed or locked in extension?
   — Are the normal spinal curves exaggerated or reversed?
   — Is the body displaced relative to the centre of gravity; for example, is the head position balanced?
   — Is there any obvious morphological asymmetry of the lateral skin surface such as scars, bruises?
3. Anterior view
   — Are the shoulder levels symmetrical at the midsternal line?
   — Is the head tilted to one side?
   — Does the normal horizontal clavicular line deviate?
   — Is the pelvic position asymmetrical (are crests level)?
   — Are the patellae deviated laterally or medially?
   — Is there any obvious morphological asymmetry of the anterior skin surface such as scars, bruises?

REFERENCES

Dinnar U, Beal M, Goodridge J et al 1982 An osteopathic method of history taking and physical examination. Journal of the American Osteopathic Association 81(5):314–321

Janda V 1988 In: Grant R (ed) Physical therapy in the cervical and thoracic spine. Churchill Livingstone, New York

Komendatov G 1945 Proprioceptivnije reflexi glaza i golovy u krolikov. Fiziologiceskij Zurnal 31:62

Mitchell F 1976 Training and measurement of sensory literacy. Journal of the American Osteopathic Association 75(6):874–884

3

Fundamentals of palpation

Viola Frymann (1963) elegantly summarises the potential which palpation offers the healing professions.

> The human hand is equipped with instruments to perceive changes in temperature, surface texture, surface humidity, to penetrate and detect successively deeper tissue textures, turgescence, elasticity and irritability. The human hand, furthermore, is designed to detect minute motion, motion which can only be detected by the most sensitive electronic pick-up devices available. This carries the art of palpation beyond the various modalities of touch into the realm of proprioception, of changes in position and tension within our own muscular system.

These words define succinctly and with feeling the tool we use and the task we perform when we palpate.

Different parts of the human hand are more or less able to discriminate variations in tissue features, such as relative tension, texture, degree of moisture, temperature and so on. This highlights the fact that an individual's overall palpatory sensitivity depends on a combination of different perceptive (and proprioceptive) qualities and abilities.

These include the ability to register temperature variations and the subtle differences which exist in a spectrum of tissue states, ranging from very soft to extremely hard, as well as the ability to register the existence and size of extremely small entities such as are found in fibrotic tissue or trigger point activity, along with the sensitivity to distinguish between many textures and ranges in tone, from flaccid to spastic, and all the variables in between. Irvin Korr (1970) helps us to understand just why the hand is so delicately able to perform its many tasks.

> Where do we find the greatest number of muscle spindles? Exactly where they logically belong. If the muscle spindle has to do with finely-tuned muscle activity, with measuring gains in extremely small lengths of muscle fibers, one would expect that for more complex movement patterns, as in the muscles of the hand, we would have a very large number of muscle spindles. And this is exactly what we find. The number of spindles per gram of muscle is only 1 in the latissimus dorsi; in the hand the number is close to 26. Functionally this is of great significance.

Physiology of touch

Palpatory perception also results in large measure from variations in the number and type (see summary in Box 3.1) of sensory neural receptors found in the skin and tissues of various anatomical regions, since this greatly influences the discriminatory capabilities of those regions.

Box 3.1 Receptors and perception

Mechanoreceptors

Light touch	Meissner's corpuscle
	Merkel's disc
	Hair-root plexus
Deep pressure	Pacinian corpuscle
Crude touch	Thought to be Krause's end-bulb
	Thought to be Ruffini's ending

Proprioception

Muscle length, tendon and limb position	Muscle spindle
	Golgi tendon organ
	Joint/kinaesthetic receptors

Nociceptors

Pain	Free nerve endings

Thermoreceptors

Warmth	Thought to be free nerve endings
Cold	Thought to be free nerve endings
Internal temperature	Hypothalamic thermostat

Light touch is generally accepted to be achieved via mechanoreceptors (such as Meissner's corpuscle and Merkel's disc, as well as hair-root plexi) lying in the skin, muscles, joints and organs. They respond to mechanical deformation resulting from pressure, stretch or hair movement. It is in the skin that the greatest number of these receptors are found. Cruder touch perception is thought to relate to Krause's end-bulb, Ruffini's ending and Pacinian corpuscles.

Sensations of heat and cold are detected by thermoreceptors which are considered to be the free nerve endings in the skin. If cold is intense, detection is by nociceptors – specialised pain detectors – which are also free nerve endings.

Kappler (1997) notes that although for some people, the palmar surface registers more efficiently, temperature variations are usually more keenly noted by the dorsum of the hand, particularly the dorsum of the second, third and fourth fingers.

Primary (afferent) sensory neurons link the target organ (in this case skin) with the spinal cord or brainstem. Sensory units of this type serve an area of skin called a receptive field. These fields may overlap; if there are many sensory units crowded close together, any tactile stimulation of such units (where there is close proximity and some degree of overlap) automatically results in signal transmission from neighbouring units to the central nervous system (CNS) being suppressed via inhibition of their synapses. This is known as lateral inhibition and serves to sharpen perception of the contrasts noted in whatever is being touched.

The degree of tactile sensitivity in any area is in direct proportion to the number of sensory units present and active in that area, as well as to the degree of overlap of their receptive fields, which vary in size.

Small receptive fields with many sensory units therefore have the highest degree of discriminatory sensitivity. This can be assessed by use of what is called a two-point discrimination test: two sharp points are touched to the area, with the distance between them being varied until the shortest distance at which it is still possible to note that two and not one point is being touched is reached (see Fig. 3.1).

Measurement of the minimum separable distance between two tactile points of stimulus proves that the greatest degree of spatial discrimination exists on the surface of the tongue, the lips and fingertips (1–3 mm). In contrast, the back of

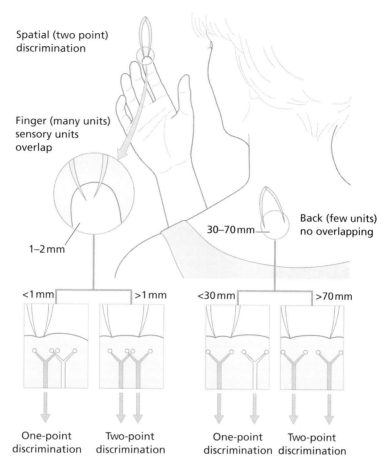

Spatial (two point)
discrimination

Finger (many units)
sensory units
overlap

1–2 mm

30–70 mm

Back (few units)
no overlapping

<1 mm   >1 mm   <30 mm   >70 mm

One-point
discrimination

Two-point
discrimination

One-point
discrimination

Two-point
discrimination

Fig. 3.1 Tactile discrimination. *Spatial discrimination*: in the two-point test, the spatial discriminative ability of the skin is determined by measuring the minimum separable distance between two tactile point stimuli. The back of the hands, the back and legs rate low (50–100 mm). The fingertips, lips and tongue rate high in this ability (1–3 mm). *Intensity discrimination*: sensitive areas are also better able to discriminate differences in the intensity of tactile stimuli. Therefore, an indentation of 6 mm on the fingertip is sufficient to extract a sensation. This threshold is four times higher in the palm.

the hands, the back and the legs have a poor degree of sensitivity to spatial discrimination (50–100 mm).

Not only is there a difference of perception relating to spatial accuracy, but also one relating to intensity. An indentation of 6 micrometres is capable of being registered on the finger pads, while 24 micrometres is needed before the sensors in the palm of the hand reach their threshold and perceive the stimulus.

Kappler (1997) notes that movements with an amplitude as small as a tenth of a millimetre (i.e. a ten thousandth of a meter, a micrometre) can be sensed by skilled palpation touch and that the most sensitive parts of the hand surface to achieve this are likely to be the pads (not tips) of the thumb and first two fingers (where more nerve endings are found than elsewhere in the hands).

The threshold on the backs of the hands, trunk and legs is some 10–20 times higher than the fingertips which, along with the tongue, are the most sensitive palpatory units available to us. It is unlikely that any clinical value can be attached to the tongue's capabilities and so the remarkable discriminatory abilities of the fingertips and pads are best used for our enhanced literacy in palpation.

This is a popular viewpoint; however, some prominent dissenters hold that proprioceptive capabilities can be harnessed to a whole-hand contact, making this the more useful contact. This will be discussed further in this chapter.

Relatively weak stimuli to the fingertips can produce brain cell activation and it is this brain–hand link which holds the key to palpatory literacy.

Variations in sensitivity – relating to both spatial and intensity factors – highlight the marked degree of variation between individuals. This may be because of anatomical differences, such as the number of receptors per sq cm, a variation which would clearly alter the degree of perception possible. In any comparative study of human (or animal) anatomy, there are clear and marked variations in size, number and position of almost all structures, not excluding neural receptors.

Physiological differences also abound in any such examination and so not everyone will have the same degree of sensitivity when they palpate. Some will find it easy to perceive delicate pulsating rhythms, whereas others may have to work long and hard to heighten their sensibilities to the point where they can do so.

Receptor adaptation

Anatomical differences are not the only factors involved in variations in palpatory sensitivity; we have to try to overcome, by constant effort, a physiological response which 'switches off' (or decreases) the rate of firing of receptors when some stimuli are maintained. This relates to what are called 'rapidly firing receptors', which tend to lose their sensitivity on any sustained contact. Those receptors related to fine touch and pressure are of just this rapidly adapting type. Under normal conditions this is thought to have value in preventing our constant awareness of whatever is touching our body (clothing, for example) but it has a nuisance value for anyone involved in palpation assessment for any length of time.

By contrast, mechanoreceptors, serving joint and muscle, are slow adapters, as are pain receptors. Some experts, such as John Upledger, suggest that use of the proprioceptive receptors should be incorporated into our palpatory endeavours. Their slow adaptation certainly adds weight to this suggestion. The alteration in sensitivity resulting from rapid adaptation to light touch is something which can be modified by practice and the exercises which follow later in this chapter will assist in this.

There is an apparent contradiction in that, while fine-touch receptor adaptation may reduce sensitivity, at times too much information is being received and a degree of discrimination, or filtering, of information is required in order to make sense of it. Kappler (1997) summarises this as follows.

> A more significant component [of palpation skills] is to be able to focus on the mass of information being perceived, paying close attention to those qualities associated with tissue texture abnormality, and bypassing many of the other palpatory clues not relevant at the time. This is a process of developing mental filters . . . The brain cannot process everything at once. By concentrating only on the portion you want, it becomes easy and fast to detect areas of significant tissue texture abnormality.

Kappler et al (1971) tested this concept and found that when they compared student examiners with experienced practitioner examiners, although the students recorded more palpation findings, the practitioners recorded more significant findings. The experienced practitioners were filtering out the unimportant, and focusing on what was meaningful, rather than being 'overwhelmed with the mass of palpatory data'.

Exercises later in this chapter will focus on learning to discriminate between different sensations.

Where do we palpate?

It seems according to many experts (see opinions below) that it is the pads of the fingers or thumbs which have the greatest discriminatory ability to measure variations in whatever is being felt. The skin surface itself, with its range of variations from hot or warm to cool or cold; thick or thin; dry, oily or moist; puffy or firm; smooth or rough and so on, is best assessed with the pads of the fingers or the palm, as a rule. As previously mentioned, the dorsum of the hand, because of its sensitivity, is thought by some to be best for measuring the skin surface for temperature and moistness variations. Some experts question this assumption because it is thought to be based mainly on histological data, suggesting that definitive tests should be carried out in which individuals who have been trained to enhance their 'temperature literacy' would have different parts of their hands assessed for sensitivity.

Assessment of the distance of structures from the surface, their depth, as well as their relative size is usually best achieved by the fingertips/pads and to some extent the palms of the hands. The palms and fingertips are also thought to be the most useful contacts for perception of variations in the status of osseous structures, through skin, fat, fascia and muscle.

Kuchera & Kuchera (1994) suggest that the coordinated involvement of the palmar surfaces of the hands and the fingers is the best tool for evaluating the shapes and contours of tissues and objects.

The whole hand including the fingers (including the proprioceptors in the forearms and wrists) is an accurate measuring instrument; the hands can be moulded to the surface in the activity of 'listening' for subtle physiological motions, such as primary respiratory motion, in cranial osteopathic terminology, or visceral motion when organ position and function are being assessed. Subtle variations in amplitude and direction of such movement, as well as the frequency of cycles of activity, can readily be assessed in this way – with practice.

Palpation of movement

If palpation is going to move beyond a simple assessment of the obvious characteristics of the tissues themselves, the hands need to register movement, pulsations and minor tremors and rhythms, along with variations in all or any of these as they respond to the palpatory processes.

The palmar finger surfaces are most efficient for picking up very fine vibration. William Walton (1971) summarised this as follows.

> Most authorities agree on two points. One is that the pads of the fingers are the most sensitive portions of the hands available to diagnosis; that part of the pad just distal to the last interphalangeal articulation is the most sensitive. The second point is that the thumb and first two fingers are the best to use. Which of these fingers or what combinations of them to use vary with the area under consideration, and the operator's own personal preference.

Sara Sutton (1977) differentiates the loci of sensitivity in the hands as follows.

> The pads of the fingers are most sensitive for fine tactile discrimination and require light touch. The dorsal surfaces of the hands are most sensitive to temperature changes, while the palmar surfaces of the metacarpo-phalangeal joints are more sensitive to vibratory changes. The center of the palm is sensitive to gross shape recognition.

John Upledger (Upledger & Vredevoogd 1983) differs markedly in his suggestions as to the ideal palpatory tool.

Most of you have been taught to palpate or touch with your fingertips . . . we, however, would urge you to palpate with your whole hand, arm, stomach or whatever part of your body comes into contact with the patient's body. The idea is to 'meld' the palpating part of your body with the body you are examining. As this melding occurs, the palpating part of your body does what the patient's body is doing. It becomes synchronised. Once melding and synchronisation have occurred, use your own proprioceptors to determine what the palpating part of your own body is doing. Your proprioceptors are those sensory receptors located in the muscles, tendons, and fascia that tell you where the parts of your body are without using your eyes.

Upledger's ideas will be expanded on and some of his exercises for enhancement of palpatory skills examined, as we progress.

Clyde Ford (1989) reminds us that we commonly 'project' our sense of touch, giving the example of writing with a pencil. We feel the texture of the page on which we are writing not at our skin surface or in our fingertips, but at the end of the pencil, thus demonstrating how our proprioceptive awareness can be projected.

Ford suggests you experiment by:

Changing the pressure with which you grasp the pencil – you'll quickly discover that you can't write. The pressure exerted to hold the pencil needs to be constant so you can extend your perception to [the] pencil tip and thereby control the complex task of writing. A good craftsperson knows this instinctively. The woodworker's sense of touch extends to the teeth of the saw, a machinist's to the end of a wrench, a surgeon's to the edge of a scalpel, an artist's to the tip of a brush.

In days gone by, when a physician had to diagnose by touch:

A good practitioner did not feel a tumour at his fingertips but he projected his vibratory and pressure sensations into the patient.

So we regularly project our sense of touch beyond our physical being and, in palpation, says Ford:

We merely make the ordinarily unconscious process available to our conscious mind. In so doing we cross the delicate boundary between self and other, to explore, to learn and ultimately to help.

Mitchell et al (1979), in their classic text, explain what they believe palpation to be aiming at.

Palpation is the art of feeling tissues with your hands in such a manner that changes in tension and position within these tissues can be readily noticed, diagnosed and treated.

This is the very simplest aim of palpation, for the method and the instrument (finger pads? whole hand?), it seems, can vary and the objectives can become ever more refined.

Mitchell, writing alone this time (Mitchell 1976), examined the subject of the training and measurement of sensory literacy (he coupled visual and palpatory literacy in the term 'sensory literacy') in a wider sense.

The necessity for projecting one's tactile senses to varying distances through an intervening medium must seem mystical and esoteric to many beginning students. The projection of the palpatory sense through varying thicknesses of tissue is actually a refinement of the sense of tension and hardness. This sense is capable of even further refinement, through perceptual eidetic imagery, to be able to recognise, characterise, and quantify potential energies in living tissues. Thus some osteopaths are able to read in the tissues the exact history of past trauma.

Achieving the ideal of skilled palpation requires mastery of a number of subtle abilities. For example, Kappler (1997) suggests we need to be able to estimate the weight of objects, the amount of pressure needed to move them, as well as the resistance being exerted against any pressure we may be applying. These skills are necessary to discriminate accurately the variations in motion of tissues, whether we are moving them or the movement is generated from the tissues themselves (muscular movement for example) or whether movement derives from some inherent motion (pulsation, etc).

Localising dysfunction: practical value of skilled palpation

As we progress through the chapters which build palpation skills, we should arrive at a point where specific dysfunctional tissues can be localised for therapeutic attention. In osteopathic medicine the locality of a dysfunctional musculoskeletal area is noted as having a number of common characteristics, summarised by the acronym ARTT (sometimes rearranged as TART). These characteristics will be further evaluated and defined in later sections of the book as they apply to skin, muscle, joints, etc.

Gibbons & Tehan (2001) explain the basis of osteopathic ARTT palpation, when assessing for somatic dysfunction (their particular focus is on spinal and joint dysfunction), as follows.

A relates to asymmetry.
DiGiovanna (1991) links the criteria of asymmetry to a positional focus stating that the 'position of the vertebra or other bone is asymmetrical'. Greenman (1996) broadens the concept of asymmetry by including functional, in addition to structural, asymmetry.

R relates to range of motion.
Alteration in range of motion can apply to a single joint, several joints or a region of the musculoskeletal system. The abnormality may be either restricted or increased mobility and includes assessment of quality of movement and 'end feel'.

T relates to tissue texture changes.
The identification of tissue texture change is important in the diagnosis of somatic dysfunction. Palpable changes may be noted in superficial, intermediate and deep tissues. It is important for clinicians to recognise normal from abnormal.

T relates to tissue tenderness.
Undue tissue tenderness may be evident. Pain provocation and reproduction of familiar symptoms are often used to localise somatic dysfunction.

Blending the elements

Denslow (1964) makes it clear that while each of these elements can be palpated for and assessed separately (tissue change, asymmetry, etc.), and that students should start the process of assessing for dysfunction by thinking of these as separate activities, over time, 'these elements will be blended into a single procedure . . . to secure, more or less simultaneously, information concerning tenderness, tissue tone, motion and alignment'.

Denslow also notes that the changes being assessed have been given a number of titles by different researchers and clinicians, including 'faulty mechanics' (Goldthwait 1937), 'trigger zones' [or points] (Travell 1951), 'segmental neuralgia', hyperalgesic zones (Lewit 1992). Additionally these changes may be described as 'subluxations' and 'facet syndrome' in chiropractic, as well as 'osteopathic lesions' and 'somatic dysfunctions' in osteopathic medicine.

If an area 'feels' different from usual and/or appears different, symmetrically speaking (one side from the other), and/or displays a restriction in normal range of motion and/or is tender to the touch, dysfunction and distress are present.

The nature of the dysfunction is not revealed, merely its presence. These elements, together with the history and presenting symptoms, can then usefully be related to the degree of acuteness or chronicity, so that tentative conclusions can be reached as to the nature of the problem and what therapeutic interventions are most appropriate.

Exercises are presented in various chapters, but particularly 5 and 9, in which ARTT characteristics are evaluated.

Specific objectives

Walton (1971), discussing physical examination as it relates to superficial and then deep palpation, points to specific objectives which should be looked for.

> There are five types of change to be noted by superficial palpation in both acute and chronic lesions: skin changes, temperature changes, superficial muscle tensions, tenderness and oedema.

And for deeper palpation:

> The operator increases the pressure on his palpating fingers sufficiently to make a contact with the tissues deep in the skin . . . six types of change may be noted: mobility, tenderness, oedema, deep muscle tension, fibrosis and interosseous changes. All but fibrosis can be perceived in both acute and chronic lesions.

In order to achieve the basic objective of being able to assess and judge such changes, education of the hands and development of heightened proprioceptive sensibility in the detection and amplification of subtle messages are required (see Exercises 3.12–3.14). This is then followed by appropriate interpretation of the information.

- *Detection* is a matter of being aware of the possible findings and practising the techniques required to expose these possibilities.
- *Amplification* requires localised concentration on a specific task and the ability to block out extraneous information.
- *Interpretation* is the ability to relate the information received via detection and amplification.

As indicated in Chapter 1, it is the detection and amplification aspects of palpation with which we are largely concerned, since what you subsequently do with any information thus gathered (i.e. how you interpret it) will largely depend upon your training and belief system.

Philip Greenman (1989) defines the three stages of palpation as being reception, transmission and interpretation. A useful warning is given that care be taken over the hands ('these sensitive diagnostic instruments') as we develop coordinated, symmetrical skills, linked with our visual sense.

> Avoidance of injury abuse is essential, hands should be clean, and nails an appropriate length. During the palpation the operator should be relaxed and comfortable to avoid extraneous interference with the transmission of the palpatory impulse. In order accurately to assess and interpret the palpatory findings it is essential that the physician concentrate on the act of palpation, the tissue being palpated, and the response of the palpating fingers and hands. All extraneous sensory stimuli should be reduced as much as possible. *Probably the most common mistake in palpation is the lack of concentration by the examiner.* [My italics]

Moving beyond the physical assessments towards the palpation of subtle circulatory and energy rhythms and patterns, as described in craniosacral therapy, 'zero balancing' and the work of various osteopathic researchers, requires that palpation skills be further refined. Where then should we begin in the process of developing and/or enhancing our proprioceptive and palpatory skills?

Exercises which can help in this task have been formulated by many experts and a good starting point would be to practise the following examples until you are comfortable with your ability to obtain the information demanded without undue difficulty. These exercises are based on the advice and work of numerous individuals who have described specific methods for the acquisition of high levels of palpatory literacy. These exercises are meant to be introduced more or less in sequence in order to gradually refine sensitivity.

Important comparative descriptors

Before starting these exercises (which are not only useful for beginners but are excellent for refreshing the skills of the more experienced therapist) it is useful to prepare a number of comparative descriptive terms for that which will be palpated. Thus, we should have a number of what Greenman (1989) calls 'paired descriptors'. These can include:

- superficial/deep
- compressible/rigid
- warm/cold
- moist or damp/dry
- painful/pain free
- local or circumscribed/diffuse or widespread
- relaxed/tense
- hypertonic/hypotonic
- normal/abnormal, and so on . . .

It is also useful to begin, when appropriate, to think in terms of whether any abnormality is acute, subacute or chronic (see Box 3.2).

In making such an assessment it is useful to couple this with information from the patient in order to confirm the accuracy or otherwise of the finding. Thus, if tissue feels chronically altered and the patient confirms that the area has been troublesome for longer than 4 weeks, an accurate 'reading' was made. (Obviously, in many instances, acute exacerbation of a chronic area may be what is being palpated, a confusing but useful palpatory exercise.) The degree of change should also be noted, using a subjective scale for conditions which appear mild, moderate or severe. A simple numerical code can be used to identify where on this scale the palpated tissues lie.

Palpation exercises

Viola Frymann (1963) summarised some very simple beginning points for developing sufficient sensitivity to commence efficient palpation of the living body. When we come to palpating tissue, she advises, quite logically, that we palpate direct, not through clothing, and that we remain as relaxed as possible

---

Box 3.2 Acute, subacute and chronic

In general terms:
- acute conditions relate to the past few weeks
- subacute to between 2 and 4 weeks
- chronic to longer than 4 weeks

during the whole process. This is important, as unnecessary tensions interfere with perception.

It is also vital that we use only sufficient weight in our contact with the region being explored and that this contact should be slowly applied to allow time for 'attunement' to the tissue being assessed.

> The gauging of tissue resistance is attained by the application of your muscle sense, your work sense. It is not merely a contact sense, a touch sense, but sensations mainly derived from work being done by the muscles. This is what is meant by proprioception.

The objective of the following series of simple exercises is to begin to refine palpation skills.

Some of Frymann's exercises will increase the sensitivity required for very light palpation needed for noting elasticity, turgor, moisture, sebaceous activity, relative warmth or coldness of tissues and so on.

It is strongly suggested that all of the exercises in the book be practised many times and that even experienced individuals, with well-evolved skills in this field, go back to some of the apparently simple exercises from time to time. It is a process which should be regarded as a voyage of discovery.

A sense of profound satisfaction awaits you when you realise just how much you can learn to read with your sense of touch.

EXERCISE 3.1: COIN PALPATION

Time suggested: several minutes at a time with each hand

Have an assortment of different denomination coins in a container and remove one at a time, with your eyes closed. Carefully feel each side of a coin and decide, by virtue of its size and weight, what value it represents. Carefully and lightly palpate and decide which is heads and which is tails.

Do the same with a number of different size/value coins.

Repeat at regular intervals until you can identify and name the coins.

EXERCISE 3.2: COIN THROUGH PAPER PALPATION

Time suggested: 2–4 minutes with each hand

Place a coin under a telephone directory and try to find it by careful palpation of the upper surface of the directory. If this is too difficult at first, do it initially with a magazine, gradually increasing the thickness of the barrier between your fingers and the coin until the telephone directory itself presents no problem.

Incorporate variations in which you use different parts of the hand to palpate for the coin.

EXERCISE 3.3: HAIR THROUGH PAPER PALPATION

Time suggested: 2–4 minutes with each hand

Place a human hair under a page of a telephone directory and palpate for it through the page, eyes closed.

Once this becomes relatively easy, place the hair under two pages and then three, doing the same thing, feeling slowly and carefully for the slight variation of the surface overlaying the hair.

Now how long does it take you to feel the hair?

Repeat until it is easy and quick.

Incorporate variations in which you use different parts of the hand to palpate for the hair.

EXERCISE 3.4: INANIMATE OBJECT DISCRIMINATION

Time suggested: 3–5 minutes with each hand

Sit at a table (blindfolded) and try to distinguish variations between objects on the table made out of different materials: wood, plastic, metal, bone and clay, for example.

Describe what you feel – shape, temperature, surface texture, resilience, flexibility, etc.

Do materials of organic and non-organic origin have a different feel? Describe any differences you noted.

EXERCISE 3.5: WOOD DENSITY PALPATION

Time suggested: 5 minutes with each hand

Van Allen (1964) developed a training method for enhancing perception of what he termed tissue 'density'. He obtained several blocks, measuring 2 × 4 × 18 inches (5 × 10 × 46 cm), of very soft wood (pine) and of progressively harder woods (cherry, walnut, maple). He states:

> Sliding one's fingers over these blocks revealed the differences in density and was a good exercise in developing tactile sensitivity. In some of these blocks I bored inch [1.9 cm] holes from the underside, half the length, to within a quarter of an inch [0.6 cm] of the upper surface, and poured the holes full of lead, peaning it solidly with a ball-pean hammer. The blocks appeared uniform as they lay face up, with the leaded ends, some one way and some another. It was not too hard for most observers to tell which end was which as they slid their fingers over them. Osteopathic physicians varied widely in their ability to do this, some detecting the differences in one sweep of the fingers, others requiring many trials.

Those who did better in the 'test' were the practitioners known for their palpatory skills.

Reproducing Van Allen's blocks, lead and all, may be somewhat difficult but obtaining blocks of wood of uniform size but of differing density should not be difficult; schools teaching manual therapy should have an array of these for their students to palpate and assess.

EXERCISE 3.6: BLACK BAG/BOX PALPATION

Time suggested: 5 minutes with each hand

Mitchell suggests different ways of performing a basic palpation exercise. He urges paired students to palpate a number of objects (unseen by the student to be tested) which are inside a box (or bag) with an opening through which the palpating student can reach to palpate.

Mitchell suggests that such a 'black box' can be used as the first stage of learning to assess temperature, texture, thickness, humidity, tension or hardness, shape (stereognosis), position, proprioception, size, motion proprioception and so on.

The hand palpates a hidden object (made of plastic, bone, metal, wood, ceramic, glass, etc.) and the student indicates the material being touched as well as what it is, before bringing it out of the bag/box.

EXERCISE 3.7: LAYER PALPATION USING INANIMATE MATERIALS

Time suggested: 5–10 minutes with each hand

An elaboration on the use of a 'black box', which Mitchell discusses, would be to enhance discriminatory faculties by including a variety of materials made of rubber, plastic, wood, metal and so on of varying thicknesses in the 'box'. Both the material as well as its relative thickness could be estimated on palpation and the results discussed.

These materials could also contain another variation in which a rough textured material, say sandpaper of different degrees of roughness, could be covered by varying thicknesses of foam. In this way multiple variations could be created for the tuning of palpatory skills: 'Layers of materials of varying tension and hardness could be superimposed. For example, somatic soft tissues overlaying bone could be simulated with stratified layers of foam padding, sheet rubber, and vinyl fabric'.

In this way, a training device with variable tensions could be constructed, says Mitchell, simulating muscular spasm, fibrotic changes, oedema and bony structures felt through varying thicknesses of soft tissue: 'It would be reasonable to expect that training with such devices would increase a student's confidence in his/her ability to tell the difference between spastic muscle and bone, or between hypertrophied muscle and contracted muscle'.

EXERCISE 3.8: PALPATION OF BONE, REAL AND PLASTIC

Time suggested: 5–7 minutes using both hands

Frymann (1963) suggests that the next objective should be to move from tools to begin to increase the student's ability to study anatomy using the hand instead of the eye. Her suggested exercise follows.

Sit, with eyes closed or wearing a blindfold, while palpating one of the cranial bones, or any other bone, real or plastic if you are unfamiliar with cranial structures.

continues

EXERCISE 3.8 (Continued)

Articular structures should be felt for and described in some detail (ideally with someone else handing the bone to you and with findings being spoken into a tape recorder for self-assessment later, when the object/bone can be studied with eyes open).

The bone should be named, sided and its particular features discussed. If you are new to cranial structures this is an excellent educational method for becoming familiar with their unique qualities.

While palpating this bone you should be asking:

- What is the nature of this object, is it plastic or bone?
- Can you discern attachment sites on the bone?

Describe the difference in feel and character between plastic and real bone. Bone, albeit no longer living, has a slight compressive resilience which plastic never has; nor can plastic achieve the detail of sutural digitation which bone contains.

Careful fingering of the unseen object would establish its shape and if anatomy is well enough understood, it could then be named and sided.

The whole process of palpating is enhanced, suggests Frymann, if the arms are supported, so that the hands and fingers are unaffected by the weight of the arms.

DISCUSSION REGARDING EXERCISES 3.1–3.8

Regular repetition, on a daily basis for a few minutes at a time, of the sort of exercises outlined above will bring a rapid increase in sensitivity and this is desirable as a prerequisite to palpating living tissue. Such exercises should continue even when you have moved on to palpating the living body.

What should emerge with repetition of these exercises is a discriminatory facility, in which the qualities and characteristics of different materials, whether organic or inorganic, as well as their slightly raised surface elevations and depressions, and their temperatures when compared with each other, are all readily noted.

After building up sensitivity in palpation using inanimate objects, it is time to move towards palpation of living tissues. The ability to know what normal tissue feels like is a most useful palpatory exercise, since anything which feels other than normal is bound to offer evidence of dysfunction.

This suggests that it is useful to perform palpation exercises with a wide range of people who are relatively young and 'normal', as well as individuals who are older, or who have suffered injury or stress in the tissues you intend palpating.

It is my personal experience that the most 'normal' muscles available for palpation are those belonging to preschool children and even this group is often already dysfunctional in terms of muscular hypertonicity.

EXERCISE 3.9: LIVING BONE PALPATION

Time suggested: 5–7 minutes with each hand

Whichever bone is used in the previous exercise (cranial or otherwise), this should be followed by a blindfolded palpation of the same bone in a live subject, with its contours, sutures (if cranial), resilience and observed (not initiated) motion being felt for and described.

The person being palpated could be lying down or seated.

When comparison is made with the live bone in this way, similarities and differences should gradually become apparent. The differences between the dead and live bone should be described and defined, ideally into a tape recorder.

Obviously, the living bone would not be palpated directly but through superficial tissue. This requires that the palpation become discriminating (Frymann (1963) talks of the 'automatic selection device of our consciousness'), filtering out information offered by soft tissues which overlie the bone that is being assessed.

If the bone chosen has superficial musculature the palpation should start lightly, just above and then on the skin, with gradual increasing pressure, to eventually have contact with the contours of the bone in question.

By applying the mind's attention to what is being palpated (for not less than 5 minutes in the early stages) subtle awareness of motion inherent in the live bone's existence might also become apparent.

If this is a cranial bone, there are three rhythms which can be felt for – pulsation, respiration and a slower rhythmic motion – and it is possible to learn to focus gradually on one or other of these at will, filtering out the others.

We will come to exercises which will improve such discrimination later.

EXERCISE 3.10: PALPATING FOR INHERENT MOTION

Time suggested: not less than 5 minutes

In order to begin to study and analyse more subtle movements, Frymann (1963) then suggests that the student of palpation should feel for a rhythmic motion, by placing one hand on a spinal segment from which stems the neurological supply to an area which is simultaneously being palpated by the other hand.

Examples include the upper thoracic spine and the heart region or the midthoracic spine and the liver.

By patiently focusing for some minutes, eyes closed, on what is being felt, she states, 'a fluid wave will eventually be established between the two hands'. Can you feel this or something which approximates to it?

EXERCISE 3.11: SIMULTANEOUS PALPATION OF NORMAL AND ABNORMAL TISSUES

Time suggested: not less than 5 minutes

Mitchell makes the somewhat bizarre (and probably unrealistic) suggestion that the blindfolded student should palpate a live arm and, simultaneously, that of a cadaver which has been warmed to body temperature. Alternatively, assuming no warm cadavers are available, he suggests that palpation be simultaneously performed on normal tissues and those of individuals affected by pathology, such as limb paralysis or inflammation, spasm or extreme hypertonicity or some other internal pathological or pathophysiological process.

The simultaneous aspect might mean literally having a hand on the normal and the abnormal tissues at the same time or palpating them sequentially, moving from one to the other and back again, seeking words to describe the differences.

Simultaneous palpation of normal and diseased, or distressed, tissues offers an educational opportunity which all practitioners and students involved in bodywork should aim to experience.

Describe the different 'feel' of normal and abnormal tissue or simply of hypertonicity and hypotonicity, for example, after palpating for several minutes.

EXERCISE 3.12: FRYMANN'S FOREARM PALPATION FOR INHERENT MOTION

Time suggested: 10 minutes

Frymann (1963) simplifies the initial palpation of living tissue, compared with non-living, sparing us the task of finding a warmed-up corpse.

In order to become familiar with an unhurried contact with living tissue, Frymann suggests that the student of palpation should sit at a table, opposite a partner, one of whose arms rests on the table, flexor surface upwards. This arm should be totally relaxed.

The student lays a hand onto that forearm with attention focused on what the palmar surface of the fingers are feeling, the other hand resting on the firm table surface. This is to provide a contrast reference as the living tissue is palpated, to help to distinguish a region in motion from one without motion.

The elbows of the palpator should rest on the table so that no stress builds up in the arm or shoulders.

With eyes closed, unhurried focus and concentration should then be projected into what the fingers and palm are feeling, attuning to the arm surface. Gradually, focus should be brought to the deeper tissues under the skin as well (without any particular increase in contact pressure from the palpating hand) and finally, to the underlying bone.

When the feel of the structure being touched and what lies below (skin, muscle, bone, etc.) has been sensed, the function of the tissues should be considered. Feel for pulsations and rhythms, periodically varying the pressure of the hand.

continues

EXERCISE 3.12 (*Continued*)

At this stage Frymann (1963) urges you to:

> Pay no attention to the structure of skin, or muscle, or bone. Wait until you become aware of motion: observe and describe that motion, its nature, its direction, its rhythm and amplitude, its consistency or its variation.

Perform the same exercise on different parts of the body and on different people, of varying body types, ages, genders.

This entire palpatory exercise should take not less than 5 minutes and ideally 10, and should be repeated with the other hand to ensure that palpation skills are not one-sided.

Remember that the objective of this exercise is to acclimatise you to evaluating inherent motion (minute pulsations, rhythms) once you have noted the structural aspect of what you are palpating.

EXERCISE 3.13: BIMANUAL INHERENT MOTION PALPATION 1

Time suggested: 5–10 minutes

When you have palpated an arm (or thigh, or indeed any other part of the body) to the point where you are clearly picking up sensations of motion and rhythmic pulsation with one hand, place your other hand on the opposite side of the same limb.

> Is this hand picking up the same motions? Are the sensations moving in the same direction, with the same rhythm previously noted, and is there the same degree of amplitude to the motion as the first sensation?

In health, they will be the same. When there is a difference it may represent 'tissue memory' of trauma or some other form of dysfunction.

Perform the same exercise on different parts of the body and on different people, of varying body types, ages, genders.

EXERCISE 3.14: BIMANUAL INHERENT MOTION PALPATION 2

Time suggested: not less than 7 minutes

Frymann (1963) suggests that on another occasion (or at the same session) you palpate one limb with one hand (say, upper arm) and another limb (say, thigh, for example) with the other and that you 'rest in stillness until you perceive the respective motions within'.

Ask yourself whether the rhythms you are feeling are synchronous and moving in the same direction.

> Are they consistent or do they undergo cyclical changes, periodically returning to the starting rhythmic pattern?

You may actually sense, she says, that the force being felt seems to carry your hands to a point beyond the confines of the body, pulling in one direction more than another, with little or no tendency to return to a balanced neutral position.

continues

> ### EXERCISE 3.14 *(Continued)*
>
> This may represent a pattern established as a result of trauma which is still manifest in the tissues. Careful questioning might confirm the nature and direction of a blow or injury in the past.
>
> Perform the same exercise on different parts of the body and on different people, of varying body types, ages, genders.
>
> As we will discover in Chapter 6, researchers such as Becker and Smith have mapped this territory well and have given us strong guidelines as to how we may move towards understanding such phenomena. Frymann's exercise is a first step in that direction.

> ### EXERCISE 3.15: UPLEDGER'S RADIAL PULSE ASSESSMENT
>
> #### Time suggested: 5–7 minutes with each hand
>
> Upledger (Upledger & Vredevoogd 1983) suggests that palpation and assessment of more obvious pulsating rhythms should be practised, for example involving the cardiovascular pulses. He describes the first stages of this learning process thus:
>
> > With the subject lying comfortably supine, palpate the radial pulses. Feel the obvious peak of the pulsation. Tune in also to the rise and fall of the pressure gradient.
> >
> > How long is diastole?
> >
> > What is the quality of the rise of pulse pressure after diastole? Is it sharp, gradual, smooth?
> >
> > How broad is the pressure peak?
> >
> > Is the pressure descent rapid, gradual, smooth or stepped?
> >
> > Memorise the feel of the subject's pulse so that you can reproduce it in your mind after you have broken actual physical contact with the subject's body. You can often sing a song after you have heard it a few times; similarly, you should be able to mentally reproduce your palpatory perception of the pulse after you have broken contact.
>
> Upledger then suggests you do the same thing with the carotid pulse and subsequently palpate both radial and carotid at the same time and compare them.

Fryman's views on pulse taking

There are some very important lessons to be learned in performing simple pulse taking. Frymann (1963) analyses some of the almost instinctive strategies we adopt if we do this well and which all should consider as they perform Exercise 3.15.

1. If the patient has a relatively normal systolic pressure (120 mmHg) light digital pressure on the pulse will obliterate it.
2. If the applied pressure is very light only a very faint sensation will be palpated, if anything at all.
3. If, however, a light initial pressure is gradually increased, a variety of pulsation sensations will be noted, until the pulse is obliterated when the digital pressure overcomes the blood pressure.

Frymann notes that this is how blood pressure was assessed before the introduction of the sphygmomanometer.

The student of palpation should experiment with variation of the degree of pressure, noting the subtle differences which are then perceived. In doing this we are learning to control the degree of applied digital pressure so that we meet that demanded by particular tissues, in order to gain optimal access to the locked-in information. Issues regarding application of pressure are discussed in Special Topic 1.

Frymann (1963) states:

> The examiner must supply the equal and opposite force to that of the tissue to be studied, [for example] the pressure in the eyeball can be estimated by attaining a balance of pressure between the examining finger and the intraocular pressure. The maturity of an abscess can be estimated similarly. Action and reaction must be equal.

This is a vital lesson in learning palpation and is echoed in later chapters when neuromuscular evaluation (NMT) methods are discussed and practised.

EXERCISE 3.16: DISCRIMINATION OF INFORMATION PALPATION

Time suggested: 3–5 minutes

Lay both hands on the upper thorax of the supine individual and palpate cardiovascular activity.

Focusing on the various characteristics of the perceived pulsations, alter your focus to the breathing pattern and its multiple motions.

Practise switching attention from the sensations associated with breathing to cardiovascular activity and back again, until you are comfortable with the idea of screening out 'background' information from that which you want to examine. To highlight the subtle cardiovascular motions, have the person being palpated hold their breath for a few seconds at a time.

Accurate evaluation of many functional and pathological states depends upon the ability to filter out that information which you require from the many other motions and sensations which are being picked up by the palpating hands. This is an exercise to revisit many times.

EXERCISE 3.17: DISCRIMINATION OF PALPATED CRANIAL SENSATIONS

Time suggested: 5–7 minutes

The person being palpated lies supine with the head approximately 12 inches (30 cm) from the end of the table, allowing space for your arms to be supported on the table surface as you rest the head on your hands, with no more than a few grams of contact pressure from your whole hand/finger contact.

The occiput should be resting on your palms and hypothenar region (see Fig. 3.2).

continues

EXERCISE 3.17 (Continued)

Sitting with your eyes closed, pay attention to cardiovascular activity (arterial pulsation, general pulsation in time with cardiac function and so on) as it is being sensed by these contacts. After a while, alter your focus to screen out cardiovascular activity and see what you can feel in relation to cranial motion, virtually coordinated with the breathing rhythm.

Can you sense a very slight motion of the neck in time with respiration? What sensations can you perceive when the person holds the breath for a few seconds at a time?

Can you describe the different rhythms and motions all demanding recognition from your hands?

Describe what you feel in your notes or into a tape recorder after 5–7 minutes of palpation.

EXERCISE 3.18: PRIMARY CRANIAL RHYTHM PALPATION

Time suggested: 5–7 minutes

Adopt precisely the same position and hand contacts as for Exercise 3.17. Screen out and attempt to ignore both cardiovascular and respiratory motions which your hands perceive and see what else you can feel.

Imagine your hands are totally bonded to the head, without more than a few grams of pressure, and with this whole hand contact shift your focus to the proprioceptors in your wrists and lower arms (which should be supported by the table, and relaxed). Sense what these are feeling.

Magnify, in this way, the very small amount of actual cranial motion available for palpation and you should gradually begin to feel as though quite a considerable degree of motion is taking place, as though the entire head were expanding and contracting laterally, to a very slow rhythm, unrelated to cardiovascular or respiratory function, perhaps 6–10 times per minute.

Trust what you feel uncritically at this stage.

Can you sense this rhythm?

Can you describe what you feel in words?

Is it a periodic 'prickling' or pressure sensation in the palms of the hand?

Is it like a 'tide coming in and then receding'?

What words would you use in your journal or on tape?

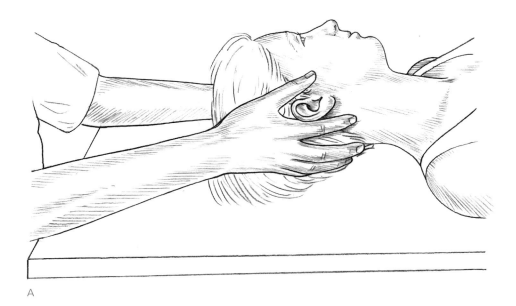

A

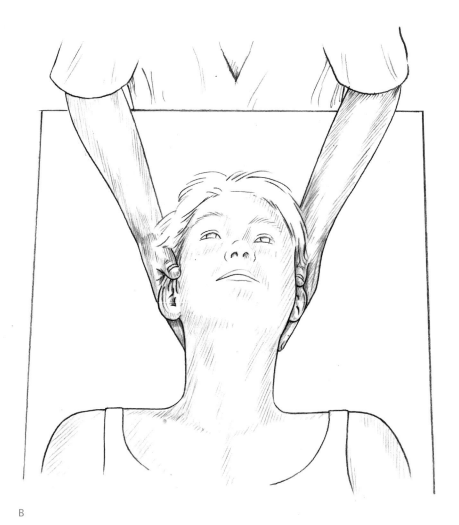

B

Fig. 3.2A, B Hand position for palpation of cardiovascular activity, inherent motion and other cranial rhythms.

EXERCISE 3.19: CRANIAL FLEXION AND EXTENSION PALPATION

Time suggested: 5–7 minutes

Holding the head as suggested in the previous two exercises, place the tips of your ring and little fingers on the occipital bones. Can you sense a very slight dipping forward of the occiput at the same time that a minute lateral expansion occurs into the palms of your hands, with a return to neutral as the head 'narrows' again?

Can you, through the available contact of your middle and index fingers (resting on the mastoid bone and temporal bone respectively), sense what is happening to these?

Describe this in your journal or onto tape.

Can you also, through your thumb contact, sense what the parietal bones are doing as these rhythmic pulsations occur?

Describe this as well.

We will return to cranial exercises in a later section where we will examine palpation of craniosacral rhythms throughout the body and reassess your initial 'findings' and descriptions.

EXERCISE 3.20: INHERENT SACRAL RHYTHM PALPATION

Time suggested: 10 minutes

Have the person to be palpated lie supine. Slide your dominant hand beneath the sacrum, so that the fingertips rest at the base of the sacrum, spreading from one sacroiliac articulation to the other. The coccyx should be gently cradled in the heel of the hand and the forearm and elbow resting comfortably on the surface of the treatment table.

Kneel or sit so that you are as comfortable as possible during the 10 minutes or so of this exercise.

With eyes closed, focus attention to all sensations reaching the palpating hand.

Can you sense a rhythm synchronous with normal respiration? If so, ask the patient to hold their breath and observe what happens to the sacral motion at this time.

Is there still a subtle motion palpable as the breath is held?

As respiration resumes, feel how this subtle motion alters again. It should be possible gradually to learn to screen the motion related to breathing from the more subtle 'cranial respiratory' rhythm.

Spend as long as possible studying these subtle variations in sacral motion. Carefully record your findings after each performance of this and similar exercises.

Greenman's palpation exercises

Philip Greenman (1989, 1996) has described some excellent exercises for both beginners and the more experienced to increase their palpation skills. These have been summarised as follows.

EXERCISE 3.21: FOREARM LAYER PALPATION (A: SKIN)

Time suggested: 7 minutes

Sit with a partner, facing each other across a narrow table. You are going to examine each other's left forearms with your right hands, so rest your left forearm on the table, palm downwards, and place your right (palpating) hand and fingers on your partner's left forearm, as he/she rests a hand and fingers on your forearm, just below the elbow.

The initial evaluation, without movement, calls for you to focus on what is being felt, noting the contours of your palpating partner's arm under the (very) light touch of your hand.

Project your thoughts to the sensors in your palpating hand, focusing initially on the attributes of the skin in touch with your contact hand, which should initially be still.

How warm/cool, dry/moist, thick/thin, rough/smooth is the palpated skin?

You and your partner should now turn the forearm over, so that the same questions can be answered regarding the volar surface.

Compare what was palpated on the dorsal surface with what was palpated on the volar surface. Evaluate and put words to the differences noted in skin texture, temperature, thickness and so on.

Now, using the lightest ('feather-like') touch of one finger pad, run this along the skin of the forearm.

Are there any areas which feel less smooth, which have an apparent roughness or moist feel, where your finger pad 'drags'?

Now, using a light pincer contact, lift a fold of skin and assess its elasticity and the speed with which it returns to normal when you release it. Do this on both surfaces of the forearm and compare these, as well as over areas of skin where 'drag' was noted when you were lightly stroking with a finger pad.

Record your findings (note: the importance and meaning of variations in skin texture will be discussed fully in the next chapter).

EXERCISE 3.22: FOREARM LAYER PALPATION (B: SKIN ON SUBCUTANEOUS FASCIA)

Time suggested: 5 minutes

In the same position, make small hand motions while a firm contact is being maintained with the skin, moving this in relation to its underlying tissues. Move the hand both longitudinally and horizontally, in relation to the forearm, and evaluate what is being palpated as you move the skin on the subcutaneous fascial tissues.

continues

EXERCISE 3.22 *(Continued)*

Try to assess its thickness and elasticity, its 'tightness or looseness'. Do the surface tissues move, glide, slide, more freely in some directions compared with others?

Compare the findings from the dorsal and volar surfaces of your partner's forearm and also compare variations in areas where skin texture, 'drag', etc. were different in the earlier palpation.

Write down or record your findings.

EXERCISE 3.23: FOREARM LAYER PALPATION (C: BLOOD VESSELS)

Time suggested: 5 minutes

With this same contact, palpate the subcutaneous fascial layer for the arteries and veins which lie in it. Use an anatomical atlas if you are rusty regarding this aspect of anatomy. In particular, find and palpate the radial artery.

Identify (i.e. name) and describe as many of the blood vessels you feel as possible, from wrist to elbow.

Assess the difference in size, texture and quality of perceived internal motion of fluids as you compare veins and arteries.

Have your palpation partner clench a fist and note what happens to the blood vessels over the course of a minute or so.

EXERCISE 3.24: FOREARM LAYER PALPATION (D: DEEPER FASCIA)

Time suggested: 5 minutes

In the same position, concentrate attention on the deeper fascia which surrounds, invests and separates muscle, by increasing your hand pressure slightly.

Use slow horizontal movements of the hands/fingers and try to identify thickened areas of fascia which act as envelopes which compartmentalise and separate muscle bundles.

It is in the subcutaneous, and deeper, fascial layers that much somatic dysfunction is found, ranging from trigger points to stress bands, relating to overuse, misuse or abuse. Look in particular for a sense of hardness, or thickening, which suggests dysfunction.

Palpate as much of the fascia between the elbow and wrist as possible and note your findings.

EXERCISE 3.25: FOREARM LAYER PALPATION (E: MUSCLE FIBRES)

Time suggested: 5–7 minutes

With the same position and contact, feel through the fascia to locate muscle bundles and fibres. Note their relative degrees of pliability or hardness and see whether you can feel their directions of action.

You and your partner should now slowly open and close the left fist in order to tense and relax the muscles being palpated. Sense the variations in tone in the muscle fibres as this takes place, particularly the difference between tissues with increased tone and relaxed tissue.

Next, you and your palpating partner should both hold your left fists closed, quite strongly, as you each palpate the hypertonic state of the forearm muscles, a most useful preparation for what will be palpated in most patients, where overuse, misuse or abuse has been operating.

Describe the textures and variations in tone which you have noted during this exercise.

EXERCISE 3.26: FOREARM LAYER PALPATION (F: MUSCULOTENDINOUS INTERFACE)

Time suggested: 5–7 minutes

The arm being palpated should now be relaxed.

Move your palpating fingers down the forearm toward the wrist and identify the interface between muscle and tendon (musculotendinous junction). Continue to palpate the tendon itself onwards towards its point of insertion, where the tendon is bound to the wrist by an overlying structure, the transverse carpal ligament.

Palpate this and see whether you can identify the various directions of fibre angle.

Which way does the tendon run?

Which way does the ligamentous structure run?

Describe in writing or on tape the characteristics and 'feel' of what you have palpated.

Review an anatomy/physiology text to help evaluate the accuracy of what you thought you were feeling.

EXERCISE 3.27: FOREARM LAYER PALPATION (G: ACTIVE ELBOW JOINT)

Time suggested: 7 minutes

Move back up to the elbow and with your middle finger resting in the hollow on the dorsal side of the elbow and your thumb on the ventral surface of the elbow, palpate the radial head. Feel its shape and texture.

How hard is it?

Does it move on slight pressure?

continues

EXERCISE 3.27 *(Continued)*

What do you feel if you move your finger and thumb slightly higher on the elbow, over the joint space itself?

You should not be able to feel the joint capsule unless there exists gross pathology of the joint. Your contact is just above the joint.

Have your partner slowly, actively, pronate and supinate the arm and note what you feel between your finger and thumb.

How does the end of range of motion vary with the action of pronation and supination?

Is it symmetrical?

Describe the end-feel (see Special topic 9 on 'End-feel', p 255).

Which end of range seems firmer/tighter (which has the harder end-feel) – supination or pronation?

Record your findings.

EXERCISE 3.28: FOREARM LAYER PALPATION (H: PASSIVE ELBOW JOINT)

Time suggested: 5 minutes

Now use your left hand to hold the hand and wrist of the arm you are palpating with your right hand.

Introduce passive supination and pronation as you palpate the joint.

Assess the total range of motion as you slowly perform these movements.

You are receiving two sets of proprioceptive information at this stage, from the palpating hand and from the one which is introducing motion.

Describe the range and the end-feel, in both supination and pronation when these are passively introduced, as well as comparing active (as in the previous exercise) with passive findings.

Does supination or pronation have the harder or softer end-feel and which seems to have the greatest range of motion?

Are you aware of the build-up of tension in the tissues ('bind') as you approach the end of the range of movement?

Are you equally aware of the sense of tissue freedom ('ease') as you move away from that barrier?

Try to become aware of 'ease' and 'bind' as you move the joint in varying directions.

Can you find a point of balance somewhere between the ends of range of motion in pronation and supination where tissues feel at their most free? If so, you have found what is called the physiological neutral point, or point of balance, which is a key feature of functional osteopathic treatment.

We will be returning to this concept and will perform more exercises involving the neutral point in later chapters (notably Chapter 8).

DISCUSSION REGARDING EXERCISES 3.9–3.28

The exercises covered in this segment have focused on enhancing perception of subtle motions, inherent movements and pulsations, which might derive from a variety of sources.

Kappler (1997) notes that:

> Inherent motion is activity unconsciously generated within the body such as respiratory motion or peristalsis, . . . [and] is postulated to occur in several ways, biochemically at the cellular or sub-cellular level; as part of multiple electrical patterns; as a combination of a number of circulatory and electrical patterns; as some periodic pattern not yet understood.

The term 'entrainment' is sometimes used to describe the way in which multiple pulsations and rhythms in the body combine to form a harmonic palpable sensation (Oschman 2001). Physicists use entrainment to describe a situation in which two rhythms that have nearly the same frequency become coupled to each other. Technically, entrainment means the mutual phase locking of two or more oscillators. There are suggestions that evidence exists of therapeutic influences from this phenomenon; for example, in a setting such as craniosacral therapy, the multiple rhythms and pulsations of the therapist might influence the more dysfunctional rhythms of the patient to return to a more normal state (Chaitow 1999, Oschman 2001).

The palpation exercises in the early part of this segment are designed to encourage awareness of subtle motions, largely outside the conscious influence of the person being assessed. In these as well as in the later exercises, especially those involving the musculoskeletal structures of the forearm, Greenman cautions that the most common errors might involve:

- a lack of concentration
- the use of excessive pressure
- too much movement.

In other words, when performing these palpations, touch lightly and slowly and above all focus on what you are feeling, if you want to palpate effectively.

Palpation skill status

These first exercises will also have helped you to gain (or enhance) an ability to differentiate (and describe) the shape, size, texture, flexibility and temperature of varying thicknesses and combinations of a variety of inorganic materials; to become able to discriminate between organic and inorganic, living and dead materials and tissues, as well as living tissues in varying states of health, and the first stages of assessment of body pulsations and rhythms, with the facility to screen one from another at will being a key stage in developing palpatory literacy.

It may also be possible for you now to sense the residual forces associated with 'tissue memory', a concept which will be examined more closely in later chapters.

These exercises can all be varied and altered to meet particular needs. They represent the ideas of some of the leading experts in the field and provide a starting point in the adventure in exploration of inner space which will follow.

REFERENCES

Chaitow L 1999 Cranial manipulation: theory and practice. Churchill Livingstone, Edinburgh

Denslow J 1964 Palpation of the musculoskeletal system. Journal of the American Osteopathic Association 63(7): 23–31

DiGiovanna E 1991 Somatic dysfunction. In: DiGiovanna E, Schiowitz S (eds) An osteopathic approach to diagnosis and treatment. JB Lippincott, Philadelphia, pp 6–12

Ford C 1989 Where healing waters meet. Station Hill Press, New York

Frymann V 1963 Palpation – its study in the workshop. Yearbook of the American Academy of Osteopathy, Newark, OH, pp 16–30

Gibbons P, Tehan P 2001 Spinal manipulation: indications, risks and benefits. Churchill Livingstone, Edinburgh

Goldthwait J 1937 Body mechanics, 2nd edn. JB Lippincott, Philadelphia

Greenman P 1989 Principles of manual medicine. Williams and Wilkins, Baltimore

Greenman P 1996 Principles of manual medicine, 2nd edn. Williams and Wilkins, Baltimore

Kappler R 1997 Palpatory skills. In: Ward R (ed) Foundations for osteopathic medicine. Williams and Wilkins, Baltimore

Kappler R, Larson N, Kelso A 1971 A comparison of osteopathic findings on hospitalized patients obtained by trained student examiners and experienced physicians. Journal of the American Osteopathic Association 70(10): 1091–1092

Korr I 1970 Physiological basis of osteopathic medicine. Postgraduate Institute of Osteopathic Medicine and Surgery, New York

Kuchera W, Kuchera M 1994 Osteopathic principles and practice, 2nd edn. Greyden Press, Columbus, OH

Lewit K 1992 Manipulative therapy in rehabilitation of the locomotor system, 3rd edn. Butterworths, London

Mitchell F 1976 Training and measuring sensory literacy. Yearbook of the American Academy of Osteopathy, Newark, OH, pp 120–127

Mitchell F, Moran P, Pruzzo N 1979 An evaluation of osteopathic muscle energy procedure. Pruzzo, Valley Park, MI

Oschman J 2001 Energy medicine. Churchill Livingstone, Edinburgh

Sutton S 1977 An osteopathic method of history taking and physical examination. Journal of the American Osteopathic Association 77(7): 845–858

Travell J 1951 Pain mechanisms in connective tissues. Transactions of 2nd Conference on Connective Tissues (Regan C ed). Josiah Macy Foundation, New York, pp 86–125

Upledger J, Vredevoogd W 1983 Craniosacral therapy. Eastland Press, Seattle

Van Allen P 1964 Improving our skills. Academy of Applied Osteopathy Yearbook, Newark, OH, pp 147–152

Walton W 1971 Palpatory diagnosis of the osteopathic lesion. Journal of the American Osteopathic Association 71: 117–131

SPECIAL TOPIC 4
The morphology of reflex and acupuncture points

Pain researchers have demonstrated beyond doubt that at least 75% of trigger points are acupuncture points, according to the traditional meridian maps (Melzack & Wall 1988, Wall & Melzack 1989). The remainder may be thought of as 'honorary' acupuncture points since, according to Traditional Chinese Medicine, all spontaneously tender areas (whether or not they lie on the meridian maps) are suitable for acupuncture (or acupressure) treatment and a trigger point is nothing if it is not spontaneously tender!

Using delicate measuring techniques, Ward (1996) examined 12 acupuncture sites which were also common trigger point sites in the trapezius and infraspinatus muscles. He found precisely the 'spike' electrical activity characteristic of an active trigger point in all of these.

Mense & Simons (2001) are less definite. 'Frequently the acupuncture point selected for the treatment of pain is also a trigger point, but sometimes it is not.'

Thermographic imaging has shown that the actual size of a trigger point is fairly small, approximately 2 mm in diameter, rather than the previously suggested 5–10 mm (Diakow 1988). Their incidence in young adults is shown to be 54% in females and 45% in males (age group 35–50).

If they usually lie in the same place as acupuncture points, what tissues are involved? Professor Jean Bossy, of the Faculty of Medicine, University of Montpellier, in France, has examined the tissues extensively (Bossy 1984) and informs us that all motor points of medical electrology are acupuncture points (which he calls 'privileged loci of the organism which allow exchanges between the inner body and the environment'). Head's maxima points, Hackett's points, visceral points, the chakra points – all are acupuncture points. He sizes them even smaller than Diakow, at between 1 and 5 mm in diameter. The skin manifestation is, he says, 'easier to feel than to see. The most superficial morphological expression is a cupule'.

And under the skin (which is a little thinner than surrounding skin) of these privileged loci, there are common features. Neurovascular bundles are commonly found and connective tissue is always a feature, with fatty tissue sometimes present. Vessels and nerves seem to be important common features, although their stimulation during treatment is usually indirect, as the result of deformation of connective tissue and consequent traction.

In some instances, tendons, periarticular structures or muscle tissues are involved, as part of the acupuncture/trigger point morphology. However, after extensive dissection, Bossy avers that, 'Fat and connective tissue are determinants for the appearance of the acupuncture sensation'.

Thus it seems that effective reflex effects only occur 'through the stimulation of multiple and various anatomical structures'.

Bossy's research has been validated by subsequent discoveries.

Acupuncture points and fascia

Staubesand & Li (1997) studied the fascia in humans using electron photomicroscopy and found smooth muscle cells embedded within collagen fibres. This research also showed that there are a great many perforations of the superficial fascial layer that are all characterised by penetration through the fascia of venous, arterial and neural structures (mainly unmyelinated vegetative nerves). Heine (1995), who also documented the existence of these perforations in the superficial fascia, was additionally involved in the study of acupuncture and established that the majority (82%) of these perforation points are topographically identical with traditional Chinese acupuncture points.

Subsequently Bauer & Heine (1998) conducted a clinical study to observe these fascial perforations in patients suffering from chronic shoulder/neck or shoulder/arm pain. They found that the perforating vessels were 'strangled' together by a thick ring of collagen fibres lying just above the perforation aperture. These were treated using microsurgery in order to loosen the distressed tissues and to achieve a freer exit of those vessels. This led to significant clinical improvements.

Schleip (2002) reports:

> Many took this [the Bauer & Heine research] as clear evidence of a new mechanical explanation model for acupuncture. Yet just a year later a back pain researcher from Spain published a study which seems to question some of Bauer & Heine's assumptions and which adds an exciting new dimension. Using a well-orchestrated double-blind study design with patients suffering from chronic low back pain, surgical staples were implanted under their skin. An interesting point was that the location of the implants was defined by their innervation (as trigger points) and was carefully chosen not to coincide with Chinese acupuncture points. The result: Kovacs' treatment led to a clear pain reduction in the majority of their patients, with at least a similar statistical improvement to those that Bauer & Heine had with their patients.
>
> Kovacs et al (1997) suggested the following explanation: most likely a class of neuropeptides, called enkephalins, are released by both treatments, which then counteract the release of substance P and other neuropeptides which are associated with pain and which support the activation of nociceptive fibres. In other words: the stimulation of certain nociceptors and/or mechanoreceptors under the skin stimulates the release of specific neuropeptides that help to depolarise already activated pain receptors which have been responsible for at least some of the chronic pain.

This sort of research into the behaviour and morphology of acupuncture (and other reflex) points helps to explain some of the common findings noted on palpation. For example, a slight 'cupule' or depression, overlaid with slightly thinner skin tissue, can usually be felt, indicating the presence of an acupuncture point (which if sensitive is 'active' and quite likely to be also a trigger point).

As we will see in Chapter 4, other palpatory signs exist, skin 'drag' and loss of elastic qualities being the most important palpatory indications of active reflex activity.

Acupuncture meridians as a 'molecular web'

Oschman (2000) quotes from the research of Manaka (1995) regarding cellular communication pathways, moving the vision of the acupuncture meridian pathways to a less mechanistic level.

> The cytoskeleton – which biologists are now referring to as the nervous system of the cell – can be fitted into . . . the meridian system, which acupuncture theory visualises as branching into every part of the organism . . . into the interiors of

every cell in the body, and even the nuclei that contain genetic material. The meridians are simply the main channels or transmission lines in the continuous molecular fabric of the body. The molecular web is more than a mechanical anatomical structure. It is a continuous vibratory network.

REFERENCES

Bauer J, Heine H 1998 Akupunkturpunkte und Fibromyalgie – M'glichkeiten chirurgischer Intervention. Biologische Medizin 6 (12): 257–261

Bossy J 1984 Morphological data concerning acupuncture points and channel networks. Acupuncture and ElectroTherapeutics Research International Journal 9

Diakow P 1988 Thermographic imaging of myofascial trigger points. Journal of Manipulative and Physiological Therapeutics 11:2

Heine H 1995 Functional anatomy of traditional Chinese acupuncture points. Acta Anatomica 152: 293

Kovacs F M et al 1997 Local and remote sustained trigger therapy for exacerbations of chronic low back pain: a randomized, double-blind, controlled, multicenter trial. Spine 22: 786–797

Manaka Y 1995 Chasing the dragon's tail: the theory and practice of acupuncture. Paradigm, Brookline, MA

Melzack R, Wall P 1988 The challenge of pain. Penguin Books, Harmondsworth

Mense S, Simons D 2001 Muscle pain. Lippincott Williams and Wilkins, Philadelphia

Oschman J 2000 Energy medicine. Churchill Livingstone, Edinburgh

Schleip 2002 Fascial plasticity – a new neurobiological explanation. Journal of Bodywork and Movement Therapies

Staubesand J, Li Y 1997 Begriff und Substrat der Faziensklerose bei chronisch-ven'ser Insuffizienz. Phlebologie 26: 72–79

Wall P, Melzack R 1989 Textbook of pain, 2nd edn. Churchill Livingstone, London

Ward A 1996 Spontaneous electrical activity at combined acupuncture and myofascial trigger point sites. Acupuncture Medicine 14 (2): 75–79

4

Palpating and assessing the skin

The significance of what is sensed when skin is palpated, in one of many ways, may not always be immediately obvious and yet this boundary, which separates the individual from the outside world, is a rich potential source of information.

Contact with someone else's skin rapidly breaks emotional and resistance barriers. Physical touch offers a unique privilege and opportunity, something which is used to great advantage by those bodyworkers who focus on both the mind and the physical condition of their patients. The body surface seems to reflect the state of the mind intimately, altering its electrical as well as its palpable physical properties.

Deane Juhan (1987) sets the scene for our understanding of the skin's importance.

> The skin is no more separated from the brain than the surface of a lake is separated from its depths; the two are different locations in a continuous medium. 'Peripheral' and 'central' are merely spatial distinctions, distinctions which do more harm than good if they lure us into forgetting that the brain is a single functional unit, from cortex to fingertips and toes. *To touch the surface is to stir the depths.* [My italics]

Learning to read changes on this surface is not easy, but contact with it provides a chance for exploration of much that is obvious and much that is deeply hidden. We will examine various concepts which relate to the mind–body link in Chapter 12. At this stage we need to look more closely at some of the physical characteristics of the skin.

As mentioned in the previous chapters, the changes which should be easily read by the palpator include the relative degree of warmth/coolness, dryness/dampness, smoothness/roughness, elasticity/rigidity, as well as the relative degree of thickness of the skin in the region. Much research and clinical experience suggests that altered skin physiology of this sort is often an end-result of dysfunction involving the sympathetic nervous system, especially as it relates to the musculoskeletal system (Gutstein 1944, Korr 1977, Lewit 1999) (see Box 4.1).

Aspects of skin physiology

In order to understand some of the dynamics involved in skin function and dysfunction, as well as some of the potential pitfalls possible in skin palpation, a brief examination of some aspects of the physiology of skin is necessary.

Credit for the main thrust of the material in this section should go to a group of researchers working in the United States. Their review (Adams et al 1982) is a clear examination of some of the main interacting elements which make the skin such a critical area in palpation.

Box 4.1 Skin as a monitor of reflexive behaviour

The skin displays evidence of reflexive change, as discussed in this chapter. Some of the clinicians and researchers who have observed these changes are quoted in this summary.

Brugger (1962) described pseudoradicular syndromes which are distinct from root syndromes and which derive from a 'nociceptive somatomotoric blocking effect' occurring in tissues such as joint capsules, tendon origins and other local (to joint) tissues. These painful reflex effects are noted in muscles and their tendinous junctions as well as the skin.

Dvorak & Dvorak (1984) include in this category of referred pain and symptoms the phenomena of viscerosomatic and somatovisceral influences in which, for example, organ dysfunction is said to produce tendomyotic changes (Korr 1975). The changes which can be observed or palpated include various patterns of vasomotor abnormality such as coldness, pallor, redness, cyanosis, etc.

Gutstein (1944) maintained that normalisation of skin secretion, and therefore of hair and skin texture and appearance, may be achieved by the removal of active trigger areas in the cervical and interscapular areas. The conditions of hyper-, hypo- and anhidrosis may accompany vasomotor and sebaceous dysfunction. Gutstein observed that abolition of excessive perspiration as well as anhidrosis followed adequate treatment.

Korr (1970, 1976, 1977) noted in early studies that readings of resistance to electricity in the paraspinal skin of an individual could show that there were often marked differences, with one side showing normal resistance and the other showing reduced resistance (facilitated area). When 'stress' was applied elsewhere in the body and the two areas of the spine were monitored, it was the area of facilitation where electrical resistance in the skin was reduced.

Beal (1985) has described this phenomenon as resulting from afferent stimuli, arising from dysfunction of a visceral nature. The reflex is initiated by afferent impulses arising from visceral receptors, which are transmitted to the dorsal horn of the spinal cord, where they synapse with interconnecting neurons. The stimuli are then conveyed to sympathetic and motor efferents, resulting in changes in the somatic tissues, such as skeletal muscle, skin and blood vessels. Abnormal stimulation of the visceral efferent neurons may result in hyperaesthesia of the skin and associated vasomotor, pilomotor and sudomotor changes. The first signs of such viscerosomatic reflexive influences are vasomotor (increased skin temperature) and sudomotor (increased moisture of the skin) reactions, skin textural changes (e.g. thickening), increased subcutaneous fluid and increased contraction of muscle. Beal (1983) suggests that investigation should pay attention to the various soft tissue layers, particularly the skin, looking for changes in texture, temperature and moisture.

Lewit (1992) also emphasises the value of light skin palpation in identifying areas of facilitation. These signs disappear if the visceral cause improves. When such changes become chronic, however, trophic alterations are noted, with increased thickening of the skin and subcutaneous tissue and localised muscular contraction. Deep musculature may become hard, tense and hypersensitive. This may involve deep splinting contractions, involving two or more segments of the spine, with associated restriction of spinal motion. The costotransverse articulations may be significantly involved in such changes.

A 5-year study involving over 5000 hospitalised patients concluded that most visceral disease appeared to influence more than one spinal region and that the number of spinal segments involved seemed to be related to the duration of the disease. Kelso (1985) noted in this study that there was an increase in the number of palpatory findings in the cervical region related to patients with sinusitis, tonsillitis, diseases of the oesophagus and liver complaints. Superficial (soft tissue and skin) changes were noted in patients with gastritis, duodenal ulceration, pyelonephritis, chronic appendicitis and cholycystitis, in the region of T5–12.

continues

Box 4.1 (*Continued*)

Skin palpation might therefore include:
- off-body scan (manual thermal diagnosis, MTD) which may offer evidence of variations in local circulation; trigger point activity is more likely in areas of greatest 'difference' (Barrell 1996). See exercises in this chapter relating to MTD
- movement of skin on fascia – resistance indicates general locality of reflexogenic activity, a 'hyperalgesic skin zone' such as a trigger point (Lewit 1992, 1999)
- local loss of skin elasticity – refines definition of the location (Lewit 1992, 1999)
- light stroke, seeking 'drag' sensation (increased hydrosis), offers pinpoint accuracy of location (Lewit 1992, 1999).

The skin contains nearly 750 000 sensory receptors which vary in the density of their presence in different regions, from 7 to 135 per sq cm. However, it is not neural endings which receive attention from these researchers; rather, they focus much of their attention onto the characteristics of human skin which derive from the activities of atrichial sweat glands, the secretions of which, apart from playing a role in temperature control, influence 'the energy and mass transfer characteristics of skin as well as altering its properties by establishing different levels of epidermal hydration and salinisation' (Adams et al 1982).

They ask us to make a clear distinction between epitrichial and atrichial sweat glands, the former being associated with hair shafts and the latter emptying directly on the skin and thus directly influencing the important phenomena of skin friction and heat transfer properties. The atrichial glands on the palmar surface of the hand (and the soles of the feet) have only a small potential for influencing heat loss but are important in being capable of modifying skin friction and pliability. It is of considerable clinical importance that the atrichial sweat glands are totally controlled by the sympathetic division of the autonomic nervous system, since this means that any palpable changes resulting from sweat production may be influenced by reflex activity, such as occurs when trigger points are active, and when emotional or stress factors are operating. The chemical mediator between the motor nerve and the secretory tubule of atrichial sweat glands is acetylcholine, a neurotransmitter which increases the tendency for muscles to contract.

The complexities of water movement through the skin need not concern us at this stage, apart from a need to emphasise that the mechanical, electrical and heat transfer properties, and characteristics, of the skin are altered by this process.

As sweating occurs, liquid is not only passed through the tubule, but diffuses laterally into surrounding peritubular drier skin areas. Even when there is no obvious sweat on the skin surface, sweat gland activity in the underlying skin continues, with some of the water which spreads into surrounding skin being reabsorbed. This mechanism is compared with the way in which the kidney tubule deals with sugar in the urine. By the same logic that it is incorrect to deduce that there is no sugar in the renal glomerular filtrate because none is detected in the urine, it is similarly incorrect to conclude that the sweat glands are inactive because there is no water on the skin surface (Adams et al 1982).

Low-level sweat gland activity has the effect of altering the degree of skin friction. Friction is low when the skin is dry and higher as it becomes moist, decreasing again when sweating becomes very intense. It is hard to turn a page with a dry finger; moisten it slightly and the task is easier but a very sweaty hand cannot grasp anything easily. We can conclude that there is a narrow range of epidermal water content that produces maximum frictional contact at the skin surface.

This knowledge may help us understand some of the reasons for the regional variations in skin friction ('skin drag') noted on palpation. Adams and his colleagues (1982) ask:

> Is it possible that regional differences in 'skin drag' perceived by the examining physician are related to segmentally active, autonomic reflexes that trigger chronic, low level, atrichial sweat gland activity, which in turn increases local epidermal hydration and skin friction at a defined body site? Do these reflexes produce, through chronic sweat gland activity, changes in the mechanical properties of the skin's surface, similar to those you might detect on the wrist skin surface when a watchband is initially removed?

Initially, after removing a watch strap (or bracelet), when the skin under it is lightly stroked, there will be a high level of epidermal water which will make the friction level high, with a great deal of skin drag. After a while this is lost and the degree of drag will be similar to the surrounding skin characteristics.

This insight into the behaviour of skin should help us to understand just why Karel Lewit (1999) is able to identify trigger point activity (or any other active reflex activity) simply by assessing the degree of elasticity in the overlying skin and comparing it with neighbouring tissue. He terms local skin areas of this type 'hyperalgesic skin zones'. This also explains why, prior to the introduction of methods of electrical detection of acupuncture points, any skilled acupuncturist could find the points very quickly indeed, by palpation, and also why measurement of the electrical resistance of the skin can now do this even more quickly (i.e. when skin is moist it conducts electricity more efficiently than when dry!).

We will examine some of Lewit's thoughts and directions later in this chapter. We also need to see how the degree of epidermal hydration (sweat) influences our perception of warmth or cold in the tissues being palpated and how the condition of our own skin affects palpation.

First, however, palpation without touch, scanning off the body in order to evaluate differences in perceived hot and cooler areas, is discussed.

Thermography in bodywork

Various forms of thermal assessment are being used clinically to identify trigger point activity and other forms of dysfunction, including infrared, electrical and liquid crystal methods (Baldry 1993), as well as manual thermal diagnosis (MTD) (Barrell 1996).

Swerdlow & Dieter (1992) found, after examining 365 patients with demonstrable trigger points in the upper back, that 'Although thermographic "hotspots" are present in the majority, the sites are not necessarily where the trigger points are located'. Is it possible that 'old' triggers lie in ischaemic, possibly fibrotic tissue, leading to 'cold spots' being identified?

Simons (1987) suggests that while hot-spots may commonly represent trigger point sites, some triggers may exist in 'normal' temperature regions and hotspots can exist for reasons other than the presence of trigger points.

Thermal examination of the reference zone (target area) to which a trigger point refers or radiates usually shows skin temperature raised, but not always. Simons attributes this anomaly to the different effects trigger points have on the autonomic nervous system. Simons (1993) explains:

> Depending upon the degree and manner in which the trigger point is modulating sympathetic control of skin circulation, the reference zone initially may be

warmer, isothermic or cooler than unaffected skin. Painful pressure on the trigger point consistently and significantly reduced the temperature in the region of the referred pain and beyond.

A 'scan' of the tissues being investigated, keeping the hand approximately 1 inch from the skin surface, is used by some practitioners (MTD) as a means of establishing areas which apparently differ from each other in temperature.

Using sophisticated equipment, French osteopath Jean–Pierre Barrell has established that areas which scan (non-touching) as 'hot' are only truly warmer/hotter than surrounding areas in 75% of instances. It seems that scanning for hot and cold areas results in the perception of greater heat being noted whenever a major difference occurs in one area compared to a neighbouring one. This means that scanning over a 'normal' then a cold area will often (usually) result in a perception that greater heat is being sensed. This does not nullify the usefulness of such approaches in attempting to identify dysfunctional tissues without being invasive, but does mean that what seems 'hot' may actually be 'cold' (ischaemic?) (Barrell 1996). Apparently when scanning manually for heat, any area which is markedly different from surrounding tissues, in temperature terms, is considered 'hot' by the brain. Manual scanning for heat is therefore an accurate way of assessing 'difference' between tissues but not their actual thermal status (see Exercise 4.5 later in this chapter).

Learning to measure skin temperature by touch

Exercises 4.1–4.9 are designed to help you to establish the basic palpation skills needed to determine heat variations in the objects and tissues being evaluated, as well as introducing you to the phenomenon of 'drag', the palpation of which is an extremely useful assessment tool.

EXERCISE 4.1: TEMPERATURE DISCRIMINATION USING INANIMATE OBJECTS

Time suggested: 10–15 seconds per object palpated

Assemble in front of you small objects made of wood, plastic, metal, china, rough-textured ceramic and paper. If possible, have several different items made of each substance. Make sure that they have all been in the same place, in the room in which you are carrying out this exercise, for at least an hour before you start. We can presume that the ambient temperature is uniform in this part of the room. Palpate each of the items individually, with each hand, sensing the relative feeling of warmth or coolness it imparts when in your hands.

Were the objects to be measured with a thermocouple, they would show almost exactly the same reading and yet you will have noted that there is a distinct difference in temperature as you feel them. Why do you think this is?

The answer will be found as you work your way through this chapter.

EXERCISE 4.2: TEMPERATURE DISCRIMINATION

Time suggested: 15 seconds

Stand barefoot on a cold tile, piece of marble or sheet of plastic. Rest one foot on the floor and the other on a rug or towel which has been in the room for some time. One foot feels cold, the other does not and yet the temperature of the floor and the rug is almost certainly the same.

What is the reason for the perceived difference?

Does this raise any questions in your mind as to the accuracy of what temperature variations we think we can 'feel' when we are palpating something or someone?

Record your thoughts in your journal.

DISCUSSION REGARDING EXERCISES 4.1 AND 4.2

The variables which influence heat flow from the object which we are feeling to the surface of the unit we are using to feel with (fingertips, hand) are related to the thermal properties of these two 'exchanging surfaces'. These thermal properties include:

- the surface areas of the exchanging surfaces
- the differences in temperature between the exchanging surfaces
- the distance over which heat is being transferred
- the intrinsic properties of heat conduction associated with the object being palpated and the palpatory unit (your hand or fingers).

A characteristic of this process, called the 'thermal conducting coefficient' (TCC), requires explanation. The TCC of a tiled floor is greater than that of the rug and this causes the thermoreceptors in your foot on the tiled floor to be more rapidly cooled than the other foot.

Your perception of one foot being 'colder' than the other is accurate, but it does not relate to any differences in the temperature of the surfaces on which you are standing.

If it can be independently verified that two objects that feel as though they have different temperatures are actually at the same temperature, then the difference sensed by your thermoreceptors (the neural receptors which transmit messages relating to heat and cold to your brain) can be attributed to a difference in thermal conductivity, or some other heat transfer property, of the object(s) being examined, but not to a difference in temperature. This is clearly of significance when it comes to making clinical judgements as to how warm or cool an area of skin feels.

A further complication becomes apparent when we examine the influence of the degree of epidermal hydration (sweat) in and on both the palpated tissues and the palpating hand.

What is the effect of sweat on our judgement of the temperature of the tissues we are palpating?

EXERCISE 4.3: THERMAL CONDUCTIVITY AND THE INFLUENCE OF MOISTURE

Time suggested: 10–15 seconds per object, per test

Take any two of the objects which you have previously palpated for temperature difference, say a pencil and a metal key or other metal object. Once again, palpate these by hand and sense the difference in thermal sensation reaching the thermoreceptors in your hand. Use the same part of your hand (palm, dorsum, fingertip, etc.) to palpate each object.

Try this first with your hands dry and then moisten the fingertips (or whatever part of the hand is being used) and repalpate the objects. Do the exercise with each hand.

Do you notice any difference in what you sense in terms of temperature when the dry hand/fingers and then the moist hand/fingers are in touch with the object?

If so, what is the difference?

Record your findings.

EXERCISE 4.4: TESTING DIFFERENT REGIONS FOR THERMAL SENSITIVITY

Time suggested: 10–15 seconds per object, per test

Next, try to see whether the thermal sensitivity of the dorsal aspect of the hand is greater than that noted by the palm or finger pad, when assessing both a wooden pencil and then a metal object.

Are you more aware of temperature differences when palpating with one or other part of your hand?

Or with one hand or the other?

Now test the same objects again, but this time use the tip of your tongue as your 'palpating' organ.

Did you sense the apparent differences in temperature more clearly with the tip of your tongue? Yes/No

DISCUSSION REGARDING EXERCISES 4.3 AND 4.4

The thermoreceptors in the palmar surface of the hand are far more densely sited than on the dorsum of the hand and are even more closely packed on the tip of the tongue (where they are close to the surface), making these regions more sensitive for palpation of heat. This means that despite the differences in epidermal thickness on the dorsum of the hand, as compared with the palmar surface, the palm is usually a better place to make contact when seeking thermal information.

Test this out for yourself, since some people seem to be more sensitive, where heat measurement is concerned, when using the dorsum of the hand and you may be one of these. This may be due to sensitisation of the palmar surface through repetitive manual contacts and the relative lack of contact of the dorsum with objects.

Note that the relative dampness or otherwise of the palpating surface influences perception of heat. This is because of better conduction when water (sweat, for example) is present, so that the temperature of the thermoreceptors is closer to that of the object being examined than it would be with a dry contact.

Variables

Your own state of hydration, your peripheral circulatory efficiency, your sympathetic nervous system activity and a number of other variables, including the ambient humidity and temperature, will influence your thermal perception as you palpate.

Adams and his colleagues (1982) summarise the problem of understanding the variables.

The thermoreceptors in an examining finger are part of a complex heat exchange system. The temperature that is felt by the examiner is directly related to the rate of action potential formation on afferent, sensory nerves arising from thermoreceptors near the dermo-epidermal junction. Their temperature is strongly dependent on heat brought to the skin (or taken away from it) by the circulating blood.

The perceived temperature is also determined by the rate of heat transfer out of, or into, the examiner's skin from the patient's skin, which relates to such factors as the area of contact, thickness of skin in both examiner and patient and the status of epidermal hydration in both, as well as heat transfer characteristics (which will be influenced by factors such as material trapped between the two skin surfaces – examiner and patient – including air, water, lotion, grease or oil, dirt, fabric and so on).

All or any of these variables will be operating each time we palpate and, to some extent at least, their net effect needs to be taken into consideration. Some of the variables affecting thermal perception are illustrated in Figure 4.1.

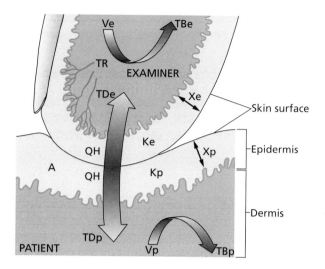

Fig. 4.1 This diagram depicts some of the physical and physiologic factors that affect the thermoreceptor (TR) discharge rate and consequently the temperature sensed in an examiner's skin in contact with a patient's skin. The temperature and its rate of change of the examiner's thermoreceptors are functions of the net effects of the time that the tissues are in contact, their contact area (A), the temperatures (TBe and TBp) and volume flow rates (Ve and Vp) of blood perfusing the examiner's and patient's skin, epidermal thickness (Xe and Xp) and thermal conductivity (Ke and Kp) of both, dermal temperature (TDe and TDp) of both, as well of the net heat exchange rate (QH) between the two tissues. QH is strongly affected by the heat transfer properties of material trapped between the two skin surfaces, for example, air, water, oil, grease, hand lotion, dirt, tissue debris, fabric (Adams et al 1982).

Palpating the skin for temperature and skin variations

Having established the need to be aware of possible misinterpretations of information gathered regarding apparent temperature differences, due to some of the many variables discussed above, it is time to begin to try to make sense of the human body as you palpate for specific characteristics available for your evaluation.

The objective of the next few exercises (4.5–4.8) is to highlight the importance of using the skin as a source of valuable information, which allows for the intelligent exploration of deeper tissues.

Try to ensure that these four exercises are done sequentially, in the same study/palpation exercise session, so that the results of each can be compared with the others, with the results of the previous test being factored into the subsequent one, and also so that they can be learned as a routine, which can be used clinically.

EXERCISE 4.5: OFF-BODY SCANNING FOR TEMPERATURE DIFFERENCES

Time suggested: 2–3 minutes maximum

Stand at waist level, with your palpation partner prone on the treatment table, exposed from the waist up. Hold your dominant hand, with palm down, close (1–3 inches/2.5–7.5 cm) to the surface of the back and make steady, deliberate sweeps of the hand to and fro, across the back, until all of it has been scanned.

As you 'scan' for temperature variations 'off the body' in this way, keep the hand moving slowly. If the hand remains still or moves too slowly, you have nothing to compare and if you move too fast, you will not perceive the slight changes as the hand passes from one area to another. Approximately 4–5 inches (10–15 cm) should be scanned per second.

As previously discussed, different aspects and areas of the hand may be more sensitive than others, so test whether your sensitivity is greater in the palm, near the wrist or on the dorsum of the hand, as you evaluate areas which feel warmer or cooler than others. These should be charted.

Make the areas which appear to you to be 'warmest' the focus for subsequent tests in this sequence, as these are the areas of greatest potential interest, remembering Barrell's (1996) evidence that the actual temperature of such areas may be cooler and that your brain will have interpreted areas which are different from each other, as you scan, as representing warmth.

Does your experience agree with the suggestion that the palmar surface is more sensitive than the dorsal surface of the hand?

Record your findings.

Viola Frymann (1963) states:

> Even passing the hand a quarter of an inch above the skin provides information on the surface temperature. An acute lesion area will be unusually warm, an area of long-standing, chronic lesion may be unusually cold as compared with the skin in other areas.

EXERCISE 4.6: DIRECT PALPATION FOR TEMPERATURE DIFFERENCES

Time suggested: 3–4 minutes for each segment of this exercise (A, B and C)

Your palpation partner should be lying prone as in the previous exercise, with the back exposed.

You should now apply hand or finger contact, without pressure, to the tissues being evaluated, which should involve those which tested as 'warm' in the previous (scan) exercise, as well as those which did not. Do not rub or press the tissues, merely mould your hand(s) to the skin surface for a few seconds, before moving to an adjacent area. In this way, slowly and carefully palpate the back for variations of skin temperature, using both hands, one at a time or both at the same time:

A when the 'patient' has been lying still for some minutes in a room of normal temperature/humidity

B when the 'patient' has actively skipped, jogged, danced or performed some other exercise for several minutes

continues

EXERCISE 4.6 *(Continued)*

C when you have performed similar exercise for some minutes.

Do you note any differences between A, B and C?

Vary your contact so that sometimes you use the palmar and sometimes the dorsal surface of the hands for this assessment under similarly variable conditions.

Is one hand more sensitive than the other?

Is one palpation contact more accurate than the other?

Do you sense differences in temperature from one area to another of the body surface and if so, how does this relate to the off-the-body scan in the previous exercise?

How does your or your partner's degree of hydration/sweating influence what you feel?

Record your findings.

EXERCISE 4.7: EVALUATING SKIN ON FASCIA RESISTANCE

Time suggested: 3–5 minutes

This palpation is based on German connective tissue massage (*Bindegewebsmassage*) named by physical therapist Elizabeth Dicke (1954). For a discussion on this method see Box 4.2. The methods used, involving patterns of repetitive dry-contact, strong friction stroke, aimed at evoking reflex responses, do not concern us in this text. However, the diagnostic methods used to identify areas (zones) suitable for treatment are significant.

Dicke's method of diagnosis is discussed by Irmgard Bischof and Ginette Elmiger (Bischof & Elmiger 1960). The subject is seated or lying prone (see Fig. 4.2). Both hands, applied flat, displace the subcutaneous tissues simultaneously against the fascia, with small to-and-fro pushes. The degree of displacement possible will depend upon tension of the tissues. It is important that symmetrical areas (i.e. both sides of the body) be examined simultaneously.

With your fingers lightly flexed and using only enough pressure to produce adherence between the fingertips and the skin (do not slide on the skin, instead slide the skin on the underlying fascia), make a series of short, deliberate, pushing motions, simultaneously with both hands, which eases the tissues (skin on fascia) to the elastic barrier on each side (see Fig. 4.2). Pay particular attention to comparing areas where 'heat' was sensed during the scan exercise.

The pattern of testing should be performed from inferior to superior, either moving the tissues superiorly or bilaterally, in an obliquely diagonal direction toward the spine.

Whether your partner is prone or seated, tissues from the buttocks to the shoulders may be tested, always comparing the sides for symmetry of range of movement of the skin to its elastic barrier.
As a palpation exercise try to identify local areas where your 'push' of skin on connective tissue reveals restriction as compared with its opposite side.

continues

EXERCISE 4.7 *(Continued)*

Dicke also suggests (Bischof & Elmiger 1960):

By pulling away a skinfold from the fascia [Fig. 4.3], the degree of tissue tension and displacement may be determined. Three different levels of displacement are distinguished:

● the most superficial displacement occurs between skin and subcutaneous tissues and is easier to find in children and in old people because the displacement is slight

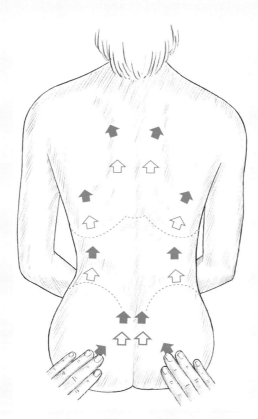

Fig. 4.2   Testing tissue mobility by bilaterally 'pushing' skin with fingerpads.

● the main displacement occurs between the subcutaneous tissue and the fascia
● the deepest displacement layer is between the fascia and the interstitial connective tissue. The movement is most evident upon large, flat areas such as the lumbosacral area, on the sacrum, and in regions of the tensor fascia lata.

By gently grasping and lifting bilateral skinfolds, see whether you can make any judgements using Dicke's comments.

Compare your findings using this method with those achieved by 'skin on fascia pushes' as described above.

continues

EXERCISE 4.7   (Continued)

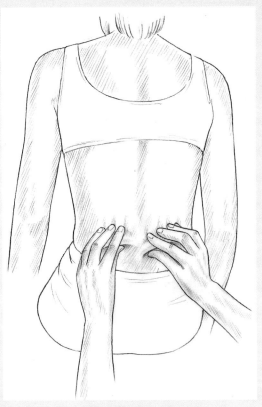

Fig. 4.3   Assessing bilateral elasticity of skin by lifting it in folds or 'rolling' it.

Box 4.2 Connective tissue massage (CTM) concepts

Apart from the diagnostic methods described in Exercise 4.7, CTM uses a further 'diagnostic stroke' which employs a two-finger contact (patient seated, as a rule) which runs longitudinally, paravertebrally, starting at the level of L5 up to the level of the seventh cervical spinous process. As the stroke (pull) starts, the upper layers of displacement are superficial and gentle; they are followed by a slower, deeper stroke which pulls on subcutaneous tissue and fascia. Displacement of the deeper tissue, as well as interstitial tissue, is accomplished by a deep and slow pull along the same 'track'.

This highlights an important point, namely that the desired depth effect is obtained by the speed of the strokes as well as the amount of pressure. This is true also of neuromuscular technique and is a most useful tip for those attempting to enhance palpatory skills.

'Slow down, the information is there, and it cannot be hurried.'

What should such strokes show? Healthy tissue elevates or 'mounds' ahead of the stroking digits (2–3 cm ahead). When an area of resistance is reached, increased tension is felt and further displacement of the skin becomes difficult or impossible. Folds of skin will be formed in front of the advancing stroke in such areas and the mass will become larger. The progress of the stroke will also become slower, as compared with the stroke across healthy tissue. Factors such as age of patient, constitutional state, posture and the area being tested will all alter the anticipated findings.

continues

Box 4.2 (*Continued*)

It is easier to displace skin against underlying tissue in slim individuals, with little fatty tissue. Obese individuals have a higher subcutaneous fat and water content, making displacement more difficult.

Dicke pointed out that even before use of the diagnostic stroke, it is often possible to see reflex areas, characterised by being retracted or elevated. Retracted bands of tissue are commonly seen in areas such as the neck, lower thoracic border and over the pelvic and gluteal areas. Depressed or flattened areas are seen over the thorax, the scapulae and between the thoracic spine and the scapula as well as over the upper iliac tissues and the sacrum. Flat elevations are visible in many cases around the seventh cervical spinous process, on the outer border of the scapulae or around the sacrum.

These raised or depressed tissue areas are not amenable to dissipation by massage and represent chronic reflex activity. They are considered to be viscerocutaneous reflexes (viscerosomatic in other words) resulting from altered blood supply leading to colloidal changes in the cells and tissues.

What is revealed by these diagnostic strokes is alteration in vascular skin reaction, tissue tension, tissue density, tissue sensitivity and often tissue displacement. Valuable clinical evidence can be gathered using these strokes and 'pushes'.

For a deeper understanding of this system, Dicke's work should be studied in depth. Fortunately this system is now taught worldwide by her followers and is much used by physical therapists, massage therapists and some doctors, osteopaths and chiropractors who employ soft tissue methods.

Note: Ideally, Exercises 4.8–4.10 should be performed in sequence, at one training/class session. Similarly, Exercises 4.11–4.13 should be performed in sequence at one training/class session.

Lewit's methods of skin evaluation

Karel Lewit has compiled a treasure-house of information (Lewit 1992, 1999). His discussion of the importance of skin palpation is worth examining (see Box 4.3).

Box 4.3 Lewit's hyperalgesic skin zones (HSZ)

Lewit (1992, 1999) points out that it was late in the 19th century that Head first reported on increased sensitivity to pinprick sensations in particular zones involved in reflex activity. Unfortunately, such a subjective symptom meant that the practitioner was dependent upon accurate feedback from the patient, for whom it was a slow and not particularly comfortable experience. Lewit also discusses the technique of 'skin rolling', in which a skinfold is lifted and rolled forwards between the fingers. Increased resistance is easily noted by the practitioner, as is the fact that, wherever reflex activity is operating, these folds of skin will also be 'thicker' (see Fig. 4.3). Unfortunately, this technique is often painful to the patient and is difficult to perform on areas where skin is tightly adherent to underlying tissue.

In the German system of connective tissue massage (CTM), a variation on this assessment method involves the skin being lightly stretched over the underlying fascia, by pressing with the fingertips in a direction away from the operator. As described in Exercise 4.7, this is usually performed bilaterally, so that variations in the degree of elasticity can be compared from one side of the body to the other, so producing evidence of reflex activity if there is a reduced degree of 'stretchability' when the two sides are compared.

continues

Box 4.3 *(Continued)*

The disadvantages of these methods lie in their fairly general indications, although this matters little to those using CTM, since they are usually attempting to identify large reflex zones which relate to organ or system dysfunction, rather than small localised areas of reflex activity required to identify, for example, myofascial trigger points.

Lewit reports that he has developed a painless and effective method which is more reliable diagnostically than those mentioned above and which transforms from diagnostic evaluation to therapeutic treatment if the process (see Exercise 4.8) is prolonged. He calls the method 'skin stretching'.

Lewit first stretches the skin with the minimum of force, in order to take up the available slack, and then takes the stretch to its end-position without force, where a slight 'springiness' is felt. He performs a similar stretch in various directions over the area being assessed.

If a hyperalgesic skin zone (HSZ) exists due to reflex input to the area, a 'stiff' resistance is felt after the slack is taken up, rather than an elastic 'end-feel'.

Like has to be compared with like and it is little use comparing the degree of elasticity available in skin overlaying, say, the lumbar paraspinal muscles with that overlaying the dorsal paraspinal tissues. The first would usually be relatively 'loose' and the other fairly 'tight', as a natural matter of course. However, if one area of dorsal paraspinal skin elasticity is compared with another area of dorsal paraspinal skin elasticity and one of these is significantly less elastic than the other, evidence is gained that reflex activity may exist below the 'tight' skin area.

Treatment of such areas, which initiates a degree of normalisation of the reflex activity which created them, is achieved by maintaining the degree of stretch for a further 10 seconds or so.

According to Lewit:

> If the therapist then holds the stretched skin in end-position [around 10 seconds is usual] resistance is felt to weaken until normal springing is restored. The hyperalgesic skin zone can then as a rule no longer be detected. If pain is due to this hyperalgesic skin zone *this method is quite as effective as needling, electrostimulation and other similar methods.* [My italics]

Lewit suggests that this method allows us to diagnose (and treat) even very small reflex areas (HSZ) lying in inaccessible or potentially painful places, such as between the toes, over bony prominences and around scars.

Just what is going on in these HSZs? They sometimes overlay areas affected by viscerosomatic reflex activity, or what is known as **segmental** facilitation, in which the neural structures in any spinal region **may** respond to repetitive stress factors, of varying types, by becoming hyperreactive. This produces undesirable consequences both locally and in the areas supplied by nerves from that spinal level. We will look at palpation methods for identifying levels of spinal segmental facilitation (other than HSZ) when we examine muscular palpation (Chapter 5).

Localised myofascial facilitation also takes place in the development of trigger points, localised areas of soft tissue disruption which have the ability to bombard distant tissues with aberrant neural impulses, often of a painful nature. HSZ will be found overlaying active (and also 'embryo' and dormant) trigger points, as well as over the target zone which the trigger point influences.

Those therapists who are interested in the acupuncture model of treatment will be aware that active points in the meridian system have an area of lowered electrical resistance overlaying them. The location of these areas is easily identified by means of Lewit's method of skin stretching (and according to him would respond therapeutically to further stretching, as they would to needling). There is more detail on the trigger point phenomenon in Chapter 5, including a summary of methods for identifying these common troublemakers, as well as a reminder of Lewit's methods.

EXERCISE 4.8: LEWIT'S SKIN-STRETCHING PALPATION (A)

Time suggested: 5–10 minutes

At first, it is necessary to practise this method slowly. Eventually it should be possible to move fairly rapidly over an area which is being searched for evidence of reflex activity (or acupuncture points).

Your palpation partner should be lying prone as in the previous few exercises. Choose two regions to be assessed, ideally areas which were 'different' on scanning and which also showed an abnormal degree of skin-on-fascia adherence in previous exercises. If possible, select an area 7.5 × 7.5 cm (3 inches by 3 inches) to the side of the dorsal spine, covering the muscular paraspinal region, as well as some of the skin over the scapula and/or ribs.

The other area should be of a similar size, in the low back/buttock area, involving far more elastic, 'loosely fitting' skin. Mark these areas with a skin pencil or felt-tip pen and begin the search.

Place your two index fingers adjacent to each other, on the skin, side by side or pointing towards each other, with no pressure at all onto the skin, just a contact touch (see Fig. 4.4A).

Lightly and slowly separate your fingers, feeling the skin stretch as you do so (see Fig. 4.4B).

Take the stretch to its 'easy' limit. In other words, do not forcibly stretch the skin, just take it to the point where resistance is first noted. This is the 'barrier of resistance' and it should be easily possible, with a little more effort, to 'spring' the skin further apart, to its absolute elastic limit.

Release this stretch and move both fingers 0.5 cm to one side of this first test site and test again in the same way and in the same direction of pull, separating the fingers. Perform exactly the same sequence over and over again until the entire area of tissue has been searched.

When performing the series of stretches, ensure that the rhythm you adopt is not too slow (it is usually impossible to retain the subtle proprioceptive memory of the previous stretch if there is too long a gap between stretches). On the other hand, if the series of stretches is performed too rapidly the individual stretch is unlikely to be to the true elastic barrier which is being assessed. My preferred recommendation is that one stretch per second be performed, if possible.

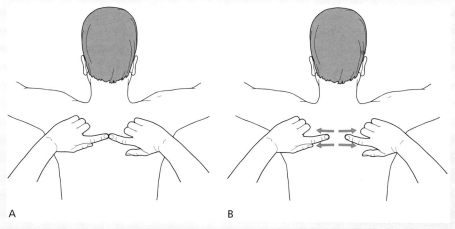

A   B

Fig. 4.4 (A) Fingers touch each other directly over skin to be tested – very light skin contact only. (B) Pull apart to assess degree of skin elasticity – compare with neighbouring skin area.

continues

EXERCISE 4.8 (Continued)

Time suggested: 5–10 minutes

In some local areas you may sense that the skin is not as elastic as it was on the previous stretch. This is a potential hyperalgesic skin zone (HSZ). Mark it with a skin pencil or felt-tip pen, for future attention.

If you were to apply light finger pressure to the centre of that small zone, you would almost always locate a sensitive contracture, which on sustained pressure may radiate sensations to a distant site (meaning that it is a trigger point, in which case add to your marking on the skin – or a record card – the direction of the radiating sensation) or may not radiate (meaning that it is either an active acupuncture point, a latent or an embryonic trigger point or some other reflex manifestation).

Record your findings.

EXERCISE 4.9: LEWIT'S SKIN-STRETCHING PALPATION (B)

Time suggested: 5–10 minutes

Now reassess precisely the same skin areas as in the previous exercise, but this time make the direction of each stretch different, perhaps going parallel to the spine rather than vertical to it, for example.

See whether you identify the same reflex areas/trigger points (HSZs) this time. Using a skin pencil or felt-tip pen, mark one or two particularly 'tight' areas (HSZs).

Record your findings.

EXERCISE 4.10: LEWIT'S SKIN-STRETCHING PALPATION (C)

Time suggested: 10 minutes

Having satisfied yourself that you can utilise skin stretching effectively to identify localised areas of dysfunction, as described in the previous two exercises, perform a search of other spinal areas which you had marked and note:

- the difference in elasticity which is available between skin overlying the dorsal area and the lumbar/gluteal area
- how it is possible to vary the direction of stretch as you move your finger contacts around the area and still be able to discriminate between elastic and less elastic skin areas
- how it is possible to begin to speed up the process, so that what took you 5 minutes of painstakingly careful stretch, followed by stretch, can now be achieved in 1 or 2 minutes, without loss of accuracy.

Record your findings.

EXERCISE 4.11: LEWIT'S SKIN-STRETCHING PALPATION (D)

Time suggested: 12 minutes

In order to develop your skills in using skin stretching diagnostically, you should now try to assess for variations in the elasticity of skin in difficult areas such as:

- the sternum/xiphoid process
- over the spinous processes
- in the webbing between the toes or fingers.

If you have no available palpation partner, perform as many of the above exercises as you can on yourself.

Using a skin pencil or felt-tip pen, mark one or two particularly 'tight' areas (HSZs).

Remember that no lubricant should be used during any of these assessments; they are best and most accurately performed 'dry'.

Be careful on hairy areas, as this could obviously cause discomfort.

Note the variations in degree of skin elasticity as you assess first one and then another anatomical site.

EXERCISE 4.12: LEWIT'S SUSTAINED SKIN STRETCH OF HSZs

Time suggested: 3–5 minutes

Now go back to a marked hyperalgesic skin zone identified in one of the previous exercises. Gently stretch the skin to its elastic barrier and hold it there for at least 10–15 seconds, without force.

Do you then feel the skin tightness gradually release so that, as you hold the elastic barrier, your fingers actually separate further?

Hold the skin in its new stretched position, at its new barrier of resistance, for a few seconds longer and then do the same to other HSZs which you identified and noted in previous assessments.

Now go back and retest the areas you have 'released' in this way and see whether these areas, which previously demonstrated reflexively restricted skin, have regained comparative elasticity.

Record your findings.

EXERCISE 4.13: LEWIT'S LARGE SKIN AREA ASSESSMENT/PALPATION

Time suggested: 2–4 minutes

Lewit describes a contact in which the ulnar borders of the cross-hands are used to assess large skin areas (such as the low back) in much the same way as the small areas were assessed by finger-induced stretching of the skin in previous exercises.

Place the palms of the hands together and then, using a firm contact, place the full length of the sides of both hands, from the little fingers to the wrist, onto an area of skin on the low back (as an example). Separate the hands slowly, stretching the skin with which they are in contact, until an elastic barrier is reached. Move to an immediately adjacent area of skin, place the hands and test as above, comparing the distance the skin stretches with the previous effort.

Do this sequentially, stretch following stretch, so that an area such as the back or thigh is covered. Identify and mark those stretches in which there seems to be restriction, as compared with neighbouring skin elasticity.

This exercise may reveal large reflexively active zones, which could relate to organ dysfunction or other neurological involvement.

Practise 'releasing' these restrictions, as in the example in Exercise 4.12, by holding the stretch at the barrier or resistance, without force, for 15–20 seconds or until an easing of tone, release of tightness, is experienced. Retest to see whether this has indeed made a difference to the elasticity of the area compared with neighbouring areas.

Record your findings.

Box 4.4 Positional release experiment

Locate an area of skin which tested as 'tight' when evaluated using Lewit's skin-stretch method. Place two or three finger pads onto the skin and slide it superiorly and then inferiorly on the underlying fascia. To which direction does the skin slide most easily?

Slide the skin in that direction and, holding it there, test the preference of the skin to slide medially and laterally. Which of these is the easiest direction?

Slide the tissue toward this second position of ease.

Now introduce a slight clockwise and anticlockwise twist to these tissues which are already being held ('stacked') in two directions of ease. Which way does the skin feel most comfortable as it rotates?

Take it in that direction, so that you are now holding the skin in three positions of ease. Hold this for not less than 20 seconds.

Release the skin and retest; it should now display a far more symmetrical preference in all the directions which were previously 'tight'.

You have already established that holding skin at its barrier (unforced) changes its function, as the skin releases (see Exercise 4.12), and now you have observed that moving tissues away from the barrier into ease can also achieve a release. This is an example of a positional release technique (Chaitow 2002).

DISCUSSION REGARDING EXERCISES 4.8–4.13

The causes of reflex activities, which manifest as hyperalgesic skin zones, may involve organic, systemic or structural dysfunction and may be local or global in their influences. They may be acute or chronic.

Thus, while identifying HSZs offers evidence of where reflexive activity may be operating, and while releasing skin tension, in the manner described by Lewit, may have some input in normalising function, this is likely to be of only temporary duration unless underlying causes are also dealt with.

The methods described above are therefore useful in identifying and localising tissues involved in reflex activity but their value in therapeutic terms should be thought of as short rather than long term.

General considerations

In this chapter some very important concepts regarding skin palpation have already been outlined. The significance of what is being noted during skin palpation has been addressed by a number of experts, for example William Walton (1971) who says:

> In superficial palpation, the operator [practitioner], using the pads of his fingers, strokes the skin gently, but firmly enough to allow perception, over the area to be examined. There are five types of change to be noted by superficial palpation in both acute and chronic lesions:
>
> - skin changes
> - temperature changes
> - superficial muscle tensions
> - tenderness and oedema.
>
>   In acute lesions an actual increase in temperature may be felt in the skin overlaying it, but evidence is vague and extremely fleeting, and not much reliance should be placed on it. The skin overlaying the lesion will feel tense and relatively immobile owing to the congestive effect of the lesion below it. In the chronic lesion, temperature changes may or may not be present . . . the skin overlaying a chronic lesion may be either normal or reduced as a result of ischaemia of the underlying tissues. This is characteristic of chronic fibrotic change.

Myron Beal (1983) has researched common paraspinal palpatory findings (mainly involving upper thoracic facilitated segments) relating to patients with acute and chronic cardiovascular disease and seems to place less importance on the reliability of superficial evidence as compared with deeper palpated changes. Skin texture and temperature changes were not apparent as consistent, strong findings, compared with the hypertonic state of the deep musculature. In one case of acute myocardial infarction there was an observable increase in the amount of subcutaneous fluid.

John Upledger, however, does not concur with Beal as to skin evidence being unreliable in such diagnosis (Upledger 1983). He describes use of the skin in localised diagnosis using a 'drag' palpation in precisely the areas in which Beal feels that deeper palpation is more reliable (see Upledger's description of this in Special topic 6 – Red, white and black reaction).

The difference of opinion between Beal and Upledger may have resulted from different palpatory methods or, more likely, simply because Beal finds the evidence from the muscles more reliable (see Chapter 5). He does, after all, say that the skin evidence is not 'as consistent' as the muscle evidence, not that skin evidence is not available or reliable.

In the next few exercises the phenomenon of increased hydrosis (sweat), and its effects on palpation, are used to remarkable effect in what is known as 'drag' palpation.

Drag palpation of the skin

EXERCISE 4.14: SKIN DRAG PALPATION

Time suggested: 5–7 minutes

Before performing this exercise do a scan of the tissues you intend to palpate, seeking apparent areas of increased warmth (as in Exercise 4.5). Also palpate directly the tissues where increased warmth was noted in the scan (as in Exercise 4.6A).

Now palpate the same skin areas, this time assessing for variations in skin friction, by lightly running a fingertip across the skin surface (no lubricant should be used), particularly comparing areas which scanned or palpated as warmer than surrounding tissues. Perform this exercise with different fingers of each hand.

The degree of pressure required is minimal – skin touching skin is all that is necessary ('feather-light touch') (see Fig. 4.5).

Movement of a single palpating digit should be purposeful, not too slow and certainly not very rapid. Around 3–5 cm (1–2 inches) per second is a satisfactory speed.

Feel for any sense of 'drag', which suggests a resistance to the easy, smooth passage of the finger across the skin surface.

A sense of 'dryness', 'sandpaper', a slightly harsh or rough texture may all indicate increased presence of sweat on, or increased fluid in, the tissues.

Variation of focus ('hills and valleys')

When performing the drag palpation exercise, attempt to modify your focus. While using precisely the same single-digit stroke, instead of thinking about the sensation of drag, attempt to appreciate a subtle rising and falling of the stroking digit, as it moves across the tissues. You are using an ancient Chinese palpation method, which allowed acupuncturists to identify active acupuncture points. When an obvious sense of rise or fall ('hill' or 'valley') was noted, in the region of a known acupuncture point site, it was considered that there was an excess of chi (hill) or a deficiency of chi (valley) and the point was treated accordingly.

Perform a light stroke precisely where you previously noted 'drag'.

Does the stroking finger seem to slightly rise or fall?

Some practitioners prefer to evaluate using this focus rather than drag. Both are equally effective, if your discriminatory focus is applied to pick up the signals.

continues

EXERCISE 4.14 *(Continued)*

After physical exercise

Once you have identified several areas of 'drag', introduce the same variables as were used in Exercise 4.6B and C, in which either you or your palpation partner will have briefly but vigorously exercised, before you repeat the 'drag' assessment.

Note your results, especially if skin friction and temperature variation noted in previous exercises (scan and direct palpation, Exercises 4.5 and 4.6) have been sensed in the same skin region.

Make a note on a chart of the findings, especially any which indicate both local skin drag/friction characteristics and also greater warmth than surrounding tissue.

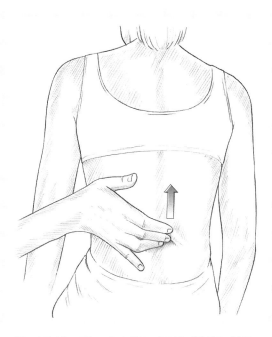

Fig. 4.5   Assessing variations in skin friction (drag, resistance).

EXERCISE 4.15   SKIN DRAG (WATCH STRAP) PALPATION

Time suggested: 10 seconds

If you are even slightly confused as to what it is that you are trying to feel in the previous exercise (4.14), remove your watch or bracelet (or have someone else remove their watch/bracelet) and lightly run a finger across the skin which was under the strap, as well as over the adjacent skin.

By running your palpating finger(s) over both 'dry' and 'moist' skin, you should easily be able to feel the difference in drag, friction and resistance.

Now wait for about 5 minutes and then, without having replaced the watch strap/bracelet, perform the exercise again. See how the drag on the skin which was under the strap is now absent, so that the previous site of 'drag' now palpates as the same as the surrounding skin. On another occasion, study perceived temperature differences in the skin under a watch strap, first immediately after it is removed and then again 5–10 minutes later, as compared with surrounding skin.

Record your findings in your journal.

DISCUSSION REGARDING EXERCISES 4.14 AND 4.15

You need to ask yourself whether an area of skin which 'feels' colder than surrounding skin is really colder (or warmer) or whether this actually relates to a higher thermal conductivity coefficient, which could be due to an increase in epidermal hydration (yours or the subject's) arising from a local or general increase in activity of the atrichial sweat glands. This in turn could be due to reflex activity, emotional distress or some other phenomenon (air conditioning, central heating?) or, as you may have discovered, exercise (Lewit 1992, 1999).

If the same skin area which scans and palpates as having a different temperature from its surrounding tissue also displays increased skin friction characteristics (drag), the likelihood of this being due to increased atrichial sweat gland activity is strong (Barrell 1996).

You also need to keep in mind your own state of physical and sympathetic activity as it relates to peripheral circulation and epidermal hydration when you palpate. Ask yourself:

● Are my hands sweating?
● Have they been sweating?
● Am I feeling anxious?

If your answer to any of these questions is in the affirmative, your thermoreceptors might be providing potentially inaccurate information as you palpate for temperature variables, a fact which would be compounded were the patient sweating or if the relative ambient humidity or temperature was high. You could also become confused in any attempt you might make to assess tissue texture changes (friction or 'skin drag') were you not aware of the possibility that similar interacting influences (hydration, humidity and so on) can alter 'skin drag' characteristics.

The phenomenon of 'drag' is commonly noted overlying active myofascial trigger points and areas of reflexogenic activity and is a superb assessment tool.

Overall palpation skill status

The successful completion of the exercises, up to this point, means that you have established an ability to discern variations in skin/surface temperature, differences in elastic qualities of skin and its relation to underlying fascia and can use the 'drag' phenomenon to locate areas of increased hydrosis.

If you are not satisfied with your degree of sensitivity in feeling temperature variations and 'drag', then repeat the exercises at regular intervals, daily if possible but several times a week at least, until you are comfortable with both the concepts and the practice of these methods.

You should also have satisfied yourself that different aspects of your hand are more sensitive than others and that a number of variables can influence the potential accuracy of what it is that you think you feel.

In the end you need to be able to compute your palpation findings along with variables such as ambient temperature, patient's (and your own) level of hydrosis, previous activity, anxiety, etc., almost instantaneously and to interpret them according to the body of knowledge you have acquired, so that the interpretation forms a part of your overall assessment of the patient's current status and requirements.

- Do you understand the physiology of the 'drag' sensation?
- Do you feel that you can discern temperature variations by means of scanning from off the body and also by direct palpation?
- Do you feel that you understand what these palpated phenomena indicate?

Review appropriate texts and note your current level of awareness relating to these topics in your journal.

Scars

Karel Lewit (1999) brings into focus yet another skin phenomenon which is often overlooked – the scar. In his discussion of conditions which are resistant to treatment or where symptoms do not seem to be explained by findings, he suggests we look for scar tissue.

> The German literature uses the term *storungsfeld* – 'focus of disturbance'. This is frequently an old scar after injury or operation, often a tonsillectomy scar. This focus-scar is usually tender on examination, with pain spots and surrounded by a hyperalgesic zone.

Such scars may act as 'saboteurs', he believes, requiring special attention. He suggests deep palpation for pain spots near scars, assessing for increased resistance ('adhesions') as well as for HSZ, by skin stretching. If release of the skin by stretching (as in Exercise 4.12) fails to resolve the situation (simple skin stretching is usually very successful with scars, says Lewit), needling (into pain spots) or local infiltration injections may be called for. When treatment has been successful, the local skin resistance, and the pain spots, should vanish and the patient's symptoms should start improving.

Upledger & Vredevoogd (1983) discuss scar tissue, illustrating its importance with the example of a patient with chronic migraine headaches which resulted from chronic fascial drag produced by an appendectomy scar.

> Deep pressure medially on the scar produced the headache; deep pressure laterally caused relief of the headache. Mobilisation of the scar was performed by sustained and deep but gentle pressure.

This resulted in freedom from headaches, according to these respected authors, who add:

Spontaneous relief of low back pain, menstrual disorders and chronic and recurrent cervical somatic dysfunction also occurred following cicatrix [scar] mobilisation.

The influence of fascia on soft tissue function and dysfunction will be considered in the next chapter.

EXERCISE 4.16: SCAR PALPATION

Time suggested: 3 minutes

Palpate a scar. Feel the scar tissue itself and see how the surrounding tissue associates with it. Is there a sense of tethering or does the scar 'float' in reasonable supple, elastic, local tissues?

If possible, palpate a recent and also a very old scar. Compare their characteristics.

See if local tenderness exists around the scar. See how the skin elasticity varies when this is the case.

Can you release the skin by sustained painless stretching?

Record your findings relating to the feel of as many scars as you come across, recent and of long standing.

EXERCISE 4.17: COMBINED SKIN PALPATION EXERCISE

Time suggested: 20–30 minutes

You should have now practised the various exercises involved in assessing temperature variations, both by scanning and directly, as well as Dicke's connective tissue method (skin on fascia 'pushes'), together with Lewit's method for identification of hyperalgesic skin zones using skin stretching, and 'skin drag'.

You should therefore now be ready to attempt an assessment in which you compare the reliability and accuracy of all these methods with each other, on one individual.

Obviously, such comparisons will only have validity if you use the same palpation partner. Try to ensure that you use all the skin assessment variations described on the same subject and compare results as you use the following palpation methods, in the following sequence.

1. Perform an off-body scan for temperature variations (remembering that cold may suggest ischaemia, hot may indicate irritation/inflammation). Note areas which are 'different'.
2. Now palpate directly, moulding your hands lightly to the tissues, to assess for temperature differences. Avoid lengthy hand contact or you will change the status of whatever you are palpating. A few seconds should be adequate.
3. Paying particular attention to those 'different' areas (from scan palpation), evaluate skin adherence to underlying fascia (using light or firm 'pushing' of assessed structures and/or skin rolling and/or tissue-lifting methods). Do such areas correspond with information gained from the scanning and palpation assessments?

continues

4. Using those areas where dysfunction has been indicated by previous assessments (1, 2 and 3 above) look for variations in local skin elasticity (Lewit's 'skin stretch'). Loss of elastic quality indicates a possible hyperalgesic zone and probable deeper dysfunction (e.g. trigger point) or pathology.
5. Finally attempt to identify reflexively active areas (triggers, etc.) by means of very light single-digit palpation, seeking the phenomenon of 'drag' (and/or 'hills and valleys'). Do these findings agree with each other? They should. If not, try again and again.

Incorporate as many of those methods which seem accurate, and with which you are comfortable, into your usual pattern of assessment.

Skilled skin palpation allows you to target areas of dysfunction below the surface and it is towards the structural information lying in the muscles themselves that our attention will next be focused.

REFERENCES

Adams T, Steinmetz J, Heisey R et al 1982 Physiologic basis for skin properties in palpatory physical diagnosis. Journal of the American Osteopathic Association

Baldry P 1993 Acupuncture, trigger points and musculoskeletal pain. Churchill Livingstone, Edinburgh

Barrell J-P 1996 Manual-thermal diagnosis. Eastland Press, Seattle

Beal M 1983 Palpatory testing of somatic dysfunction in patients with cardiovascular disease. Journal of the American Osteopathic Association July

Beal M 1985 Viscerosomatic reflexes: a review. Journal of the American Osteopathic Association 85(12): 786–801

Bischof I, Elmiger G 1960 Connective tissue massage. In: Licht S (ed) Massage, manipulation and traction. Licht, New Haven, Connecticut

Brugger A 1962 Pseudoradikulare syndrome. Acta Rheumatologica 19: 1

Chaitow L 2002 Positional release techniques' 2nd edn. Churchill Livingstone, Edinburgh

Dicke E 1954 Meine Bindegewebsmassage. Stuttgart

Dvorak J, Dvorak V 1984 Manual medicine diagnostics. Georg Thieme Verlag, Stuttgart

Gutstein R 1944 A review of myodysneuria (fibrositis). American Practitioner and Digest of Treatments 6(4): 114–124

Juhan D 1987 Job's body. Station Hill Press, New York

Kelso AF 1985 Viscerosomatic reflexes: a review. Journal of the American Osteopathic Association 85(12): 786–801

Korr I 1970 Physiological basis of osteopathic medicine. Postgraduate Institute of Osteopathic Medicine and Surgery, New York

Korr I 1975 Proprioceptors and somatic dysfunction. Journal of the American Osteopathic Association 74: 638

Korr I 1976 Spinal cord as organiser of disease process. Academy of Applied Osteopathy Yearbook, Newark, OH

Korr I (ed) 1977 Neurobiological mechanisms in manipulation. Plenum Press, New York

Lewit K 1992 Manipulative therapy in rehabilitation of the locomotor system, 2nd edn. Butterworths, London

Lewit K 1999 Manipulative therapy in rehabilitation of the locomotor system, 3rd edn. Butterworths, London

Simons D 1987 Myofascial pain due to trigger points. International Rehabilitation Medicine Association

Simons D 1993 Myofascial pain and dysfunction review. Journal of Musculoskeletal Pain 1(2): 131

Swerdlow B, Dieter N 1992 Evaluation of thermography. Pain 48: 205–213

Upledger J 1983 Craniosacral therapy – beyond the dura. Eastland Press, Seattle

Upledger J, Vredevoogd W 1983 Craniosacral therapy. Eastland Press, Seattle

Walton W 1971 Palpatory diagnosis of the osteopathic lesion. Journal of the American Osteopathic Association 71: 117–131

SPECIAL TOPIC 5
Is it a muscle or a joint problem?

Is the patient's pain a soft tissue or a joint problem? How can we rapidly make this differentiation?

There are several simple screening tests we can apply in answer to these questions, based on the work of Professor Freddy Kaltenborn, of Norway (Kaltenborn 1980).

1. Does passive stretching (traction) of the painful area increase the level of pain? If so, it is probably of soft tissue origin (extraarticular).

2. Does compression of the painful area increase the pain? If so, it is probably of joint origin (intraarticular), involving tissues belonging to that anatomical joint.

3. If active (controlled by the patient) movement in one direction produces pain (and/or is restricted), while passive (controlled by the therapist) movement in the opposite direction also produces pain (and/or is restricted), the contractile tissues (muscle, ligament, etc.) are implicated. This can be confirmed by resisted tests, described below.

4. If active movement and passive movement in the same direction produce pain (and/or restriction), joint dysfunction is probable. This can be confirmed by use of traction and compression (and gliding) tests of the joint (see Special topic 9 on joint play).

Resisted tests are used to assess both strength and painful responses to muscle contraction, either from the muscle or its tendinous attachment. This involves producing a maximal contraction of the suspected muscle while the joint is kept immobile somewhere near the midrange position. No joint motion should be allowed to occur. This is done after Test 3 above, to confirm a soft tissue dysfunction rather than a joint involvement. Before doing the resisted test it is wise to perform the compression test to clear any suspicion of joint involvement.

Cyriax's test

If on resisted testing (Cyriax 1962) the muscle seems strong and also painful, there is no more than a minor lesion/dysfunction of the muscle or its tendon. If it is weak and painful, there is a more serious lesion/dysfunction of the muscle or tendon. If it is weak and painless, there may be a neurological lesion or the tendon has ruptured. A normal muscle tests strong and pain free.

It is suggested that you test all these statements on painful conditions of known origin.

Obviously, in many instances, soft tissue dysfunction will accompany (precede or follow on from) joint dysfunction. Joint involvement is less likely in the early stages of soft tissue dysfunction than (for example) in the chronic stages of muscle shortening. There are few joint conditions, acute or chronic, without some soft tissue involvement.

The tests described above will give a strong indication, though, as to whether the major involvement in such a situation is of soft or osseous structures.

Compression

An example of a joint assessment involving compression would be that described by Blower & Griffin (1984) for sacroiliac dysfunction. This showed that pressure applied over the lower half of the sacrum, or over the anterior superior iliac spines, was diagnostic of sacroiliac problems (possibly indicating ankylosing spondylitis) if pain is produced in the sacrum and buttocks. Soft tissue dysfunction would not produce painful responses with this type of compression test. (Note that lumbar pain is not thought to be significant if it occurs on sacral pressure, as this action causes movement of the lumbosacral joint, as well as some motion throughout the whole lumbar spine.)

Joint or muscle dysfunction – which is primary?

Janda (1988) answers this question when he says that it is not known whether dysfunction of muscles causes joint dysfunction or vice versa. He points out, however, that since clinical evidence abounds that joint mobilisation (thrust or gentle mobilisation) influences the muscles which are in anatomic or functional relationships with the joint, it may well be that normalisation of the muscles' excessive tone in this way is what is providing the benefit and that, by implication, normalisation of the muscle tone by other means (such as MET) would produce a beneficial outcome and joint normalisation. Since reduction in muscle spasm/contraction commonly results in a reduction in joint pain, the answer to many such problems would seem to lie in appropriate soft tissue attention.

Liebenson (1990) takes a view with a chiropractic bias.

> The chief abnormalities of (musculoskeletal) function include muscular hypertonicity and joint blockage. Since these abnormalities are functional rather than structural they are reversible in nature . . . Once a particular joint has lost its normal range of motion, the muscles around that joint will attempt to minimise stress at the involved segment.

After describing the processes of progressive compensation as some muscles become hypertonic while inhibiting their antagonists, he continues:

> What may begin as a simple restriction of movement in a joint can lead to the development of muscular imbalances and postural change. This chain of events is an example of what we try to prevent through adjustments of subluxations.

We are left, then, with one view which suggests that muscle release will frequently normalise joint restrictions and another which holds the opposite, that joint normalisation sorts out soft tissue problems, leaving direct work on muscles for rehabilitation settings and for attention if joint mobilisation fails to deal with long-term changes (fibrosis, etc.).

It is possible that both are to some extent correct; however, the certainty is that what is required is anything but a purely local focus, as Janda helps us to understand.

SPECIAL TOPIC EXERCISE 5.1: EVALUATING SOFT TISSUE AND JOINT INVOLVEMENT

Time suggested: 5–10 minutes

You will require palpation partners with known soft tissue and joint dysfunction to perform this evaluation adequately.

Test the various guidelines described above (i.e. performing active and passive movement in the same and in different directions; as well as compression-distraction) to establish whether what you are dealing with is purely of joint or purely of soft tissue origin. Decide whether these methods are accurate.

Remember that it is common for both a joint and associated soft tissues to be distressed simultaneously, which might provide you with conflicting evidence (i.e. both joint and soft tissue involvement). If this is the case, knowledge that there is joint involvement may influence your therapeutic approach.

REFERENCES

Blower, Griffin 1984 Annals of Rheumatic Disease 43: 192–195
Cyriax J 1962 Textbook of orthopaedic medicine. Cassell, London
Janda V 1988 In: Grant R (ed) Physical therapy of the cervical and thoracic spine. Churchill Livingstone, New York
Kaltenborn F 1980 Mobilization of the extremity joints. Olaf Novlis Bokhandel, Oslo
Liebenson C 1990 AMRT, part 1. Journal of Manipulative and Physiological Therapeutics 13(1): 2–6

5

Palpating for changes in muscle structure

Unlike the skin, which is there for us to see as well as touch, once we begin to explore the inner regions of the body and try to deduce just what state the soft tissues are in, far greater skills are required if we are to successfully gather clinically useful information. General guidance can be given as to what superficial muscular tissues should feel like under given conditions and it is not difficult to learn to read such information by gentle palpation.

But it is not just the relative state of tone, tension, contraction, flaccidity and so on which need to be assessed, important though these factors are; there are also fluid fluctuations through connective tissue, and other rhythmic patterns, which indicate the degree of normality, or otherwise, of the soft tissues, as well as possibly having wider implications. In order to make sense of these fluid movements when it comes to palpating at greater depth – or understanding more subtle energy – fairly refined skills are required.

Some of these have been well explored and explained by diligent researchers, among them John Upledger (1987), who discusses the mechanics which govern vital physiological motions in some of the exercises in Chapter 2; Rollin Becker, in his articles on 'Diagnostic touch' (Becker 1963, 1964, 1965); Fritz Smith (1986); and Stanley Lief, the prime developer of neuromuscular technique (Chaitow 1988, 1996a, Chaitow & DeLany 2000).

The techniques and exercises based on the work of these and other developers of the art and science of palpation have expanded the potential for skilful assessment of the pathophysiological state of muscles and other soft tissues. In this chapter we will be reviewing methods aimed at determining structural changes in the soft tissues (increased tone, shortening, fibrous development, periosteal pain points, trigger points and so on) and in the next chapter the palpation of those functional changes which can be 'read' through muscles and other soft tissues will be considered.

How and why changes occur in the soft tissues

Before we delve into methods of palpation of soft tissue structures, we should briefly review the reasons why the changes we are trying to evaluate occur. A host of interacting factors have the ability to increase muscular tone, including stress response, postural anomalies and overload, repetitive physical actions (sport, occupation, hobbies, and so on), emotional distress, trauma, structural factors (congenital short leg, cranial distortion at birth), visceral and other reflex activity. These can be summarised as overuse, misuse and abuse of the musculoskeletal structures.

When tone in a muscle is initially increased for any length of time, a degree of local irritation results, due to two factors.

1. Local tissue hypoxia or ischaemia, involving inadequate oxygenation of the tissues due to increases in tone and demand.
2. Relative inadequacy of drainage and removal of metabolic waste products.

This combination leads first to fatigue, then to irritation and in some instances to inflammation over time. This might be termed the 'acute' phase of the body response to any persistent increase in tone. During this stage, discomfort is probable and pain possible, creating a cycle in which even greater tone and therefore more pain would be likely. Palpation would indicate the tissues to be warmer than surrounding tissue, possibly oedematous and usually very sensitive.

If these changes occur in response to a single or short-term adaptive demand, (for example, playing tennis for the first time after a long break, digging the garden in the spring or any one-off, unaccustomed effort), self-regulatory mechanisms ensure that the stiffness and soreness fade away after a few days. However, if the adaptive demands are repeated, different effects are likely.

Local adaptation syndrome

This phase may be equated with the alarm stage in Selye's (1984) general adaptation syndrome (GAS). Indeed, all elements of the GAS can be scaled down to a local level (a single muscle or joint, for example) in which the same stages are passed through (alarm, adaptation, collapse). This is then referred to as the local adaptation syndrome (LAS).

As would be expected according to both the GAS and LAS, after the acute phase would come the phase of adaptation. In the muscular sense this means that if increased tone is maintained for longer than a few weeks, a chronic stage evolves. This is characterised by indications of structural changes in the supporting tissues with the development of fibrotic modification.

Some see these alterations as an 'organising' response, in which sustained tone is replaced by concrete, supportive bands. The body is seen to be adapting to the seemingly permanent demand for increased tone in the musculature (Lewit 1999).

The degree of relative ischaemia, hypoxia and toxic debris retention increases at this stage, varying from person to person (and region to region) in relation to features such as age, exercise, nutritional status, and so on. Any pain noted would probably have a deep, aching quality and palpation would reveal a fibrous, stringy texture along with other palpable changes, perhaps involving oedema; it is during this adaptation stage that early signs would be noted of myofascial trigger point development, in which discrete areas of the affected soft tissues would evolve into localised areas of facilitation (Kuchera et al 1990, Norris 1998).

Highly sensitive, discrete and palpable tissue changes evolve which are themselves capable of sending noxious impulses to distant target areas where pain and new 'crops' of embryonic trigger points develop. Bands of stress fibres commonly become evident in the hypertonic tissues and the muscles affected in this way begin to place increasing degrees of tension on their tendons and osseous insertions (Mense & Simons 2001, Simons et al 1999). (See also notes on connective tissue diagnostic methods in Chapter 4 for commentary on palpable bands and zones.)

As all this occurs, tendon changes begin, at first evoking an acute and later an adaptation response which progresses on to degenerative changes. As these stresses begin to affect the tendons and as these begin to adapt, it is usually possible to palpate very tender periosteal pain points (PPP) or to note early signs of joint dysfunction (Lewit 1999).

The natural sequence described by Selye (1984), in which tissues progress from an acute phase to an adaptation phase (which can last many years) and ultimately (when adaptive capabilities are exhausted) to the final phase of degeneration and disease, is the natural consequence of any unrelieved chronic hypertonicity. The end result could take the form of arthritic joint changes or chronic muscular or other soft tissue dysfunction (Lewit 1999, Murphy 2000, Ward 1997).

Postural muscles react differently to phasic muscles

As will become clear, the abbreviated pattern of LAS, outlined above, has quite different effects in postural (stabilising) muscles as compared to what takes place in active phasic muscles similarly stressed.

The clinical and research work of Lewit (1999), Janda (1982, 1983, 1996) and others has shown that postural muscles (see later in this chapter for a fuller explanation of this phenomenon) when chronically abused, misused or overused will tend to shorten and eventually to contract. Phasic muscles, however, when faced with the same insults, will tend to weaken but will not shorten.

Palpation tasks

The palpating hand(s) needs to uncover the locality, nature, degree and if possible the age of soft tissue changes which take place in the sequence outlined above. As we palpate we need to ask:

- Is this palpable change acute or chronic (or, as is often the case, an acute phase of a chronic condition)?
- If acute, is the inflammation associated with the changes?
- How do these palpable soft tissue changes relate to the patient's symptom pattern?
- Are these palpable changes part of a pattern of stress-induced change which can be mapped and understood?
- Are these soft tissue changes painful and if so, what is the nature of that pain?
- Are these palpable changes active reflexively and if so, are they active or latent trigger points (do they refer symptoms elsewhere and does the patient recognise the pain as part of their symptom picture)?
- Are the palpable changes the result of trigger points elsewhere or of other reflex activity (see discussion of viscerosomatic reflex activity later in this chapter)?
- Are these changes present in a postural or phasic muscle group? (See later in this chapter for methods of assessing shortened postural muscles.)
- Are these palpable changes the result of joint restriction ('blockage', subluxation, lesion) or are they contributing to such dysfunction?

In other words, we need to ask ourselves 'What am I feeling, and what does it mean?'.

Viola Frymann (1963) suggests the need for some thought as to how deeper palpation might be carried out as we search for such changes, acute or chronic:

> A slightly firmer approach brings the examiner into communication with the superficial muscles to determine their tone, their turgor, their metabolic state. Penetrating more deeply, similar study of the deeper muscle layers is possible [and] the state of the fascial sheaths and condensations may be noted.

Light and variable touch needed

The words 'firmer' and 'penetrating more deeply', if taken too literally, could lead to 'counterproductive' palpation. If these recommendations were to involve a noticeable increase in applied pressure, two negative possibilities might occur.

First, there could be a defensive retraction of the palpated tissues, tensing superficial musculature, making assessment difficult or its interpretation invalid; and second, there is likely to be a lessening of sensitivity as pressure increases on the surface of the palpating digit or hand, especially if it is sustained for more than a short time, greatly affecting the accuracy of perception.

Palpation solutions

Different solutions have been found to overcome these problems. In Lief's system of neuromuscular evaluation, which will be outlined later in this chapter, these problems are largely overcome by use of what is termed 'variable' pressure, in which the digital contact matches the resistance it meets from the tissues. A subtle and effective method is therefore available for fairly deep assessment of soft tissue status, with little evidence of protective tensing by the tissues or of much loss of sensitivity in the thumb or finger contact.

Others have approached this problem differently, most notably John Upledger, with his 'melding' and synchronisation approach, which leads to the palpating hand or digits doing 'exactly what the patient's body is doing and would otherwise be doing, even if you weren't there'.

Rollin Becker (1963) uses what he describes as a 'fulcrum' palpation technique, which increases perception of tissues at depth without greatly increasing direct pressure on the skin surface.

Fritz Smith (1986) makes his assessments in yet another way, using, among other methods, what he terms a 'half-moon' vector contact.

The first section of this chapter will look at palpation of structure. One aspect of identification of structural change is to observe its behaviour, its function, and several examples of Janda's functional assessments will be incorporated into exercises in this chapter. These functional exercises, which, for example, evaluate the firing sequence of muscles as normal movements are performed, are not to be confused with the palpation of function, which involves the assessment of subtle rhythmic fluctuations and pulses, which are discussed and evaluated in Chapter 6. The exercises which follow in this chapter incorporate various ideas and recommendations for palpation of the soft tissues, derived from a number of prominent physicians and researchers from various schools and disciplines, including Janda, Magoun, Tilley, Lief, Nimmo, Lewit and Beal. This will be followed by a summary of recommended methods for sequential assessment of shortened postural muscles, the importance of which will be explained as we progress.

Interspersed amongst this review material will be a number of exercises which can enhance sensitivity when practising one or other of these methods. There is inevitably going to be a degree of overlap in the concepts of these innovators of palpatory (and therapeutic) technique, but each has a unique insight into the needs of the practitioner who is trying to make sense of physical problems as they 'read' the body.

It is suggested that all the methods outlined in this and the next chapter be attempted, practised and assessed for their individual degree of usefulness. Many therapists use all these methods (and others) in appropriate settings.

Palpation and assessment of structure

Jiri and Vaclav Dvorak outline their basic requirements for sound palpation of structures of the musculoskeletal system (Dvorak & Dvorak 1984). They insist that a healthy anatomical structure cannot be differentiated from surrounding structures, whereas 'a pathologically altered structure, however, can be exactly differentiated from the surrounding healthy tissue'.

Rolf (1962) reminds us of the importance of keeping fascia in mind when we try to make sense of what we are palpating.

> Our ignorance of the role of fascia is profound. Therefore even in theory it is easy to overlook the possibility that far-reaching changes may be made not only in structural contour, but also in functional manifestation, through better organisation of the layer of superficial fascia which enwraps the body . . . Osteopathic manipulators have observed and recorded the extent to which all degenerative changes in the body, be they muscular, nervous, circulatory or organic, reflect in superficial fascia. Any degree of degeneration, however minor, changes the bulk of the fascia, modifies its thickness and draws it into ridges in areas overlying deeper tensions and rigidities.

Apart from starting to palpate from the site where the patient localises the symptom (usually pain), the Dvoraks' other major emphasis is on the therapist having a 'three-dimensional anatomical perception' of what is being palpated, a useful description to emphasise the need for a sound anatomical knowledge.

Such knowledge leads, they suggest, to the application of 'adequate pressure with regard to area, force and direction' as 'the muscles, ligaments and other structures are located above and next to each other in the specific topographical region'.

They suggest beginning at the site of pain, localising this and palpating precisely for hard, bony structures and along tendons for information about the insertion; making comparisons not with symmetrically placed sites but with 'locations with the same anatomical arrangement and sites undergoing no changes'; differentiating from similar changes in adjacent structures, by palpating the course, shape and opposite poles of attachment (origin and insertion) of such structures; identification of myotendinosis by use of stroking and pressing palpation, performed perpendicular to the direction of the fibres, until origins and insertions are reached.

It is suggested that you compare this description with the diagnostic methods of Lief's neuromuscular technique and Nimmo's methods, as outlined later in this chapter (see Box 5.2), and decide which approach best suits your way of working.

The facilitated segment

Harold Magoun is renowned as one of the giants of osteopathic medicine, both clinically and theoretically. Writing in the *Journal of the American Osteopathic Association*, Magoun (1948) made an important contribution to our understanding of the structural analysis of muscular tissues. Describing what the searching practitioner will uncover, he says:

> What should palpation reveal? First he finds that the soft tissues are abnormal. Then he must determine if the condition is a primary lesion (local) or a viscerosomatic reflex. While these are often combined, especially if not recent, the differential diagnosis is most important.

He makes the distinction between what will be palpated if the cause of altered soft tissue feel is a local problem or if it is of reflex origin:

> The primary lesion involves mainly the deep muscles, producing an inert and irregular rigor; if of long standing, the superficial tissues may be atonic or stringy. The hypersensitivity is usually limited to the deeper tissues.

Magoun points out that there may be oedema in the connective tissue and that if the condition is years old:

> Fibrous degeneration takes place, with overgrowth of connective tissue, calcification, thickening of the periosteum, and so on.

He then differentiates the above description from what would be found if the cause of tissue changes were of reflex (organ disease) origin:

> The uncomplicated viscerosomatic reflex is manifested by a concentration of both superficial and deep tissues, both of which are hypersensitive to the same degree [only deep tissues are expected to be sensitive in primary lesion condition]. *This continuous contraction, or exaggerated tone, makes the tissues hard and tense in a regular homogeneous manner.* [my italics]

Compare this description with the research findings of Beal (1983), some 35 years later, when he makes clear the difference in general somatic effect of such a reflex change in which:

> There is no change in the nutrition such as brings about a wasting or ropy condition of the muscles; there is no change in the circulation so as to produce haemorrhage or oedema; there is no ligamentous thickening or fibrositis or oedema about the joint.

Beal rightly directs attention to correction of viscerosomatic reflex activity by dealing with the causes of the dysfunction of the affected organ, which might involve nutritional, manipulative or surgical intervention.

According to Lewit (1999) the first signs of viscerosomatic reflexive influences are vasomotor (increased skin temperature) and sudomotor (increased moisture of the skin) reactions, skin textural changes (e.g. thickening), increased subcutaneous fluid and increased contraction of muscle. The value of light skin palpation in identifying such areas of facilitation, as described in the previous chapter, cannot be too strongly emphasised.

Tilley and Korr on the facilitated segment

R McFarlane Tilley (1961) summarised his ideas on digital palpation of the spine as follows.

1. Light palpation to discover areas of increased moisture on the skin surface, indicating increased sweat gland activity.
2. Moderate friction of the skin by heavier stroking to elicit 'red reaction' [see Special topic 6].
3. Deep palpation to elicit muscular tension and tenderness of tissues upon pressure.

He follows these observations with an examination of the topics of range of motion and restriction. Stress patterns may develop for any number of physical or emotional reasons, he states, as a result of which spinal nerve pathways and cord centres become facilitated (hyperreactive). When this occurs related spinal musculature becomes palpably stressed; reflex relationships may be involved, including both viscerosomatic (organ to body tissues) and somaticovisceral (body tissues to organ) pathways.

Professor Irvin Korr (1976) has compared any facilitated area of the spine to a 'neurological lens', in which stress factors which impinge upon any aspect of the body or mind are automatically targeted through the facilitated segment, further focusing and intensifying activity through its neurological structures.

A simple diagnostic palpation method for 'compressing' or 'springing' the paraspinal tissues is outlined below (see Exercise 5.2 p 118). This method can readily confirm the presence of a facilitated segment.

Key palpatory features of the facilitated segment

The common palpatory feature of segmental facilitation, as it manifests in the paraspinal musculature, is of a feeling of relative rigidity and tenderness, as compared with the segments above and below. As a rule this will involve two or more adjacent segments, rather than just one local segment.

There is likely to be both a loss of full range of motion at the affected segment(s) as well as an asymmetry, one side or other being more affected. If the paraspinal rigidity results from visceral pathology, it will fail to respond – other than for a very short time – to any manual treatment applied to the muscles or joints involved.

These rigid muscular states can, however, be a useful prognostic indicator of change, for better or worse, as therapy is applied to the dysfunctioning organ in question.

The palpation criteria discussed in Chapter 3, under the acronym 'ARTT', will therefore apply: asymmetry, restricted range of motion, tenderness and tissue changes.

Tilley (1961) lists the possible implications of segmental facilitation, in various spinal regions, based on osteopathic clinical observations.

- Myocardial ischaemia: rigid musculature in any two adjacent segments between T1 and T4 (usually left, but not essentially so).
- Cardiopulmonary pathology: any two adjacent segments of muscular paraspinal rigidity in the upper thoracic spine, either side or bilaterally.
- Duodenal pathology: any two adjacent segments of muscular paraspinal rigidity and tenderness, right side thoracic spine, levels 6, 7 and 8.
- Pancreatic dysfunction: any two adjacent segments of muscular paraspinal rigidity and tenderness, bilaterally, thoracics 6, 7, 8 and 9.
- Liver and gall bladder: any two adjacent segments of muscular paraspinal rigidity and tenderness, right side thoracics 8, 9 and 10.
- Chronic fatigue related to 'adrenal exhaustion' or stress: any two adjacent segments of muscular paraspinal rigidity and tenderness in thoracics 9, 10, 11 and 12.
- Renal disease: tenderness and painful on pressure, aggravated by percussion, thoracics 11, 12 and lumbars 1, 2.
- Female and male reproductive organ problems: lumbosacral area tenderness or rigidity.

Note: It is important to differentiate between segmental facilitation and spinal 'splinting', which occurs as a result of underlying pathology such as TB spine, vertebral metastasis (primary or secondary) and osteoporosis. Splinting such as this will usually be more widespread than the two adjacent segments associated with segmental facilitation. No attempt should be made to reduce such splinting, which is protective.

How accurate is ARTT palpation?

A study compared Jones' (1981) palpation methods (see page 137 discussion of Jones' strain/counterstrain (SCS) later in this chapter) with standard osteopathic palpation procedures (i.e. ARTT) methods. McPartland & Goodridge (1997) state:

This study addresses five questions:
What is the inter-examiner reliability of diagnostic tests used in strain–counterstrain technique?
How does this compare with the reliability of the traditional osteopathic examination (ARTT exam)?
How reliable are different aspects of the ARTT exam?
Do positive findings of Jones's points correlate with positive findings of spinal dysfunction?
Are osteopathic students more reliable with SCS diagnosis or ARTT tests?

The examiners palpated for tender points which corresponded to those listed by Jones (1981) for the first three cervical segments. These points were located by means of their anatomical position, as described in Jones' original textbook, and were characterised as being areas of 'tight' nodular myofascial tissue.

The ARTT exam comprised assessment for:

● tender paraspinal muscles
● asymmetry of joints
● restriction in ROM
● tissue texture abnormalities.

Of these, zygapophyseal joint tenderness and tissue texture changes were the most accurate. In Jones' methodology the location of the tender point is meant to

EXERCISE 5.1: ARTT PALPATION

Time suggested: 5–10 minutes

If possible, examine a person with known visceral (cardiovascular, digestive, liver, etc.) disease.

Targeting only spinal and paraspinal tissues (i.e. no further away from the spine than the tips of the transverse processes), palpate the skin (using the elements suggested in the previous chapter of scanning, skin-on-fascia pushes, skin stretches and drag palpation) in order to evaluate the efficiency of these methods in identifying suspicious areas for further, deeper investigation by palpation.

Now palpate the superficial and deeper musculature paraspinally (see layer palpation Exercises 3.21–3.26 in Chapter 3) in order to see whether a local segment (i.e. involving at least two adjacent vertebrae) can be identified which matches the description given by Magoun earlier in this chapter, i.e. if involved in viscerosomatic adaptation the tissues will display homogeneous tension/hardness (and possibly fibrotic thickening), as well as hypersensitivity in both superficial and deeper layers.

There should therefore be superficial and deep contraction of tissues, on one or both sides of the spine, at an appropriate segmental level (see previous page for Tilley's suggested paraspinal sites).

If possible, compare your palpation findings with those adjacent to a known structural (spinal) problem where only the deeper tissues should be contracted and sensitive. Also compare your findings with the feel of 'normal' paraspinal tissues.

Can you locate a segment in which asymmetrical evidence exists of tissue change and abnormal tenderness (range-of-motion restriction is not included at this stage, as this topic is not covered until Chapter 9).

Record your findings in your journal.

define the nature of the dysfunction. However, McPartland & Goodridge found that: 'Few Jones points correlated well with the cervical articulations that they presumably represent'.

They did find that overall use of Jones' tender points (i.e. soft tissue tenderness) was a more accurate method of localising dysfunction, in symptomatic patients, than use of joint tenderness evaluation, in the ARTT exam, and that 'students performed much better at SCS diagnosis than TART diagnosis'.

Both methods are valuable and have stood the test of time. It is for you to see which offers you the best way to identify dysfunction.

Identifying segmental facilitation by palpation

Myron Beal, Professor in the Department of Family Medicine at Michigan State University College of Osteopathic Medicine, conducted a study in which over 100 patients with diagnosed cardiovascular disease were examined for patterns of spinal segment involvement (Beal 1983). Around 90% had 'segmental dysfunction in two or more adjacent vertebrae from T1 to T5, on the left side'. More than half also had left side C2 dysfunction.

Beal reports that the estimation of the intensity of the spinal dysfunction correlated strongly with the degree of pathology noted (ranging from myocardial infarction, ischaemic heart disease and hypertensive cardiovascular disease to coronary artery disease). He further reports that the greatest intensity of the cardiac reflex occurred at T2 and T3 on the left.

The texture of the soft tissues, as described by Beal, is of interest:

> Skin and temperature changes were not apparent as consistent strong findings compared with the hypertonic state of the deep musculature.

The major palpatory finding for muscle was of hypertonicity of the superficial and deep paraspinal muscles with fibrotic thickening. Tenderness was usually obvious, although this was not specifically assessed in this study. Superficial hypertonicity lessened when the patient was supine, making assessment of deeper tissue states easier in that position.

Beal's palpation method for identifying thoracic areas of segmental facilitation

With the patient supine, the thoracic spine is examined by the practitioner sliding the fingers under the transverse processes and applying an anterior (toward the ceiling) compressive force, assessing the status of the superficial and deep paraspinal tissues, as well as the response of the transverse process to an anterior, compressive, springing force (hence Beal's term of 'compression test' for this method) (see Fig. 5.1).

This compression is performed, one segment at a time, progressively down the spine, until control becomes difficult or tissues inaccessible. It is also possible to perform the test with the patient seated or side-lying, though neither is as effective as the supine position.

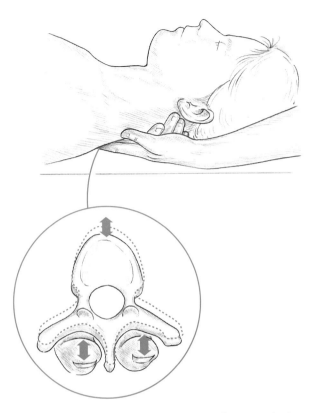

Fig. 5.1 Beal's 'springing' assessment for paraspinal facilitation rigidity associated with segmental facilitation.

EXERCISE 5.2: BEAL'S COMPRESSION PALPATION

Time suggested: 5–7 minutes

As an exercise in developing this particular skill, it is suggested that some time be spent carefully springing the thoracic paraspinal tissues (and transverse processes) with a supine partner precisely as described by Beal in the previous paragraph.

If possible, try to perform such palpation on people with and without known cardiovascular (or other visceral) dysfunction, in order to develop a degree of discrimination between normal and abnormal tissue states.

Your palpation model is supine and you are seated at the head of the table. Slide one hand under the spine of the patient, so that fingers are placed precisely as shown in Figure 5.1, at the level of T1–2.

Using minimal force, ease the contact fingers toward the transverse processes, taking out available tissue slack. Spring the compressed tissues toward the ceiling to evaluate the degree of 'give' or elasticity.

Repeat the spring/compression evaluation until easy access is lost at around T6–7.

Compare and record your findings with those gathered when you performed Exercise 5.1.

EXERCISE 5.3: COMBINED VISCEROSOMATIC REFLEX PALPATION

Time suggested: 10–12 minutes

Use all the elements in Exercises 5.1 and 5.2 on the same patient at the same time, and see which methods produce the most reliable evidence of viscerosomatic reflex activity.

Descriptions of palpatory findings

It may be useful to consider how the physicians performing similar palpation to those in Beal's exercise described what they actually felt. The terms most commonly used to describe their palpatory findings, in viscerosomatic conditions, in a study of palpatory reliability by Rosero and colleagues (1987) were selected from 16 descriptive terms provided for their use. Only five were consistently used to indicate what they were feeling on palpation.

- 'Resistant' (firm, tense)
- 'Temperature/warm'
- 'Ropiness' (cord-like)
- 'Heavy musculature' (increased density)
- 'Oedematous'

Of these, 'resistant' and 'temperature/warm' were the descriptions most commonly used.

Did you feel the 'resistant and warm' tissues when doing Exercises 5.1, 5.2 and 5.3? If not, perhaps you should repeat the exercises.

Muscles and facilitation

When considering paraspinal soft tissues we must not forget the very small intersegmental muscles in this area, which would be dramatically affected by such facilitation. Korr (1976) reminds us:

> Intersegmental mobility is very finely tuned by the small and easily forgotten muscles that run from segment to segment. Their critical role is not always appreciated in considerations of longstanding degenerative changes. We can see that the large muscles, for example the erector spinae group, initiate large movements, but which mediates the translation of forces from one segment to the next? What concentrates the force of a particular motion at one particular locality, not once but a hundred thousand times in 20 years or so?
> The intersegmental muscles are the conditioning agents and if their function is disturbed the result may be a change in the tracking characteristics at that particular junction, which in time will show impaired function.

Korr also reminds us that the more active a muscle is in fine movement, the greater the number of muscle spindles there will be present (as in the hands). He continues:

> Studies such as those involving the deep occipital muscles have indicated roughly the same ratio between spindles in the small and large muscles [as in the hand, i.e. 26:1.5]. *Although disturbances here are not apparent on routine examination they are detectable when the clinician has a well developed palpatory sense.* [My italics] Locating these disorders, and modifying or removing them, insofar as possible, is a most logical and important element in preventive medicine.

Supportive Chinese evidence

Paraspinally, in Traditional Chinese Medicine, lie the Bladder Meridian points. In a study of 33 patients with gastric or duodenal ulceration, some significant findings were produced.

This group of patients was scheduled for subtotal gastrectomy (Cunxin et al 1986) but before operation they were palpated paraspinally. The patients lay on their sides and were palpated two or three times with the physician's thumb along the medial line of the Urinary Bladder Channel of Foot Taiyang (1.5 of the subject's thumbwidths lateral to, and parallel with, spinous processes) from above downward. The location of any tender spots (hereafter referred to as reaction spots) and the shape and location of any palpable mass under the reaction point were recorded.

The researchers recorded the degree of pressure required to elicit tenderness on these points and also applied pressure 10 cm (4 inches) lateral to the reaction points as a means of establishing a control for comparison.

A week after surgery to remove the organ or the area of ulceration, the same reaction points (and the control points) were reassessed. (See Special topic 1 on the subject of measuring precise pressure levels when palpating.)

Before surgery 89.4% of the patients with peptic ulcer had reaction points overlaying traditional acupuncture points Pishu (UB 20) and Weishu (UB 21), at spinal levels T9–12. The palpated findings at that time are described as 'mainly cord-like in shape, soft and mobile', averaging 1.19 sq cm in size.

At the time of reassessment (after surgery) these were scarcely palpable and required far greater pressure to elicit tenderness – from a mean of 1.89 kg of pressure to a mean of 3.22 kg of pressure. The pressure required to 'hurt' the control points hardly varied pre- and postoperatively, at around 3.5 kg.

The significance of these findings is that:

- somatic reference points resulting from visceral pathology are palpable
- the findings may range from rigidity, if segmental facilitation is operating, to 'soft and cord-like' if it is not
- both the sensitivity and the structural changes alter, or vanish, in tandem with changes or disappearance of the visceral disease (or of the whole organ).

Such palpatory findings therefore have prognostic value.

The Chinese study also examined the effect of needling similar reactive points, relating to stomach pain, unrelated to ulceration, in over 100 patients. They achieved a 93.8% response rate (improvement or 'cure') which led them to claim:

DISCUSSION OF PALPATORY PROGRESS INVOLVING EXERCISES 5.1–5.3

By applying the ARTT palpation sequence (albeit without range-of-motion evaluation at this stage) and palpating for the changes described by Beal and, most importantly, by understanding the mechanisms involved in facilitation and viscerosomatic influence, you will have begun to discriminate between primary biomechanical dysfunctions (overuse, strains, etc.) and reflexogenically induced changes. ARTT palpation can of course be used to locate dysfunction of many types, including those of mechanical or overuse origin. However, combining the sequence with the compression method (Exercise 5.2) allows you to focus on the phenomena described by Beal and others.

Anomalies of internal viscera are manifested on the body surface, and needling these surface reaction points (acupuncture points) produces regulating effects on visceral functions, and so can correct the anomaly.

Whether this claim can be substantiated or not is debatable, since causes (*Helicobacter pylori* activity, smoking, stress, diet and so on) are unlikely to be corrected by acupuncture alone. However, a beneficial influence can certainly be claimed for the methods described.

Palpation skills can therefore provide evidence, from the paraspinal muscles, of visceral dysfunction and we have Beal's 'compression' test as a guide to what to anticipate if pathology is marked, and involves the spinal segment itself.

Neuromuscular technique

Neuromuscular technique (NMT) evolved in Europe in the 1930s as a blend of traditional Ayurvedic (Indian) techniques and methods derived from other sources. The therapist who created this method of combined diagnostic and therapeutic value was Stanley Lief. He and his son Peter (a graduate of the National College of Chiropractic, Chicago) and his cousin Boris Chaitow (also a National graduate) developed the techniques now known as NMT into an excellent and economical diagnostic (and therapeutic) tool. Our attention will be focused on the palpatory, assessment/diagnostic potential of NMT, for this is a system which allows methodical, sequential, systematic, controlled combing of the major accessible (to palpating digits) sites of trigger points and other forms of localised soft tissue dysfunction (Chaitow 1991, 1996a).

Nimmo's contribution

Other methods commonly used in seeking out trigger points, such as those advocated by Raymond Nimmo (taught in the United States as 'receptor-tonus technique' and incorporated into another form of NMT, neuromuscular therapy, in the USA), do not always have this feature of systematic, sequential, comprehensive pattern of search, which leaves little to chance. Increasingly, the two versions of NMT are being blended, however, so that if there are trigger points present, NMT (Lief's or American version) will probably identify them.

Nimmo's contribution to the understanding of local myofascial dysfunction is outlined later in this chapter, with specific detail in Box 5.2.

Many 'point' systems

Within shortened muscles (see p 158 for a discussion of assessment for short muscles) and within weakened ones as well, there is often an abundant crop of palpable, localised, discrete, sensitive areas of altered structure, which may or may not be active trigger points but which are all potential trigger points.

All palpable, sensitive, tissue changes are of importance in palpatory analysis. Some will be trigger points but even if such 'points' are not referring symptoms elsewhere, they are of potential diagnostic value. They could, as examples, be points described in some other system, such as Chapman's neurolymphatic reflexes, Bennet's neurovascular reflexes, active acupuncture points or Jones' 'tender' points. All such points are characterised by the overlying skin being less elastic than surrounding tissue (see Chapter 4) or by having a measurable degree of lowered electrical resistance.

One simple definition of a trigger point is that it is a palpable, sensitive, localised structure within the soft tissues which, when active, is sending aberrant, noxious, neurological impulses to a distant site and which, on pressure, refers symptoms – usually involving pain but with other symptoms possible – to that predictable target area.

Travell & Simons, authors of the finest exposition on myofascial trigger points to date (Simons et al 1999, Travell & Simons 1992), give a broader definition of trigger points, which is summarised later in this chapter.

Lief's methods

The major sites of these self-perpetuating troublemakers (trigger points) are often close to the origins and insertions of muscles and this is where NMT probes for information more effectively than most other systems.

There are numerous ways of finding such localised areas of dysfunction, as witness the methods advocated by Travell, Pruden and Nimmo, as described in this chapter, and others. However, many practitioners in the UK and US have come to the conclusion that few other forms of trigger point assessment measure up to Lief's original methods in terms of ease of application, economy of time and effort and efficiency of result.

Lief advocated that the exact same sequence of contacts be followed on each occasion, whether assessing or treating, the difference between these modes being merely one of repetition of the strokes, with some degree of added pressure when treating. Lief's recommendation did not, however, mean that the same treatment was given each time, for the essence of NMT is that the pressure applied, both in diagnosis and in therapy, is variable and that this variability is determined by the tissues themselves.

Thus, while repetition of a diagnostic or therapeutic stroke might appear identical to its predecessor, it would differ depending upon the state of the tissues it was passing through. This concept will become clearer as we progress.

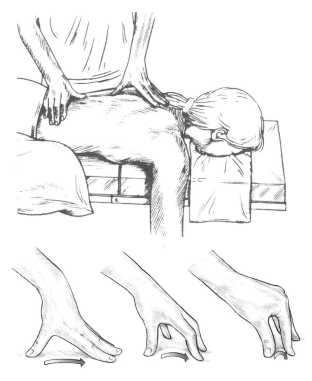

Fig. 5.2   Neuromuscular thumb technique. The practitioner uses the medial tip (ideally) of the thumb to sequentially 'meet and match' tissue density/tension and to insinuate the digit through the tissues seeking local dysfunction.

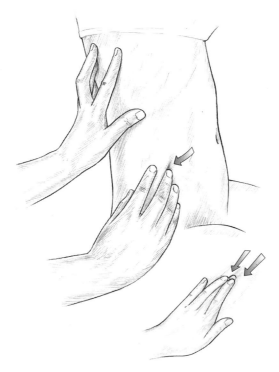

Fig. 5.3 Neuromuscular finger technique. The practitioner utilises index or middle finger, supported by a neighbouring digit (or two), to palpate and assess the tissues between the ribs for local dysfunction. This contact is used instead of the thumb if it is unable to maintain the required pressure.

Palpating digit

A light lubricant is always used in NMT, to avoid skin drag; the main contact is made with the tip of the thumb(s), more precisely the medial aspect of the tip, as a rule (see Fig. 5.2).

In some regions the tip of the index or middle finger is used instead (see Fig. 5.3), as these allow easier insertion between the ribs for assessment (or treatment) of, for example, intercostal musculature. This 'finger contact' is identical with that suggested in *bindegewebsmassage*, except that in the German system no lubricant is used.

Practitioner's body mechanics

The practitioner's posture and positioning are particularly important when applying NMT, as the correct application of forces dramatically reduces the energy expended and the time taken to perform the assessment/treatment.

The examination table should be at a height which allows the therapist to stand erect, legs separated for ease of weight transference, with the assessing arm straight at the elbow. This allows the practitioner's bodyweight to be transferred down the extended arm through the thumb, imparting any degree of force required, from extremely light to quite substantial, simply by leaning on the arm. (This presents a problem for a small number of practitioners whose thumbs are too flexible or unstable. A solution is for them to use only the finger contact described below.)

Weight transference from the back to the leading leg, with knees slightly flexed, is a sound way of controlling accurately the degree of pressure being applied while saving energy.

It is important that the fingers of the assessing/treating hand act as a fulcrum and that they lie at the front of the contact, allowing the stroke made by the

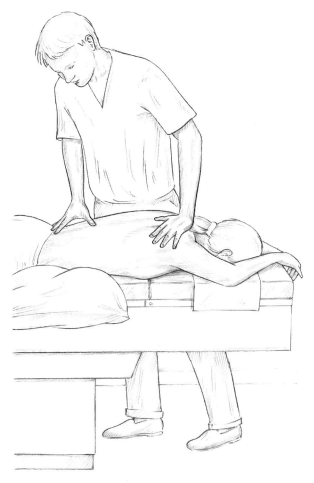

Fig. 5.4   Practitioner using neuromuscular technique. Note position of feet; straight right arm; right hand position; thumb position.

thumb to run across the palm of the hand, towards the ring or small finger as the stroke progresses (see Fig. 5.4).

Achieving control and delicacy of touch

The way the hand and body are used in NMT, as described above, produces numerous benefits, the most important being control. Were the thumb merely pushed along through the tissues it would lack the delicacy of fine control, which Lief's NMT demands.

The finger/fulcrum remains stationary as the thumb draws intelligently towards it, across the palm. This is quite different from a usual massage stroke, in which the whole hand moves. Here the hand is stationary and only the thumb moves.

Each stroke, whether it be diagnostic or therapeutic, extends for approximately 4–5 cm before the thumb ceases its motion, at which time the fulcrum/fingers can be moved further ahead in the direction the thumb needs to travel.

The thumb stroke then continues, feeling and searching through the tissues.

Variable pressure – the key to successful NMT

Another vital ingredient, indeed the very essence of the thumb contact, is its application of variable pressure (diagnostic pressure is in tens of grams initially) which allows it to 'insinuate' and tease its way through whatever fibrous, indurated or contracted structures it meets.

The degree of resistance or obstruction presented by the tissues determines the degree of effort required. Thus, in heavily tensed tissues, kilos of pressure may be needed for a subsequent diagnostic stroke.

Tense, contracted or fibrous tissues are never simply overcome by force, as this would irritate and add to dysfunction. Rather, the fibres are 'worked through', using substantial pressure at times but in a constantly varying manner in which both angles of application of pressure and degrees of pressure are constantly altered to meet the particular demands of the tissues.

The intelligent thumb or fingertip

A degree of vibrational contact, as well as the variable pressure, allows the stroke and the contact to have an 'intelligent' feel and seldom risk traumatising or bruising tissues even when heavy pressure is used.

As in the advice quoted in previous chapters, it is a requirement of NMT palpation/assessment that the thumb tip be seen as an extension of the brain, that an intelligent quality be added to the mechanical nature of its travels over and through tissue.

The patient picks this up rapidly and senses that the approach is not just a mechanical process but an intimate response to the needs of her pain or dysfunction.

As in much palpation, it is usual to suggest that NMT be applied with eyes closed.

A 'nice hurt' is all that is usually complained of, even when pressure is fairly deep.

It is helpful to try to get the medial tip of the thumb to be the precise contact and, as a rule, this is achieved after a little practice, unless there is hypermobility of the thumb joints preventing a stable contact of this sort.

Relax the working arm

Whether thumb or finger contact is used (see below for discussion on finger contact), it is of some importance, in terms of both energy conservation and ease of application of NMT, that the arm and even the hand which is doing the work remain relatively relaxed.

This may seem to be a contradiction in terms but it requires some emphasis. If the muscles of the forearm are tensed unduly or if the fingers which form the fulcrum towards which the thumbs move are rigid, an inordinate amount of energy will be wasted, the arm will tire rapidly, control will diminish and the 'feel' to the patient will be harsh rather than gentle. Perception will be dulled in the process unless a relatively relaxed state is maintained throughout.

The finger-fulcrum does not grasp, or 'dig into', the tissues on which it rests. It merely alights and rests there, with minimal pressure, as the thumb travels towards it.

Effort, if any is required in terms of added pressure, is achieved by shifting bodyweight through the almost straight arm, not by using arm or hand strength.

Finger stroke

When a finger contact is used instead of the thumb (which always travels away from the practitioner in a controlled manner, towards the finger-fulcrum at the end of the extended arm), the hand is drawn towards the practitioner's body, with the treating finger slightly hooked, as in the methods of *bindegewebsmassage*. This allows for control of the hand and the use of bodyweight in a different manner to that applied when the thumb is employed.

Unlike the thumb stroke, in which the rest of the hand is stationary, with the finger stroke the whole hand (and sometimes the whole arm) moves.

Another major area where finger contact is useful, apart from the intercostal structures, is the lateral pelvic region and lateral thigh.

As the palpating hand is brought toward you, over a curved surface, its main usefulness will be perceived.

By leaning backwards, weight on the back leg, and allowing the hooked finger to be pulled through the tissues in a controlled manner, a moderate degree of counterweight from the patient's inertia can be utilised, increasing depth of penetration, with minimal effort for the practitioner.

Standing on the side opposite the one being treated, the hooked finger – supported by its neighbouring digit if possible – can be inserted deeply into the intercostal space, or the lateral pelvic musculature, above the trochanter, and as the practitioner leans back and allows the weight of the patient to apply drag, the fingers are slowly drawn through these tissues, thus assessing the nature of dysfunction in this region (or applying cross-fibre or inhibitory contacts, if these contacts are being used therapeutically rather than diagnostically).

Palpation using NMT

The pattern of strokes which Lief and Chaitow evolved allows maximum access to potential dysfunction in the shortest time and with least demand for altered position and wasted effort. These strokes are illustrated, together with the suggested practitioner foot positions for each spinal region (see Figs 5.5–5.9).

Diagnostic assessment involves one superficial and one moderately deep contact only. If treatment is decided on at that time then several more strokes, applied from varying angles, would be used to relax the structures, to stretch them, to inhibit contraction or to deal with trigger points elicited in the examination phase.

Trigger point treatment is possible by use of direct inhibitory pressure followed by stretching of the affected musculature. (This is fully described in Chaitow 1991, 1996a, Chaitow & Delany 2000.)

NMT for particular areas

In assessing (or treating) joint dysfunction or problems involving the extremities, it is suggested that all the muscles associated with a joint receive NMT attention to origins and insertions and that the bellies of the muscles be assessed for trigger points and other dysfunction.

In this way, not only the apparently affected joint receives attention but, at the very least, the ones above and below it.

A full spinal NMT assessment should be accomplished in approximately 15 minutes with ease, once the method is mastered. (Treatment of those areas which demand extra attention would add perhaps another 5–10 minutes.)

It is suggested that every patient receive full spinal and abdominal (including thoracic) neuromuscular assessment, at least once at the outset of any treatment programme, and that this should be repeated periodically to evaluate changes brought about by whatever additional treatment is decided upon. It is, of course, not necessary to do a full assessment at each visit. A diagnostic evaluation of a localised region, accompanied by other diagnostic and assessment modalities and methods, might be all that is necessary.

By following a pattern which does not vary, involving the regions illustrated, and most importantly by recording whatever findings there are each time, a clear individual pattern of dysfunction and localised structural changes can be established for each patient and progress or lack of it readily noted.

With effective use of NMT, not only would localised, discrete 'points' be discovered but also patterns of stress bands, altered soft tissue mechanics, contractions and shortenings. Beal's rigid paraspinal tissues (see Exercise 5.2) would be readily identified, as would the difference between changes resulting from viscerosomatic activity and localised dysfunction, as described by Magoun earlier in this chapter.

NMT, in its therapeutic mode, has proved itself as an adjunct to manipulation, as well as often being able to obviate the need for other soft tissue or osseous approaches. Even if only the diagnostic approach is adopted, the patient will still have had a 'treatment' and will usually report marked benefits.

Is the term 'neuromuscular technique' accurate?

Knowledge of the function of the neural 'reporting' stations, such as the various components of the muscle spindle and Golgi tendon organs, has allowed us to understand how NMT may achieve its results.

When used near origins and insertions, the load detectors – the Golgi tendon organs – are clearly receiving mechanical input, especially if the direction of the stroke is towards the belly of the muscle. The effect of any degree of pressure away from the origin and insertion, towards the belly, would be initially to increase tone and, if sustained, would produce reflex relaxation of the muscle (Walther 1988).

If pressure is away from the belly of the muscle, near both the origin and insertion simultaneously, there will be a tendency for muscle to lose tone. The muscle spindles register length of muscle and rate of change of that length, and pressure via NMT would alter length locally, as well as having an inhibitory effect on neural discharge.

Pressure inhibition of neural discharge is the main NMT contribution to trigger point treatment. The overall effect of NMT via neural mediation is one in which reduced tone is created in hypertonic structures, over and above the purely mechanical effects introduced by stretching, friction and drainage of fluids and toxic wastes.

Many hours of patient NMT work are required before achieving the degree of sensitivity which allows the smallest local area of dysfunction to be identified. It is this idea of optimum palpatory literacy which should be the objective of those who utilise NMT.

EXERCISE 5.4: FINGER AND THUMB NMT STROKES

Time suggested: 15 minutes

Begin to practise NMT by concentrating on your body position.

Make sure your treatment surface is of a height which will allow you to stand in the manner illustrated and described (Fig. 5.4), without hunching or stretching unduly. This position must allow a straight arm position (when the thumb contact is being used), as well as the ability to transfer weight in order to increase pressure without arm muscle strength being employed.

continues

EXERCISE 5.4 *(Continued)*

Time suggested: 15 minutes

After applying a light lubricant, position yourself and place your treating hand according to the illustration (Fig. 5.2) and description, with your fingers acting as a fulcrum, thumb (medial tip) feeling through the tissues, slowly and with variable pressure. Practise this, in no particular sequence of strokes, until the mechanics of the body-arm-hand-thumb positions are comfortable and require no thought.

Pay attention to varying the pressure, to meeting and matching tissues and to using bodyweight transferred through a straight arm to increase penetration when needed.

Also practise the use of the finger stroke, especially on curved areas, by drawing the slightly hooked and supported (by one of its neighbouring digits) finger toward yourself, in a slow, deliberate, searching manner (see Fig. 5.3).

EXERCISE 5.5: APPLICATION OF NMT IN ASSESSMENT MODE

Time suggested: 10–15 minutes per segment (Figs 5.5–5.10 each represent a segment)

Choose any of the illustrated NMT sequences from Figures 5.5–5.10 (5.7A or B would be an ideal uncomplicated starting sequence for practice; however, over time practise all the sequences) and follow the strokes precisely as illustrated, although the direction of strokes need not follow arrow directions. The objective is to obtain information, without causing excessive discomfort to the patient and without stressing your palpating hands. NMT in its treatment mode involves greater pressure in order to modify dysfunctional tissues but in these sequences you are 'information gathering' only, not treating. In time, with practice, treatment and assessment meld seamlessly together, with one feeding the other.

Chart any findings you make – tender areas, stress bands, contracted fibres, oedematous areas, nodular structures, hypertonic regions, trigger points and so on. If trigger points are located, note their target area as well.

In this sequence (Fig. 5.7A&B) intercostal strokes are illustrated and you should use the hooked finger contact to search these regions. For example, stand on the left side of the patient to assess right intercostals.

Record any findings.

Work slowly and try to follow the descriptions given above, regarding the way the thumb insinuates its way through the tissues, never overwhelming them, never gouging or pushing unfeelingly.

continues

EXERCISE 5.5 (Continued)

Time suggested: 10–15 minutes per segment (Figs 5.5–5.10 each represent a segment)

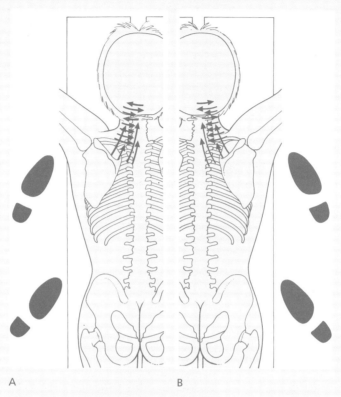

A   B

Fig. 5.5A, B   Neuromuscular technique for commencing upper thoracic and cervical region. Illustrating position of practitioner and lines of application.

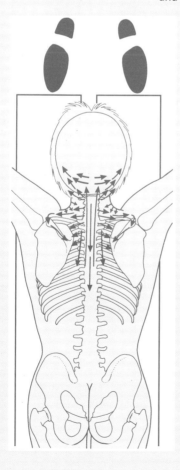

Fig. 5.6   Neuromuscular technique working from head of patient to address upper trapezius and cervical region. Illustrating position of practitioner and lines of application.

continues

Time suggested: 10–15 minutes per segment (Figs 5.5–5.10 each represent a segment)

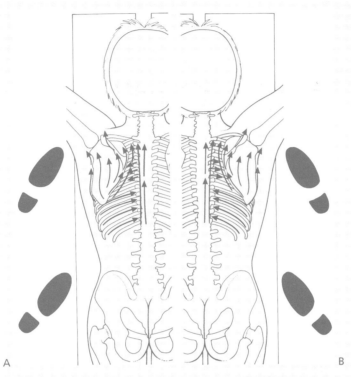

Fig. 5.7A, B   Neuromuscular technique for the mid-thoracic region. Illustrating position of practitioner and lines of application.

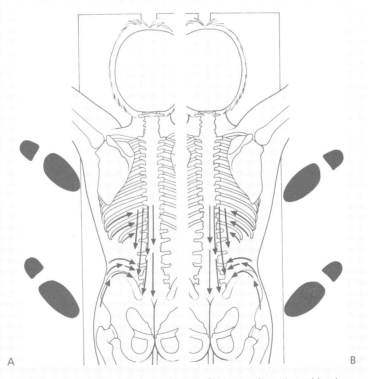

Fig. 5.8A, B   Neuromuscular technique for lower thoracic and lumbar region. illustrating position of practitioner and lines of application.

continues

Time suggested: 10–15 minutes per segment (Figs 5.5–5.10 each represent a segment)

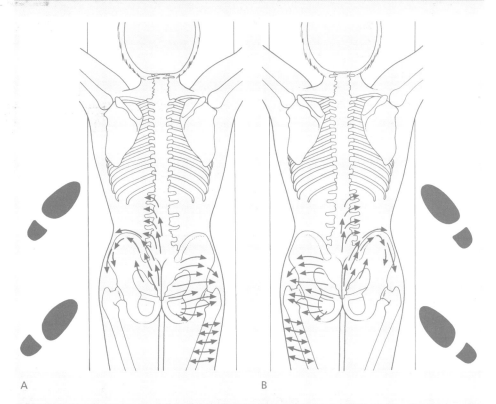

A   B

Fig. 5.9A, B   Neuromuscular technique for gluteal and upper thigh region. Illustrating position of practitioner and lines of application.

Time suggested: 20–30 minutes for abdominal segment

Allow your palpating contact to be your eyes. Try to work with your eyes closed so that sensory focus is heightened.

Record your feelings and findings in your journal, noting both your positive and negative feelings about this novel way of using your hands (which can take some weeks of regular use to become second nature).

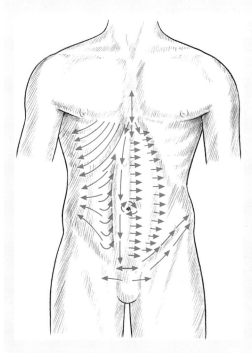

Fig. 5.10   Neuromuscular general abdominal technique. Lines of application.

Abdominal assessment using NMT

When assessing the abdominal area for soft tissue dysfunction, junctional tissues should receive particular attention (Simons et al 1999). For example, you should be aware of the anatomical position and relationships of the following, by the time you start to assess the abdominal area.

- The central tendon
- The lateral aspect of the rectal muscle sheaths
- The insertion of the recti muscles and external oblique muscles into the ribs
- The xiphisternal ligament, as well as the lower insertions of the internal and external oblique muscles
- The intercostal areas from fifth to twelfth ribs

It is also important to pay attention to scars from previous surgeries which may be the sites of formation of connective tissue trigger points (Simons et al 1999). After sufficient healing has taken place, these incision sites can be examined by gently pinching, compressing and rolling the scar tissue between the thumb and finger, to examine for evidence of trigger points (Chaitow & DeLany 2000).

Is the palpated pain in a muscle or an organ?

Since, when palpating the abdominal region, there is no underlying osseous structure available to allow compression of the musculature, there is a need for a particular strategy which helps to decide whether palpated pain is deriving from superficial tissues or from internal structures.

When a local area of pain is noted using NMT or any other palpation method, it should be firmly compressed by the palpating digit, sufficient to produce pain/referred pain (if a trigger is involved) but not enough to cause distress. The supine patient should then be asked to raise both (straight) legs from the table (heels must be raised several inches). As this happens there will be a contraction of the abdominal muscles which produces a compression of any palpated trigger point between the muscle and the finger/thumb, and pain may increase.

If pain decreases on the raising of the legs, the site of the pain is beneath the muscle and probably involves a visceral problem (Thomson & Francis 1977). It is of course possible for there to be a problem in the viscera and also in the abdominal wall, in which case this test would be in error in ascribing all symptoms of pain to a muscle wall lesion. The superficial musculature may be receiving distress sensations from an inflamed or irritated organ. The test described above therefore gives a clue, but not an absolute finding, as to the locality of the problem causing the pain.

Anterior intercostal and abdominal palpation assessment

The initial objective of the NMT strokes described below is to evaluate for soft tissue changes (active or latent trigger points, tissue texture changes, asymmetry, tenderness, etc.) with a finger contact which 'meets and matches' tissue tension.

You should be facing the supine patient at their waist level and be half-turned towards the head, with legs apart for an even distribution of weight and with knees flexed to facilitate the transfer of pressure through the arms.

Since many of the manoeuvres in the intercostal area, and on the abdomen itself, involve finger and thumb movements of a light nature, the arms can be fairly relaxed during assessment. However, if deep pressure is called for, and especially when this is applied via the thumb, the same criterion of weight transference, from the shoulder through the thumb, applies and the straight arm is used when applying NMT to the low back for the economic and efficient use of energy.

A series of strokes is applied with the tip of the thumb, along the course of the intercostal spaces, from the sternum laterally (see Fig. 5.10). It is important that the attachments of the internal and external muscles receive attention. The margins of the ribs, both inferior and superior aspects, should receive firm gliding pressure from the distal phalanx of the thumb or the middle or index finger. If there is too little space to allow such a degree of differentiated pressure, then a simple stroke along the available intercostal space has to suffice. If the thumb cannot be insinuated between the ribs a finger (side of finger) contact can be used, in which this is drawn towards the practitioner from the side, contralateral to that being treated, toward the sternum.

The intercostals, from the fifth rib to the costal margin below the 12th rib, should receive a series of two or three deep, slow-moving, gliding, sensitive strokes on each side, with special reference to points of particular congestion or sensitivity.

It is useful to note the possible presence, in the intercostal spaces close to the sternum, of neurolymphatic (Chapman's) reflex points, which are discussed and illustrated in detail later in this chapter (see Figs 5.12–5.17). These points require only light circular pressure when being contacted in order to assess for their status. If a localised area of dysfunction is found, which refers pain or other symptoms which are familiar to the patient, an active trigger point will have been located. Gentle probing on the sternum itself may elicit sensitivity in the rudimentary sternalis muscle, which has been found to house trigger points. It is not necessary to change sides during the assessment of the intercostals, unless it is found to be more comfortable to do so.

Having palpated and assessed the intercostal musculature and connective tissue, and having charted any trigger points you may have located, use either a deep thumb pressure or the pads of the fingertips to apply a series of short strokes, in a combination of oblique lateral and inferior directions from the xiphoid process.

Caution: pulsations

If, during palpation, any large pulsating mass is noted in the abdominal midline, between the xiphoid and the umbilicus, caution should be exercised. Kuchera (1997) notes:

> A normal abdominal aorta in an adult should not be wider than an inch [2.5 cm]. Pulsations occurring anteriorly are normal, but lateral pulsations from the aorta suggest a weak vessel wall, or aneurysm. Palpate [also] the inguinal area for a good pulse and compare the right and left sides. If a decreased pulse is found on one or both sides, ask the patient about claudication and then palpate and evaluate the pulse at the popliteal, postero-tibial, and dorsal pedis arteries, in that leg, and compare [these] to pulses in the opposite leg.

Palpating the rectal sheath

Your thumbs or fingers may then be used to apply a series of deep slow palpation strokes, along and under the costal margins (see Fig. 5.10). Whether diaphragmatic attachments can be located is questionable but sustained, firm (but not invasively aggressive) pressure allows gradual access to an area which can reveal trigger points of exquisite sensitivity, with often surprising areas of referral. Many seem to produce sensations internally, while others

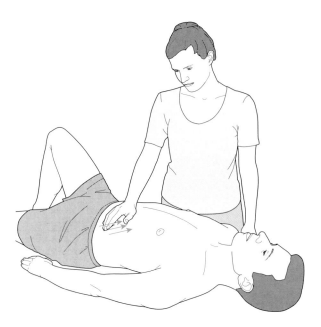

Fig. 5.11　Suggested directions of movement in assessment (and treatment) of intestinal mesenteries (after Kuchera, in Ward 1997).

create sensations in the lower extremities or in the throat, upper chest and shoulders.

A series of short palpation strokes using fairly deep, but not painful, pressure is then applied by the thumb, from the midline up to the lateral rectal sheath. This series starts just inferior to the xiphoid and concludes at the pubic promontory. It may be repeated on each side several times, depending upon the degree of tension, congestion and sensitivity noted.

It is useful, when applying these palpation strokes, to be aware of the mesenteric attachments as described by Wallace et al (1997) and Kuchera (1997) (see Fig. 5.11).

A similar pattern of assessment is followed (using the thumb if working ipsilaterally and fingers if working contralaterally), across the lateral border of the rectal sheath.

A series of short, deep, slow-moving (usually thumb) palpation strokes should be applied from just inferior to the costal margin of the rectal sheath, until the inguinal ligament is reached. Both sides are assessed in this way.

A series of similar strokes is then applied on the one side and then the other laterally, from the lateral border of the rectal sheath (see Fig. 5.10). These strokes follow the contour of the trunk, so that the upper strokes travel in a slightly inferior curve whilst moving laterally (following the curve of the lower ribs), and the lower strokes have a superior inclination (following the curve of the crest of the pelvis), as the hand moves laterally. A total of five or six strokes should be adequate to complete these palpation movements, before performing the same strokes on the opposite side. You are seeking evidence of local soft tissue changes, as well as any underlying sense of tension or 'drag' on supporting tissues.

In palpating/assessing the side on which you are standing, it may be more comfortable to apply the stroke via the flexed fingertips, which are drawn towards you, or the usual thumb stroke may be used. In palpating/assessing the opposite side, thumb pressure can more easily be applied, as in spinal technique, with the fingers acting as a fulcrum and the thumb gliding towards them in a series of 2 or 3 inch-long strokes. The sensing of contracted, gangliform areas of dysfunction is more difficult in abdominal work and requires great sensitivity of touch and great concentration on your part.

Palpation of the symphysis pubis

The sheaths of the rectus abdominis muscles, from the costal margins downwards to the pubic bones, are evaluated by finger or thumb strokes. Attention should be paid to the soft tissue component of, as well as the insertions into, the iliac fossa, the public bones and the symphysis pubis, including the inguinal ligaments (see Fig. 5.10).

Commencing at the ASIS, palpation strokes should be made which attempt to evaluate the attachments of internal and external obliques and transversus abdominis.

A deep but not painful stroke, employing the pad of the thumb, should be applied to the superior aspect of the pubic crest. This should start at the symphysis pubis and move laterally, first in one direction and, after repeating it once or twice, then the other.

A similar series of palpation strokes, starting at the centre and moving laterally, should then be applied over the anterior aspect of the pubic bone. Great care should be taken not to use undue pressure as the area is sensitive at the best of times and may be acutely so if there is dysfunction associated with the insertions into these structures.

A series of deep slow movements should then be performed, with the thumb, along the superior and inferior aspects of the inguinal ligament, starting at the pubic bone and running up to and beyond the iliac crest.

Palpation of the lateral rectus sheath

Your thumbs or fingertips may then be insinuated beneath the lateral rectus border, at its lower margins, and deep pressure applied towards the midline. Your hand or thumb should then slowly move cephalad, in short stages, whilst maintaining this medial pressure. This lifts the connective tissue from its underlying attachments and helps to normalise localised contractures and fibrous infiltrations.

Palpating in the region of the umbilicus

A series of strokes should then be applied around the umbilicus. Using thumb or flexed fingertips, a number of stretching movements should be performed, in which the non-active hand stabilises the tissue at the start of the palpation stroke, which firstly runs from approximately 1 inch (2.5 cm) superior and lateral to the umbilicus on the right side, to the same level on the left side.

The non-active hand then stabilises the tissues at this end-point of the stroke and a further stretching and probing stroke is applied interiorly to a point about 1 inch (2.5 cm) inferior and lateral to the umbilicus, on the left side. This area is then stabilised and the stroke is applied to a similar point on the right.

The circle is completed by a further stroke upwards, to end at the point at which the series began.

Note that the superior mesenteric attachment, which supports the small intestine, is located 1 inch (2.5 cm) superior and 1 inch (2.5 cm) laterally to the left of the umbilicus (see Fig. 5.11). Additional strokes may be applied along the midline and the sheaths of the recti muscles from the costal margins downwards.

Palpation of the linea alba

Additional strokes should be applied along the midline, on the linea alba itself, while searching for evidence of contractions, adhesions, fibrotic nodules, oedema and sensitivity.

Caution is always required to avoid deep pressure on the linea alba, especially if the patient has weakened this muscular interface via pregnancy, surgery or trauma. It should also be recalled that the linea alba is a place of attachment of the external obliques as well as transversus abdominis (Braggins 2000).

EXERCISE 5.6: ANTERIOR THORACIC AND ABDOMINAL NMT PALPATION

Time suggested: 20–30 minutes initially, but aim to reduce this to 10 minutes with practice

Practise the abdominal/lower rib cage sequence as described above and illustrated in Figure 5.10.

Remember to use lighter contacts than would have been appropriate for paraspinal musculature.

See what soft tissue changes you can discover in these tissues, especially near origins and insertions, below the thoracic cage, near the pelvic and pubic insertions, in the lower intercostal structures.

If there are scars, search diligently around these for sensitive and tight structures.

For greater guidance on this and other NMT sequences, see *Modern neuromuscular techniques* (Chaitow 2002a).

EXERCISE 5.7: COMPREHENSIVE NMT EVALUATION

Time suggested: 30–60 minutes

Over a period of several weeks, work your way through the individually illustrated segments of the spinal NMT assessment, several times each (taking 20 minutes for each segment at first, reducing with practice to 8–10 minutes and then around 5–6 minutes each).

Then put them all together, doing a full spinal assessment, charting everything you find. At first this will take up to an hour. With practice it can be effectively and thoroughly done in 20–30 minutes.

Always chart and record your findings.

DISCUSSION REGARDING EXERCISES 5.4–5.7

Neuromuscular technique in its palpation mode (as opposed to treatment mode) is a delicate, efficient and above all proven (by over 65 years of use) method for assessment of soft tissue dysfunction. It is only by repetitious practice that skill can be achieved and the exercises are designed to give you that opportunity.

Jones' strain/counterstrain palpation

Lawrence Jones (1981) described the evolution of his therapeutic methods, which he called strain/counterstrain, which partly depend upon identification of 'tender' points found in the soft tissues associated with joints which have been stretched, strained or traumatised. These are identified, according to Dvorak & Dvorak (1984), as 'swollen, flat regions in specific parts of the body'.

They are usually located in soft tissues which were shortened at the time of the strain or trauma (i.e. in the antagonists to those which were stretched during the process of injury). For example, in spinal problems resulting from a forward-bending strain, in which back pain is complained of, the appropriate 'tender' point would be found on the anterior surface of the body. The same process can take place in slow motion, so to speak, where chronic adaptation occurs rather than sudden strain. In such cases, once again, the tender points would be located in shortened structures rather than in those which have lengthened. Tender points would be exquisitely sensitive on palpation but usually painless otherwise. Once identified, such points are used as monitors (explained below) as the area, or the whole body, is repositioned ('fine tuned') until the palpated pain disappears or reduces substantially.

Tissue tension almost always eases at the same time as the easing of pain in the palpated point. If the 'position of ease' is held for some 90 seconds, there is often a resolution of, or at least marked improvement in, the dysfunction which resulted from the trauma.

This method is fully explained in Jones' book (1981) and a modified version is described in my book *Positional release techniques* (Chaitow 2002b). The reason for its inclusion in this survey of palpation is that awareness of its principles helps the therapist to account for unexplained and previously unreported sensitive areas, uncovered during palpation, whether or not Jones' methods of treatment are subsequently used.

EXERCISE 5.8A: JONES' TENDER POINT PALPATION – USING PALPATION PARTNER

Time suggested: 5–10 minutes per strain or point

When available, palpate the musculotendinous tissues which are antagonists to those stretched during a joint or spinal trauma or strain.

These should be in an area not complained of as being painful: any localised, extremely tender area in such tissue may be a 'Jones tender point'.

Apply sufficient pressure to the point to cause mild discomfort and then slowly position the joint or area in such a way as to remove the tenderness from the point. Creating 'ease' in the tissues housing the point usually involves producing some degree of increased slack in the palpated tissues.

Hold this position for 90 seconds and then slowly return to a neutral position and repalpate.

Has the tenderness reduced, vanished?

Are the tissues more relaxed?

Record your findings and continue to attempt to use this approach a number of times until the concept becomes imprinted.

If no suitable patient is available on which to evaluate the validity of Jones' 'strain' concept, use yourself as a model.

Find by palpation (using one of the simple skin methods described in Chapter 4, such as 'drag') a painful tender area in your upper left chest region, just below the clavicle (almost everyone is sensitive to pressure in this area).

Sit in an upright chair and apply sufficient finger pressure to cause yourself mild pain. Rate this pain as a '10' where '0' is equal to no pain at all.

Take your head and neck into flexion, approximating your chin with your chest. Does the palpated pain reduce? What is the 'pain score' now?

By trial and error find out what degree of neck flexion eases the pain the most and then add also some degree of side bending and then rotation of the neck and head, away from the pain side (to the right, in this example). Does the pain get easier or worse? Locate that position of the head/neck where pain in the palpated point is least. Do the palpated tissues feel less or more tense?

Now, with your neck still flexed forward, side bend and rotate the head toward the pain side (to the left, in this example). Does the pain get easier or worse? Locate that position of the head/neck where pain in the palpated point is least. Do the palpated tissues feel less or more tense?

Based on these directions of movement (flexion, side bending, rotation to the right and then left) decide which movements reduce the pain score the most. Do the tissues being pressed feel 'slacker', more 'easy' when the pain is most reduced or not?

Usually, not always, the position of maximum ease for a tender area in the upper left chest will involve neck flexion and side bending/rotation toward the left – the side of pain.

And usually, almost always, the position which reduces the pain score the most is accompanied by palpated softening, slackening, of the painful tissues (Jones 1981).

Similarly any pain points you locate on the back of your body, say behind the shoulder, will require (usually) extension and 'fine tuning' using other variables of side bending and rotation, to ease pain and tension.

Record your findings and experiment with other areas of the body to see whether you can ease painful points by positioning, using these guidelines.

The palpation aspects of this exercise involve:

- locating tender points by skin or other assessment
- noting changes in palpated tension in the tissues as fine tuning is performed to ease the pain.

Such points are similar to Ah Shi points (spontaneously tender points) as reported in Traditional Chinese Medicine (TCM) for several thousands of years. In TCM, however, they are not used in the manner described above but are considered to be amenable to acupuncture or acupressure methods for as long as they remain sensitive. These points are sometimes also trigger points, in that they may refer pain to a distant target (Baldry 1993).

Trigger point (TP) palpation

Travell & Simons (1992) and Simons et al (1999), medical pioneers of our understanding of trigger points, describe specific characteristics which identify them from other myofascial changes.

1. A TP which is active causes pain to be referred to a predictable site, producing symptoms recognisable to the patient.
2. The trigger point itself is seldom located where the patient complains of pain.
3. There will be taut fibres (palpable bands) in the muscles which house TPs and pressure or tension applied to such a band (pressing or stretching the muscle actively or passively) will usually refer pain to the target area.
4. There will be a palpable ropiness, or nodularity, in muscles which house TPs and the muscle will have a reduced range of motion.
5. A TP will be found at the site of the greatest sensitivity/tenderness in any taut band of muscle fibres.
6. If the tissue housing the TP is 'rolled' briskly by fingers or thumb so that there is a sudden change of pressure on it, a 'twitch' response may be observed.
7. Sustained digital pressure on the TP (or insertion into it of a needle) usually reproduces the referred pain pattern for which it is responsible.
8. Other autonomic phenomena may also be evoked, apart from pain.

Travell maintains that the high intensity of nerve impulses from an active trigger point can, by reflex, produce vasoconstriction, a reduction of the blood supply to

---

Box 5.1 Possible trigger point symptoms

Pain
Over- or undersecretion of glands
Numbness
Itching
Localised coldness
Oversensitivity to normal stimuli
Paleness
Redness of tissues
Spasm
Menopausal hot flashes
Twitching
Altered texture of skin (very oily, very dry)
Weakness and trembling of muscles
Increased sweat production

In triggers found in the abdominal and thoracic muscles:
Halitosis (bad breath)
Heartburn
Vomiting
Distension
Nervous diarrhoea and constipation
Disordered vision
Respiratory symptoms
Skin sensitivity

specific areas of the brain, spinal cord and nervous system, thus provoking a wide range of symptoms capable of affecting almost any part of the body. Among symptoms reported by Travell, and others, as a direct result of trigger point activity (as proved by their disappearance when the triggers were dealt with) are those listed in Box 5.1.

Trigger point compression guidelines (Chaitow & DeLany 2000, 2002)

Central trigger points are usually palpable either with flat palpation (digital pressure against underlying structures using a thumb or finger) or with pincer compression (tissue held more precisely between thumb and fingers like a C-clamp, or held more broadly, with fingers extended like a clothes pin) (see Fig. 5.12).

Flat palpation into the tissues, using the thumb for example, should be slowly achieved, teasing and searching with the thumb tip, as tissues are slowly compressed toward underlying structures.

Compressions may be applied wherever the tissue may be lifted without compressing neurovascular bundles.

A more specific compression of individual fibres is possible by using the more precise pincer compression using the tips of the digits or flat palpation against underlying structures, both of which methods entrap specific bands of tissue.

Compression between fingers and thumb has the advantage of offering information from two or more of the examiner's digits simultaneously, whereas flat palpation against underlying tissues offers a more solid and stable background against which to assess the tissue.

Once compressed by flat or pincer palpation, the patient/model is asked whether the pain is local, referring, radiating and if radiating or referring, what the target area is and whether the pain is familiar, a common symptom experience, in which case it is an active trigger. All other triggers are 'latent' and of less importance clinically. Additionally, the tissue can be rolled between

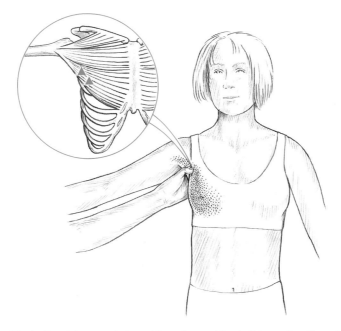

Fig. 5.12 Illustrating trigger points and target area (shaded) in pectoralis major muscle (sternocostal fibres) and ideal palpation method in this area (as well as trapezius, sternomastoid and scalenes). Pincer palpation of trigger points in the sternocostal fibres of the pectoralis major muscle. Referred pain patterns and trigger points (small triangle) in the left pectoralis major muscle. Solid area shows essential areas of referred pain and stippled area shows the spillover pain areas. The lateral free margin of the muscle, which includes fibres of the costal and abdominal sections, forms the anterior axillary fold.

EXERCISE 5.9: TRIGGER POINT PALPATION

Time suggested: 15 minutes

Find, on yourself or on a suitable palpation partner, a number of trigger points, using NMT or other palpation method such as 'skin drag' and the compression guidelines outlined above.

A good place to start looking is upper trapezius, between the angle of the neck and the shoulder joint, where most adults have trigger points, although these are not always active.

Establish precisely the 'target' or reference area to which pain is being referred, when each trigger point is compressed. If located in the sternomastoid, scalene or upper trapezius muscles, the points should be lightly 'squeezed' or 'pinched' rather than pressed by a single-digit contact.

Go through the Simons/Travell guidelines to evaluate whether any of the other possible trigger effects are present, as listed in Box 5.1.

Record your findings.

fingers and thumb to assess quality, density, fluidity and other characteristics which may offer information to the discerning touch.

Nimmo's perspective on trigger points

Raymond Nimmo developed a system which he called 'receptor tonus', which systematically uncovered trigger points and then 'deactivated' them by inhibitory pressure, followed by stretching of the muscles involved if they were hypertonic or strengthening if they were hypotonic.

He also applied himself to what he termed 'noxious' points in ligaments. He diagnosed all noxious points by their sensitivity, claiming that properly applied pressure would elicit painful points in all hypertonic and hypotonic muscles.

He summarised his approach by saying: 'We have three things with which to deal, to wit: noxious or trigger points, ligament and tonus'.

His method of identification of trigger or noxious points can be understood if we examine the following quote from his lecture notes (Nimmo 1966) which covers examination of the subscapular area for trigger points affecting the shoulder:

Look about 2.5 inches [6.5 cm] to left of spinous processes, on a level with the lower scapula border. Let the fingers glide along until a slight difference is found in the small muscles. If such a point is sensitive it should be treated.

After describing his method for dealing with the trigger (5 seconds sustained pressure, repeated if necessary) he continues:

After holding pressure on a point, say on the level of the lower scapula border, move in a straight line upwards along the internal margin of the scapula about one inch [2.5 cm]. Here, usually, another point may be found. Treat it in the same manner and move upward about another inch [2.5 cm] and look for another point.

Nimmo states that 90% of all patients will have trigger points in one of these sites and referred pain will be to the shoulder or head from these. He continues by suggesting the practitioner search the body in the sites listed in Box 5.2, where the given percentages (Nimmo's figures) demonstrate active, sensitive, 'noxious' points. Only sensitive points are treated, never non-painful ones.

1. Superior angle of scapula, on tendon of *levator scapulae*. This refers to head, face, neck and shoulders: 90% incidence reported.
2. Between and on the ribs, between the transverse processes and around rib heads. Triggers here indicate an imbalance between *paraspinal musculature* due to Davis's Law which states: 'If hypertonus exists on one side, tonus is released on the other side'. Affects most people.
3. Inferior angle of scapula, on inner insertions of *infraspinatus*. Also along inner border until spine of scapula is reached, working outwards until insertion of infraspinatus on humerus is palpated. 'After this, search the space toward the lateral edge of the scapula, letting thumb fall off outwardly, then flipping it back on, pressing partly against infraspinatus and partly against fascia beneath and also on teres minor. Here is a favourite place for trouble. It will usually refer to the back of the arms and to the 4th and 5th fingers. Upper infraspinatus refers to front of shoulders.' 90% of patients have triggers here.
4. Press on internal aspect of *supraspinatus*, moving laterally towards its insertion. Triggers here are a common cause of 'tired' shoulders. A 40% incidence of triggers at this site is reported.
5. Search outer border of scapula for *teres major* points. Triggers are common if patient cannot raise arm behind back. 60% of patients were found by Nimmo to have triggers in these muscles.
6. *Upper trapezius* is searched by squeezing it between fingers and thumb, moving slowly from shoulder region towards spine until triggers are found. Pain refers to mastoid area or to forehead. Very common – 90%.
7. Pressure ('firm', says Nimmo) on superior border of sacrum, between iliac spine and sacral spinous process, produces pressure on *SI ligament*. Move contact superiorly and inferiorly searching for sensitivity. Triggers here are involved in all low back syndromes and 50% of all patients, according to Nimmo. As in all descriptions given, it is suggested that you search both sides.
8. Press just superiorly to sacral base adjacent to spine medial to PSIS. This is the *iliolumbar ligament*. Heavy pressure is required to find triggers which are involved in most low back problems. Search both sides. 90% incidence reported.
9. Hook thumb under *sacrosciatic* and *sacrotuberous ligaments* medial and inferior to ischial tuberosity, lifting and stretching laterally if painful. Nimmo reports a 30% incidence of triggers in these sites.
   Note: Nimmo used a palm-held, rubber-tipped wooden T-bar, in order to apply pressure to areas requiring high poundage such as iliolumbar ligament.
10. Medial pressure is applied by the thumb to lateral border of *quadratus lumborum*, avoiding pressure on tips of transverse processes, starting below last rib down to pelvic rim. A 'gummy' feel will be noted if contracture exists (plus sensitivity) in contrast to resilient, homogeneous feel of normal muscle. Often associated with low back problems. If *latissimus dorsi* is also involved, pain may radiate to shoulder or arm. 80% of patients show trigger activity in these muscles, according to Nimmo's research.
11. Search area below posterior aspect of ilia for noxious points associated with *gluteal muscles* generally.
12. Search central region of belly of *gluteus medius* for triggers which can produce sciatic-type pain. 90% incidence.
13. Search midway between trochanters and superior crest of ilium, in central portion of *gluteus minimus* where trigger affecting lateral aspect of leg or foot, or duplicating sciatic-type pain, is common. This also has a 90% incidence of triggers, as opposed to gluteus maximus, which produces active triggers in only 4% of patients.

continues

Box 5.2 (*Continued*)

14. The point of intersection, where imaginary lines drawn from the PSIS and the trochanter, and the ischium and the ASIS meet, is the access point for contact with the insertion of the *piriformis muscle*. If the line from the ASIS is taken to the coccyx, the intersection is over the belly of piriformis. These two points should be palpated; if sensitivity is noted, the muscle requires treatment. Sciatic-type pain distribution to the knee is a common referred symptom. A 40% incidence of triggers is reported by Nimmo.
15. *Hamstring* trigger points lie about a hand's width above the knee joint in about 20% of patients.
16. Trigger points in *abductor magnus muscle* lie close to its origins and insertions, notably near the tendinous insertion, and close to the ischium.
17. The area *posterior* to the *tibia* is a site for trigger points relating to calf pain. 90% of patients display triggers here, according to Nimmo.
18. Triggers abound in the region of the *external malleolus*, especially if recurrent ankle strains have occurred.
19. With patient side-lying and practitioner standing facing patient at chest level, reach across with cephalad hand to ease scapula into maximum abduction while thumb of the caudad hand is inserted under scapula to try to contact *serratus magnum* and *subscapularis muscles* (both have 90% incidence of triggers). Careful probing allows contact with triggers and restrictions, which occur in 90% of individuals.
20. Search for triggers in the *upper cervical muscles* with patient face upwards and practitioner's thumb applying pressure against these muscles, medially and upwards (to ceiling) along length of lamina groove from occiput to base of neck. 90% of patients have triggers in these muscles.
21. Same position, right hand under and cupping lower neck, thumb anterior to *trapezius* fibres, rotate head to right allowing hand to slowly glide towards floor. Thumb can descend into 'pocket' created by the head position (Fig. 5.13). When thumb has reached as far as possible, pressure towards the opposite nipple allows contact to be made with insertion of splenius capitus muscle (around second thoracic vertebra). Referred pain to base of neck is a common symptom. Again, 90% of people have triggers here.
22. Standing at head of patient, place right thumb just superior to clavicle, lateral to outer margin of *sternomastoid*; flex neck by raising head with other hand, allowing right thumb to enter area below clavicle over attachment of *anterior scalene muscle*. Patient's head is turned right, bringing *scalene* directly under thumb. Pressure laterally with thumb finds triggers located here, a common (90%) finding.
23. *Anterior cervical muscles* are palpated for changes and trigger points by facing seated patient and inserting thumbs under jawline to contact anterior surface of upper transverse processes. Gliding thumbs inferiorly allows contact with *longus capitus, coli,* and so on (70% trigger point incidence). Care is required as to degree of pressure and time spent in the region of carotid body.
24. *Sternomastoid* palpation is performed with patient face upwards, head turned towards side being assessed. Contact is by 'squeezing' between finger(s) and thumb as direct pressure is avoided in this muscle (as in scalene, apart from its insertions).
25. Triggers lying in *masseter* and *external pterygoid muscles* are found with practitioner sitting at head of supine patient. Triggers here relate to TMJ dysfunction, tinnitus and salivary gland dysfunction.
26. Functional disturbances of the eyes may stem from active triggers in the *temporalis muscle*, which is palpated from same position as 25.
27. Standing to side of supine patient, grasp wrist with cephalad hand and abduct the arm; other hand contacts coracoid process and thumb contact glides towards sternum, assessing *subclavius muscle*. A similar stroke from coracoid process towards xiphoid assesses *pectoralis minor* (Nimmo reports a 90% incidence of triggers in both muscles, only 10% in *pectoralis major*).

continues

Box 5.2 (*Continued*)

28. Thumb pressure should be applied to the *biceps tendon* insertion for a distance of 2.5 cm or so below its insertion in search of a trigger which would relate to shoulder problems (90% incidence).

29. Trigger points are found on the sternum in the rudimentary *sternalis muscle* (40% incidence of triggers) as well as in *cartilaginous attachments* of ribs on sternum.

30. With supine patient, knees flexed, contact is flat of hand (fingers more than palm) with other hand on top of it, applying pressure from just inferior to rib margins, going under these as far as possible to approach triggers lying in *upper abdominal musculature* (90%). Finger pads are stroked in a series of movements from the most superior point reached under the ribs, towards the umbilicus. Tight bands will be felt, in which triggers reside.

31. *Serratus magnus* is searched with flat of hand stretching it towards its attachments (90% incidence).

32. Patient in the same position. Practitioner standing on side opposite that to be assessed and starting some 7.5 cm below umbilicus on a line from it to the ASIS, a firm flat hand contact is made; this is taken inferior and then medial, allowing contact to be made *anterior to fourth and fifth lumbar vertebrae* (site of hypogastric plexus and ganglionated cord). This is likely to be an area of referred sensitivity (upwards to chest) in 70% of patients. This contact could be avoided in the elderly, the obese or patients with aneurysms or sclerotic aortas.

33. Patient in same position, Practitioner standing on side to be examined. Place finger pads just superior to ASIS, pressing towards floor and then towards feet, allowing access under the pelvic crest to contact *iliacus muscle*. A gliding contact followed by flexing of the contact fingers allows searching of this area for triggers (90%).

34. Access to the *psoas muscle* is suggested from lateral margin of *rectus abdominis*, allowing finger contact to pass under the sigmoid on the left and under the caecum on the right. This accesses the belly of psoas in non-obese patients. Another access is directly towards the spine from the midline (patient with flexed knees) some 7.5 cm below umbilicus. On approaching the spine (denser feel), finger pad contact slides laterally over body of lumbar vertebrae (2, 3 or 4) to opposite side. This will contact origin of psoas, a common site for triggers (50–70%).

35. *Abductor longus* and *pectineus* can be contacted with patient in same position, as thumbs glide along abductor towards pubic attachment and then laterally to contact pectineus. 50% of patients have triggers in this muscle.

36. *Quadriceps* can be contacted and searched with thumbs, heel of hand or fingers, with patient supine. Triggers abound in both *rectus femoris* (90% incidence) and the *vasti* (70%).

37. *Tensor fascia lata* is best contacted with patient side-lying, affected leg straight, supported by flexed other leg. Triggers here can produce sciatic-type pain (70%).

38. *Gracilis* attachment into the knee region (via its tendon) is a major trigger site (90%). The muscle itself should be assessed from tibial attachment to the pubis.

39. *Anterior tibialis muscle* may rarely contain triggers affecting feet or toes.

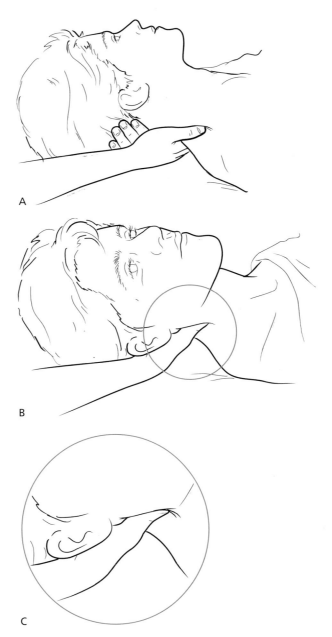

Fig. 5.13 The thumb slides into a 'pocket' formed anterior to the trapezius while remaining posterior to the transverse process to directly palpate a portion of lower splenii.

Read through the text of Box 5.2 carefully and select particular aspects or work steadily in sequence through Nimmo's suggested trigger point location protocols. For example, to start with, take description 1 or 2 (levator scapula attachment and posterior rib attachment areas) and see whether you can find active trigger points using Lief's NMT assessment method (thumb or finger contact) and/or one of the skin palpation methods described in Chapter 4 ('drag', elasticity, etc.) to evaluate the accuracy of these methods in locating triggers in the areas suggested by Nimmo.

See whether any of the triggers you locate are associated with joint and other restrictions as described by Lewit (see below). This will be assisted by use of the joint palpation methods as described in Chapter 9.

Over time, attempt to evaluate all of Nimmo's target sites. It is important to include in this search methods previously covered in this and other chapters, notably skin evaluation, NMT and layer palpation.

Note your findings in your palpation journal and compare your results with those suggested as likely by Nimmo (based on his percentages).

Lewit's view of trigger point significance

Karel Lewit (1992, 1999) suggests that, apart from their local significance in terms of pain and their influence on target areas, trigger points can have a clinical significance due to their links with certain pathologies. For example, triggers in:

- the thigh adductors indicate hip pathology
- iliacus indicate lesions of segments L5–S1 (coccyx)
- piriformis indicate lesions of segment L4–5 (coccyx)
- rectus femoris indicate lesions of L3–4 (hip)
- psoas indicate lesions of thoracolumbar junction (T10–L1)
- erector spinae muscles indicate lesions of corresponding spinal level
- rectus abdominis indicate problems at xiphoid, pubis or low back
- pectoralis indicate problems of upper ribs or thoracic viscera
- subscapularis are common in 'frozen shoulder'
- middle trapezius indicate radicular syndrome of the upper extremity
- upper trapezius indicate cervical lesion
- sternomastoid indicate lesion of CO–1 and C2–3
- masticatory muscles relate to headache and facial pain.

Periosteal pain points (PPP)

Lewit also interprets periosteal pain points as relating to specific functional or structural problems.

As tonus increases and becomes chronically entrenched, leading to changes in the structure of the soft tissues, with increased fibrous tissue and decreased elastic content becoming palpably apparent, so do stresses build up on the tendons and their osseous insertions into the periosteum. Many are characteristic of certain lesions, making them useful as diagnostic aids.

The feel of periosteal pain points varies; however, a frequently palpated common feature is of a sensitive 'soft bump' at the point of attachment of tendons and ligaments. This is often observed on spinous processes where one side is tender, relating to tension or spasm in the muscles on that side, which also prevents easy rotation of the body of that vertebra to that side. Intervertebral joints can be palpated directly in some areas; for example, the cervical joints are accessible when the patient is supine. Greater pressure is required through paraspinal tissues with the patient prone for access to other spinal joints (for example, using NMT approaches as described above).

Many extremity joints are available for direct palpation. The hip attachments can be reached via the groin if care is taken. Acromioclavicular and sterno-clavicular joints are easily accessed, as is the TMJ anterior to the tragus.

Table 5.1 gives the sites of some PPP and the significance accorded to them by Lewit (1999).

Table 5.1 Some PPP and their significance according to Lewit (1999)

PPP	Significance
Head of metatarsals	Metatarsalgia (flat foot)
Calcaneal spur (a classic PPP)	Tension in plantar aponeurosis
Tubercle of tibia	Tension in long adductors, possibly hip lesion
Attachments of collateral knee ligaments	Lesion of the corresponding meniscus
Fibula head	Tension in the biceps femoris or restriction of the head of the fibula
PSIS	Common, but no specific indication
Lateral aspect of symphysis pubis	Tension in the adductors, SI joint restriction or a hip lesion
Coccyx	Tension in the gluteus maximus, levator ani or piriformis
Iliac crest	Gluteus medius or quadratus lumborum tension or dysfunction at thoracolumbar junction
Greater trochanter	Tension in the abductors or a hip lesion
T5–6 spinous process	Lesion of the lower cervical spine
Spinous process of C2	Lesion at C1–2 or C2–3 or tension in levator scapulae
Xiphoid process	Tension in rectus abdominis or 6th, 7th or 8th rib dysfunction
Ribs in mammary or axillary line	Tension in pectoralis attachments or a visceral disorder
Sternocostal junction of upper ribs	Tension in scalene muscles
Sternum, close to the clavicle	Tension in sternomastoid muscle
Transverse process of atlas	Lesion of the atlas/occiput segment or tension in either rectus capitis lateralis or sternomastoid
Styloid process of the radius	Elbow lesion
Epicondyles	Elbow lesion or tension in muscles attaching to epicondyles
Attachment of deltoid	Scapulohumeral joint lesion
Condyle of the mandible	TMJ lesion or tension in masticatory muscles

EXERCISE 5.11: PALPATION FOR PPPS

Time suggested: 3–5 minutes per PPP and associated muscle

Work your way through palpating the PPP points, as described in Table 5.1, and see how many are present as sensitive, palpable structures in your palpation partner.

Try to assess the potentially involved soft tissues, as indicated in the descriptions in the table. Are they indeed involved?

Try to establish the connection between a PPP and the soft tissue dysfunction associated with it, by evaluating the tone and general 'feel' of attaching muscles.

This will become increasingly pertinent if you incorporate tests for shortness of such muscles, as outlined later in this chapter, which are specifically linked to PPPs, according to Lewit's research (1992, 1999).

Record your findings.

DISCUSSION OF PALPATORY PROGRESS INVOLVING EXERCISES 5.8–5.11

Assessment using skills covered in earlier exercises/chapters allows the localisation of trigger points, Jones' tender points and periosteal pain points. These differently named 'points' may in the end all represent the same phenomena, viewed and labelled differently. It matters little what we call particular reflex areas, as long as we can find them and evaluate their influence on the individual and the symptoms being complained of. The palpation skills which reveal something as 'different', as not 'normal', relate to variations in texture, tone, fluid content, etc. And by seeing these different perspectives (Nimmo, Simons, Travell, Jones, Lewit, etc.) and practising the identification through touch of the points/zones/areas they describe, your skills will advance.

In the next segment of this complex chapter, you will meet yet another type of point – the neurolymphatic (Chapman's) point (which may also be a trigger point, a Jones' point, etc.). By understanding how and where to locate these your skills will continue to develop.

Chapman's neurolymphatic reflex points

We have seen that viscerosomatic reflex activity is commonly associated with the development of facilitated spinal segments (Exercises 5.1, 5.2 and 5.3) and that another form of localised facilitation is associated with trigger point evolution.

The soft tissue changes which result are palpable, both via the skin and directly in the muscles and other soft tissues affected. Additional soft tissue changes which might be picked up during palpation include Jones' (1981) tender points, associated with joint strain or trauma, and trigger points as described by Travell (Travell & Simons 1992) and others.

We now need to examine, albeit briefly, another reflex system which is assessed by careful palpation. In the 1930s, osteopathic physician Frank Chapman and, subsequently, his brother-in-law Charles Owens charted a group of palpable reflex changes which they termed neurolymphatic reflexes. Owens (1963) described the palpable changes consistently associated with the same viscera which are found in the fascia.

> These extremely localised tissue changes (gangliform contractions) are located anteriorly in the intercostal spaces near the sternum. They may vary in size from one half the size of a shotgun pellet to that of a small bean and occasionally are multiple. This type of change is apparent in some of the reflexes found on the pelvis, but the ones found on the lower extremity (colon, broad ligament and prostate) vary in character. Here there may be areas of 'amorphous shotty plaques' or 'stringy masses'.

Patriquin (1997) describes the characteristics of Chapman's reflexes as:

> small, smooth, firm, discretely palpable, approximately 2–3 mm in diameter. Sometimes described as feeling like small pearls of tapioca, lying, partially fixed, on the deep aponeurosis or fascia.

The variations in tissue texture probably result from a combination of both the nature and severity of the visceral involvement and the constitution of the patient. The degree of tenderness noted on palpation differentiates these from what Chapman terms 'fat globules'. In some areas, such as in the rectus femoris muscle, reflexes (from the suprarenal gland) have the feel of acute contraction. Posterior reflexes are found mainly between the spinous processes and the tips of the transverse processes, where they have more of an oedematous, swollen feel and sometimes are 'stringy' in nature, on deeper palpation.

Beryl Arbuckle (1977) discussed Chapman's initial discovery of these reflexes in her fine collection *Selected writings of Beryl Arbuckle*.

> Chapman found highly congested points in different regions of the fascia, and with certain very definite groupings he found to exist a definite entity of disease or, reversely, with a particular disease he always found a definite pattern in these regions. These findings led him to conclude that the states of hypercongestion were due to a lymph stasis, in viscus, or gland, which was manifested by soreness or tenderness at the distal ends of the spinal nerves. To understand this reasoning one must have a knowledge of the lymphatic system, the autonomic nervous system, and the interrelation of the endocrine glands, and the embryologic segmentation of the body.

Arbuckle cites, in support of Chapman's concepts, the research of Speransky (1944), which demonstrated that CSF travels through the lymphatic structures to all areas of the body. This fact, reinforced by Erlinghauser's (1959) research into CSF circulation through tubular connective tissue fibrils (described in Chapter 6), combined with knowledge of the many nutrient substances carried by nerve axons, strongly supports Chapman's concept of neurolymphatic reflexes (Korr 1967).

Charts and details for the manual treatment of these reflexes are to be found in *An endocrine interpretation of Chapman's reflexes* (Owens 1963), as well as in *Modern neuromuscular techniques* (Chaitow 1996a, 2002a). The illustrations in this chapter and the accompanying tables in the Appendix (p 379) are meant to be be used for palpation purposes.

Arbuckle says:

> Trained, seeing, sensing, feeling fingers . . . are able to 'open some of the windows and doors' for the correction of perverted circulation of fluids.

How easy is it to achieve this? Owens says:

> You may not at first be able readily to locate the gangliform contractions with ease, but with practice you will acquire a readiness of tactile perception that will greatly facilitate your work. Do not use excessive pressure on either anterior or posterior.

(See Figs 5.14–5.19.)

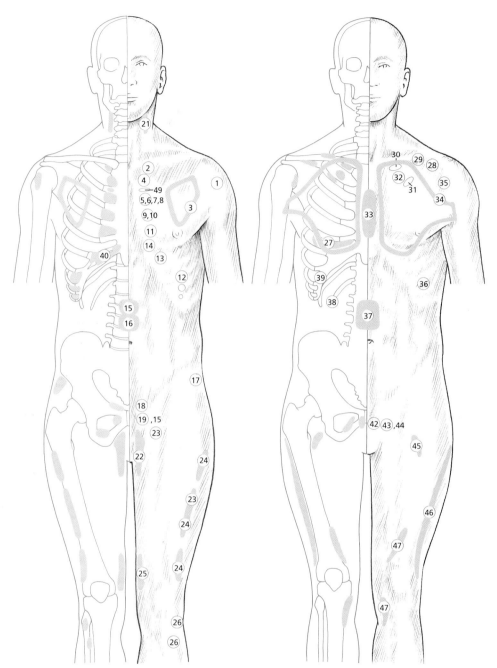

Fig. 5.14   Chapman's neurolymphatic
reflexes – anterior surface (1).

Fig. 5.15   Chapman's neurolymphatic
reflexes – anterior surface (2).

Clinical value of the reflexes

Since the location of these palpable tissue changes is relatively constant in relation to specific viscera, it may be possible to establish the location of pathology without knowing its nature. The value of these reflexes is threefold.

1. As diagnostic aids. Patriquin (1997) points out that some of the reflexes, such as that for appendix (tip of 12th rib on the right – see point 38 on Figure 5.14) are invaluable in helping with differential diagnosis when faced with right lower abdominal pain. 'Today, Chapman's reflexes are more likely to be used as an integral part of [osteopathic] physical examination, than as a specific therapeutic intervention.'

2. They can be utilised to influence the motion of fluids, mostly lymph.

3. Visceral function can be influenced through the nervous system.

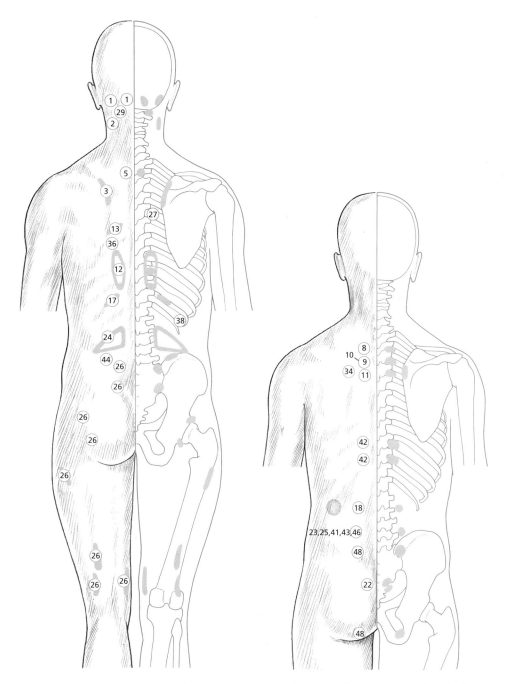

Fig. 5.16 Chapman's neurolymphatic reflexes – posterior surface (1).

Fig. 5.17 Chapman's neurolymphatic reflexes – posterior surface (2).

[The] reflexes can be clinically manipulated to specifically reduce adverse sympathetic influence on a particular organ or visceral system . . . patients with frequent bowel movements from the effects of IBS report they have normal or near normal function for days to months after soft tissue treatment over the iliotibial bands and/or the lumbosacral paraspinal tissues and associated Chapman's reflexes (Patriquin 1997).

Chapman, Owens and Arbuckle suggest that these points are only active – and therefore of use for treatment purposes – when both the anterior and posterior points of a pair are active, as evidenced by both being at the same time palpable and sensitive. The degree of sensitivity of the anterior of the pair indicates the degree of associated lymphatic congestion.

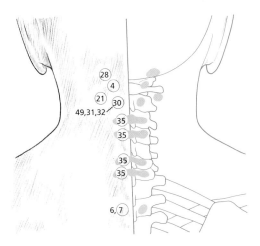

Fig. 5.18 Chapman's neurolymphatic reflexes – posterior cervical surface.

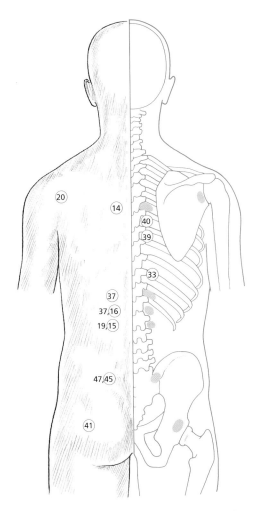

Fig. 5.19 Chapman's neurolymphatic reflexes – posterior surface (3).

The sequence suggested by these researchers is that a start be made by palpating the anterior reflexes. If any are found to be active by virtue of being easily palpable and sensitive, the pair of this reflex is then examined posteriorly. If this is also palpable and sensitive, treatment commences on the anterior reflex point.

Gentle rotary pressure is used in the treatment phase, dosage being determined by palpation. The aim is to procure a decrease in oedema, dissolution of the gangliform contracture in the deep fascia and subsidence of the tenderness in the anterior reflex areas. The actual time involved in treating a point may be from 20 seconds to 2 minutes.

Rechecking for sensitivity by gentle palpation is suggested. This is said to give a strong indication of the success or otherwise of the effort thus far. Since these are reflex areas, the skin overlaying them would be subject to the influences discussed in Chapter 4. These points can therefore be found by looking for them specifically, once you have knowledge of their existence, or by skin stretching, 'drag' palpation or via a systematic soft tissue assessment, such as Lief advocated.

EXERCISE 5.12: PALPATING CHAPMAN'S REFLEX AREAS/POINTS

Time suggested: 4–6 minutes to evaluate and 'treat' a pair of reflex points

If this system interests you, spend some time palpating for pairs of neurolymphatic points as illustrated (Figs 5.14–5.19) and described above.

See the tables in the Appendix (p 379) for captions relating to these figures. Record your findings.

Altered muscle structure and function

The final segment of this section deals with a sequence in which postural muscles may be assessed for relative shortness. Before this sequence, three 'functional assessments' will be outlined, which examine the way in which muscles are firing when particular actions are performed by the patient/model. Muscle-firing sequences offer evidence of normality or dysfunction and, depending on the region, can point to the probability of particular muscles being short or inhibited.

Janda (1983) has shown that postural muscles have a tendency to shorten, not only under pathological conditions but often under normal circumstances. Postural muscles are genetically older; they have different physiological and probably biochemical qualities compared with phasic muscles, which normally weaken and exhibit signs of inhibition in response to stress or pathology.

Most problems of the musculoskeletal system involve, as part of their aetiology, dysfunction related to aspects of muscle shortening (Janda 1978, 1983, Lewit 1999, Liebenson 1996). Where weakness (lack of tone) is apparently a major element, it will often be found that antagonists are shortened, reciprocally inhibiting their tone, and that prior to any effort to strengthen weak muscles, hypertonic antagonists should be dealt with by appropriate means, after which spontaneous toning occurs in the previously hypotonic or relatively weak muscles. If tone remains reduced then, and only then, should exercise and/or isotonic muscle energy technique procedures be brought in (Chaitow 2001, Janda 1978).

Firing sequences and functional assessment

The following simple observation and palpation tests allow for a rapid gathering of information with a minimum of effort. They are based on the work of Janda (1983) and interpretations of this by Liebenson (1996). After a description of each test, a palpation exercise will be outlined.

Prone hip extension test

The patient lies prone and the practitioner stands at waist level with hands placed so that the cephalad one spans the lower erector spinae on both sides, and the caudad hand rests with the thenar eminence on gluteus maximus and the fingertips on the hamstrings. The patient is asked to raise the leg into extension of the hip. The normal activation sequence is gluteus maximus and hamstrings, mor or less simultaneously, followed by erector spinae (contralateral then ipsilateral).

If the hamstrings and/or the erectors adopt the role of gluteus, as indicated by their firing first, they are working inappropriately, are therefore 'stressed' and will by implication have shortened.

EXERCISE 5.13: HIP EXTENSION FIRING SEQUENCE (see Fig. 5.20)

Time suggested: 3 minutes

Your palpation partner lies prone. You stand at waist level, with your cephalad hand spanning the low back so that the pads of your fingers touch one side of the erector spinae and the heel of your hand touches the other. Your caudad hand is placed so that the heel is on gluteus maximus and the finger pads are on the upper hamstrings.

Ask your partner to raise the leg into extension. Note the firing sequence. Have your partner relax and perform the palpation test again several times.

Do the gluteals fire first (they should)? Do the hamstrings come in very fast, with gluteals much later (they shouldn't)?

Most worryingly of all, do one or other of the erectors fire first? If the hamstrings or erectors fire early, then these are likely to have shortened and this will be demonstrable in the tests later in the chapter.).

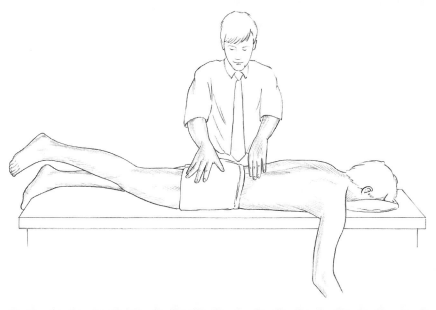

Fig. 5.20   Hip extension test. The normal activation sequence is gluteus maximus, hamstrings, contralateral erector spinae, ipsilateral erector spinae.

Hip abduction test – observation (Fig. 5.21) and palpation (Fig. 5.22)

The patient lies on the side with lower leg flexed to provide support and the upper leg straight, in line with the trunk. The practitioner stands in front of the patient at the level of the feet and observes (no hands on) as the patient is asked to abduct the leg slowly.

- Normal – hip abduction to 45°.
- Abnormal – if hip flexion occurs (indicating TFL shortness) and/or leg externally rotates (indicating piriformis shortening) and/or 'hiking' of the hip occurs at the outset of the movement (indicating quadratus overactivity and therefore, by implication, shortness) (Fig. 5.21).

The test should be repeated with the practitioner standing behind the patient at waist level, with a finger pad on the lateral margin of quadratus lumborum. As the leg is abducted, if quadratus fires strongly and first (before gluteus medius), a twitch or push will be felt by the palpating finger, indicating overactivity and probable shortness of quadratus lumborum (this would show visually as a 'hip-hike', as mentioned in the first part of the test).

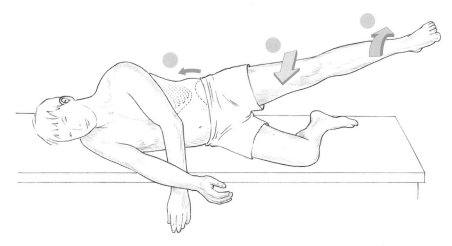

Fig. 5.21 Hip abduction observation test. Normal firing sequence is gluteus medius or TFL first and second, followed by quadratus lumborum. If QL fires first it is overactive and will be short. If TFL is short the leg will drift into flexion on abduction. If piriformis is short the leg and foot will externally rotate during abduction.

EXERCISE 5.14: HIP ABDUCTION FIRING SEQUENCE TEST (see Figs 5.21 and 5.22)

Time suggested: 3–4 minutes

Your palpation partner should lie on his side, lower leg flexed, upper leg straight, in line with the trunk.

You stand in front, at the level of the feet and observe (no hands on yet) as your partner is asked to abduct the leg slowly.

Observe the area just above the crest of the pelvis – does it 'jump' at the outset of the abduction or at least obviously activate before a 25° abduction has taken place? If so, QL is overactive and probably short.

Have your partner relax completely and repeat the abduction. Does the leg drift anteriorly during abduction? If so, TFL is probably short. Does the leg and foot turn outward (externally rotate)? If so, piriformis is probably short (see Fig. 5.21).

Now, standing behind your side-lying palpation partner, place one or two finger pads of your cephalad hand lightly on the tissues overlying QL, approximately 2 inches (5 cm) lateral to the spinous process of L3 (Fig. 5.22). Place your caudad hand so that the heel rests on gluteus medius and the finger pads on TFL. Assess the firing sequence during hip abduction. If QL fires early (you will feel a strong twitch or 'jump' against your palpating fingers), it is overactive and short.

The ideal sequence is TFL – gluteus medius – QL (but not before about 20–25° of abduction).

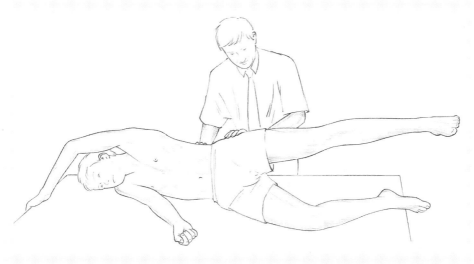

Fig. 5.22   Palpation assessment for quadratus lumborum overactivity. The muscle is palpated, as is the gluteus medius and TFL, during abduction of the leg. The correct firing sequence should be gluteus and TFL, followed at around 25° elevation by quadratus. If there is an immediate 'grabbing' action by quadratus it indicates overactivity, and therefore stress, so shortness can be assumed.

Scapulohumeral rhythm test

This is an important assessment which can give information as to the status of some of the most important upper fixators of the shoulder.

The patient is seated with the arm at the side, elbow flexed and facing forwards. The practitioner stands behind and observes as the patient is asked to raise the elbow towards the horizontal.

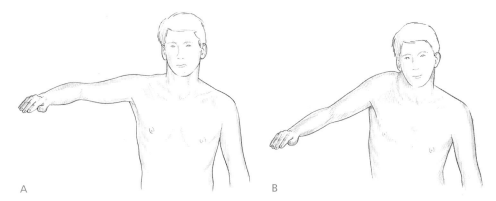

Fig. 5.23 Scapulohumeral rhythm test. A. Normal – elevation of the shoulder after 60° of abduction. B. Abnormal – elevation of the shoulder before 60° of abduction.

- Normal – elevation of shoulder only after 60° of arm abduction.
- Abnormal – if elevation of the shoulder or obvious 'bunching' occurs between shoulder and neck or winging of the scapulae occurs within the first 60° of shoulder abduction (indicating levator scapulae and upper trapezius tightness, and lower and middle trapezius as well as serratus anterior weakness) (see Fig. 5.23).

This pattern, of weak lower fixators and overworked and probably shortened upper fixators, is common in postural patterns involving a forward head carriage with round-shouldered stance.

EXERCISE 5.15: ASSESSING SCAPULOHUMERAL RHYTHM (see Fig. 5.23)

Follow the description of the scapulohumeral rhythm test described above. This is a purely observational assessment, without touching.

If the test is positive, seen as a bunching of upper trapezius before the abduction of the humerus has reached 60°, the implicated muscles (levator scapulae, upper trapezius) should be tested for shortness (see below).

DISCUSSION OF PALPATORY PROGRESS INVOLVING EXERCISES 5.12–5.15

In these last few palpation and observation exercises the interface between structure and function has been reached, particularly with Janda's functional assessments. In those you were able to feel and observe inappropriate behaviour and to link that to likely structural modification, in this instance shortness. These clues to structural change can then be confirmed by the sort of tests and assessments which form the remainder of this chapter. The palpation of neurolymphatic 'points' was also a link between structure (the soft tissue changes) and function (the modified lymphatic flow). It is in this type of exercise that the clinical usefulness of such evaluations becomes obvious, as this impinges on the real world of people's problems, involving pain and restriction, and your role in trying to make sense of what has happened and what can be treated.

Assessing muscles for shortness

As part of a comprehensive palpation protocol, it is desirable to learn to assess short, tight muscles in a standardised manner. Janda (1983) suggests that to obtain a reliable evaluation of muscle shortness the following criteria be observed.

- The starting position, method of fixation and direction of movement must be observed carefully.
- The prime mover must not be exposed to external pressure.
- If possible, the force exerted on the tested muscle must not work over two joints.
- The examiner should perform at an even speed a slow movement that brakes slowly at the end of the range.
- The examiner should keep the stretch and the muscle irritability about equal and the movement must not be jerky.
- Pressure or pull must always act in the required direction of movement.
- Muscle shortening can only be correctly evaluated if the joint range is not decreased, as might be the case should an osseous limitation or joint blockage exist.

It is in shortened muscle fibres, as a rule, that reflex activity is noted. This takes the form of local dysfunction variously called trigger points, tender points, zones of irritability, neurovascular and neurolymphatic reflexes, etc. Localising these is possible via normal palpatory methods (NMT, 'drag', skin elasticity, etc.) or as part of neuromuscular diagnostic treatment. Identification of tight muscles may also be systematically carried out as described below. Note that the assessment methods presented are not themselves diagnostic but provide strong indications of probable shortness of the muscles being tested.

See Special topic 9 on 'end-feel' for descriptions of different end-feel characteristics.

The following tests are derived from the work of Janda (1983), Kendall et al (1952) and a variety of other sources.

Tests for postural muscle shortening
Ease and bind

Before commencing a muscle-by-muscle sequence in which postural muscles are evaluated for relative shortness, one such test makes a useful teaching aid for establishing a sense of 'tension', 'bind' or resistance, occurring as a muscle or other soft tissue structure is moved towards a barrier of resistance. The concept and reality of tissues providing palpating hands or fingers with a sense of their relative 'bind' as opposed to their state of 'ease' is one which needs to be grasped. There can never be enough focus on these two characteristics which allow the tissues to reveal their current degree of comfort or distress.

Osteopathic pioneer HV Hoover (1969) describes 'ease' as a state of equilibrium or 'neutral' which the practitioner senses by having at least one completely passive, 'listening' contact, either of the whole hand or a single or several fingers or thumb, in touch with the tissues being assessed.

Bind is, of course, the opposite of ease and can most easily be noted by lightly palpating the tissues surrounding, or associated with, a joint as this is taken towards its end of range of movement, its resistance barrier.

In order to 'read' hypertonicity, palpation skills need to be refined and as a first step John Goodridge (1981) suggests the following test, which examines medial hamstring and short abductor status, as a means of becoming comfortable with the reality of ease and bind in a practical manner.

EXERCISE 5.16A: GOODRIDGE'S 'RESISTANCE' PALPATION

Time suggested: 5 minutes

This palpation exercise evaluates the concept of 'ease and bind' during assessment of adductors of the thigh (see Fig. 5.24).

Before starting, ensure that your palpation partner lies supine, so that the non-tested leg is abducted slightly, heel over the end of the table. The leg to be tested is close to the edge of the table.

Ensure that the tested leg is in the anatomically correct position, knee in full extension and with no external rotation of the leg, which would negate the test.

After grasping the supine patient's foot and ankle, in order to abduct the lower limb, close your eyes during the abduction and feel, in your own body, from the hand through the forearm into the upper arm, the beginning of a sense of resistance. Stop when you feel it, open your eyes and note how many degrees in an arc the limb has travelled.

What Goodridge is trying to establish is that you learn to recognise the very beginning of the end of range of free movement, where easy motion ceases and effort begins. This 'barrier' is not a pathological one but represents the first sign of resistance, the place at which tissues require some degree of passive effort in order to move them.

This is also the place at which a sense of 'bind' should be palpated, in the next part of this exercise, below. It is suggested that the process be attempted several times, so that you get a sense of where resistance begins, before doing the next part of this exercise sequence. Then do the exercise again, but this time as described in Exercise 5.16B.

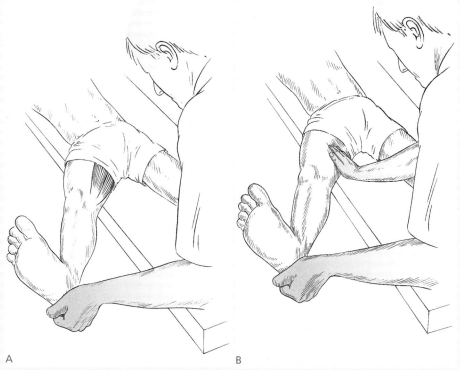

A   B

Fig. 5.24A, B Assessment of 'bind'/restriction barrier with the first sign of resistance in the adductors (medial hamstrings) of the right leg. (**A**) The practitioner's perception of the transition point, where easy movement alters to demand some degree of effort, is regarded as the barrier. (**B**) The barrier is identified when the palpating hand notes a sense of bind in tissues which were relaxed (at ease) up to that point.

EXERCISE 5.16B: GOODRIDGE'S EASE AND BIND PALPATION

Time suggested: 5 minutes

Stand between your palpation partner's partially abducted leg and the table, facing the head of the table, so that all control of the tested leg is achieved by using your lateral arm/hand, which holds and supports the leg at the ankle, while your table-side hand rests on the inner thigh, palpating the muscles which are being tested.

This palpating hand (often called a 'listening' hand in osteopathy) must be in touch with the skin, moulded to the contours of the tissues being assessed, but should exert no pressure and should be completely relaxed.

Abduction of the tested leg from its neutral resting position is introduced passively by the outside hand/arm, until the first sign of resistance is noted by the hand which is providing the motive force, i.e. the one holding the leg. As you approach this point of resistance (as noted in the previous exercise), can you sense a tightening of the tissues in the mid-inner thigh, which your table-side, listening hand is touching? This sensation is known as 'bind'.

If this sensation is not clear, then take the leg back towards the table and out again, but this time go past the point where easy movement is lost and effort begins and towards its end of range. Here you will certainly sense bind.

As you once more take the leg back towards the table you will note a softening, a relaxation, an 'ease' in these same tissues.

Go through the same sequence with the other leg, becoming increasingly familiar with the sense of these two extremes (ease and bind), and try to note the very moment at which you can palpate the transition from one to the other, not to its extreme but where it begins, whether you are moving from ease to bind or the other way.

Normal excursion of the straight leg into abduction is around 45°, and by testing both legs in the manner described, you can evaluate whether the twos sets of adductors are both tight and short or whether one is and the other is not. Even if both are tight and short one may be more restricted than the other and this may be the one to treat first.

Note: It is suggested that you practise performing palpation exercises for ease and bind on many other muscles, as listed below for example, when they are being both actively and passively moved, until you are comfortable with your skill in reading this change in tone.

The point at which you feel bind (or where the hand carrying the leg feels the first sign that effort is required) is the resistance barrier where a muscle energy isometric contraction commences, in application of MET to acutely taut structures.

Record your experience, using the two methods of evaluating shortness in this muscle (Exercises 5.16A and 5.16B), and try wherever possible to use a directly palpating hand to assess bind as you perform the following exercises.

For each of the following exercises, involving assessment of individual muscle shortness, it is suggested that around 5 minutes be spent practising each side, at first. This should, with practice, be reduced to around 2–3 minutes. The muscles included here are representative ones (hamstrings, piriformis, erector spinae, upper trapezius).

For a wider range of assessment guidelines see Janda's *Muscle function testing* (1983), Lewit's *Manipulation in rehabilitation of the locomotor system* (1999) or Chaitow's *Muscle energy techniques* (2001).

EXERCISE 5.17A: PALPATION FOR HAMSTRING SHORTNESS – UPPER FIBRES

Time suggested: 5 minutes

In order to assess for shortened hamstrings (biceps, femoris, semitendinosus and semimembranosus), your palpation partner should lie supine with the leg to be tested outstretched and the other leg flexed at knee and hip, to relax the low back.

In order to assess tightness in the left leg hamstrings (upper fibres), you should be standing at the side of the leg to be tested, facing the head of the table.

The lower leg is supported by your caudad hand, keeping the knee of that leg in light extension and if possible resting the heel of that leg in the bend of the elbow to prevent lateral rotation. The cephalad hand can then rest on the hamstrings, around mid-thigh, to evaluate for bind as elevation takes place.

The range of movement into hip flexion should (with a supple hamstring group) allow elevation of the tested leg to about 80° before bind is noted. Does the first sign of resistance, bind, occur before 80°? If so, hamstrings are shortened.

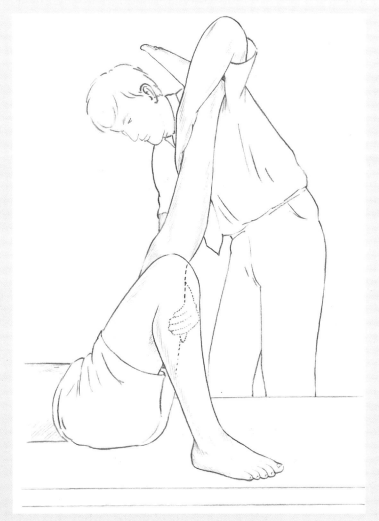

Fig. 5.25 Assessment for shortness of hamstring, upper fibres, by palpation during leg raising.

continues

EXERCISE 5.17A *(Continued)*

Repeat the palpation exercise while your palpation partner lies with the head and neck turned fully away from the side you are testing and then again fully turned toward the side you are testing. Was there any difference in the degree of elevation of the leg before bind was noticed when the neck was turned?

There could be because of the tonic neck reflex in which cervical rotation increases ipsilateral extensor tone and contralateral flexor tone, while it decreases contralateral extensor and ipsilateral flexor tone. Simply put, this means that when the neck is turned away from the side being tested, the hamstrings should be more relaxed. And when the neck is turned toward the side being tested, they should test as tighter than previously (Murphy 2000). Was this apparent during the test?

EXERCISE 5.17B: PALPATION FOR HAMSTRING SHORTNESS – LOWER FIBRES

Time suggested: 3–5 minutes

To make this assessment the tested leg is taken into full hip flexion (helped by the patient holding the upper thigh with both hands (see Fig. 5.26)).

You should place a hand onto the fibres just inferior to the popliteal space to assess for bind as the leg straightens. The knee is then passively straightened until resistance is felt or bind is noted by this palpation hand resting on the lower hamstrings.

If the knee cannot easily straighten with the hip flexed, this indicates shortness in the lower hamstring fibres and a degree of pull behind the knee and lower thigh will be reported, during any attempt to straighten the leg.

If the knee is capable of being straightened with the hip flexed, having previously not been capable of achieving an 80°, straight-leg raise, then the lower fibres are cleared of shortness and it is the upper hamstring fibres which require attention.

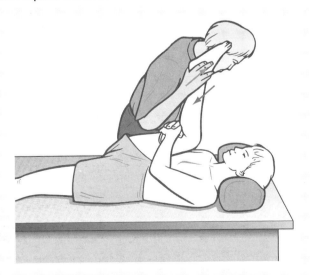

Fig. 5.26   Assessment for shortness of hamstring, lower fibres, by palpation during leg straightening.

EXERCISE 5.18: PALPATING FOR SHORTNESS OF PIRIFORMIS

Time suggested: 3–4 minutes

When short, piriformis will cause the affected side leg of the supine individual to appear to be short and externally rotated.

Have your palpation partner side-lying, tested side uppermost. You should stand in front of and facing the pelvis.

In order to contact the insertion of piriformis, draw two imaginary lines: one runs from the ASIS to the ischial tuberosity and the other from the PSIS to the most prominent point of the trochanter (see Fig. 5.27). Where these lines cross, just posterior to the trochanter, is the insertion of the muscle and pressure here will produce marked discomfort if the structure is short or irritated.

In order to locate the most common trigger point site, in the belly of the muscle, the line from the ASIS should be taken to the tip of the coccyx rather than the ischial tuberosity. The other line from the PSIS to the trochanter prominence is the same.

Pressure where one line crosses the other will access the mid-point of the belly of piriformis, where trigger points are common.

Light compression here which produces a painful response is indicative of a stressed and probably shortened muscle.

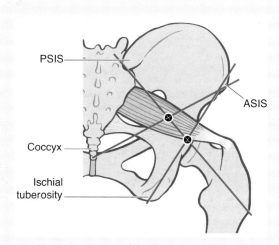

Fig. 5.27 Landmarks are used as coordinates to locate the attachment of piriformis at the hip, and also the site of major trigger point activity in the belly of the muscle.

EXERCISE 5.19: PARAVERTEBRAL MUSCLE PALPATION

Time suggested: 3 minutes for observation, up to 15 minutes if additional palpation methods are introduced

5.19A
Your palpation partner should be seated on the treatment table, legs extended, pelvis vertical.

Flexion is introduced in order to approximate the forehead to the knees without strain. An even curve should be observed and a distance of about 10 cm from the knees achieved by the forehead. No knee flexion should occur and the movement should be a spinal one, not involving pelvic tilting (see Fig. 5.28).

continues

EXERCISE 5.19 *(Continued)*

Time suggested: 3 minutes for observation, up to 15 minutes if additional palpation methods are introduced

5.19B

Your palpation partner should be seated at the edge of the table, knees flexed and lower legs hanging over the edge, relaxing the hamstrings.

Forward bending is introduced so that the forehead approximates the knees. If flexion of the trunk is greater in this position than in 5.19B above, then there is probably tilting of the pelvis and shortened hamstring involvement.

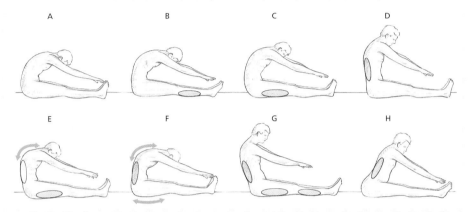

Fig. 5.28 Tests for shortness of the erector spinae and associated postural muscles. (A) Normal length of erector spinae muscles and posterior thigh muscles. (B) Tight gastrocnemius and soleus; the inability to dorsiflex the feet indicates tightness of the plantarflexor group. (C) Tight hamstring muscles, which cause the pelvis to tilt posteriorly. (D) Tight low back erector spinae muscles. (E) Tight hamstring; slightly tight low back muscles and overstretched upper back muscles. (F) Slightly shortened lower back muscles, stretched upper back muscles and slightly stretched hamstrings. (G) Tight low back muscles, hamstrings and gastrocnemius/soleus. (H) Very tight low back muscles, with lordosis maintained even in flexion.

Locating and palpating areas of 'spinal flatness' during Exercises 5.19A & B

During these assessments there should be a uniform degree of flexion throughout the spine, with a 'C' curve apparent when looked at from the side. However, all too commonly areas of shortening in the spinal muscles may be observed, particularly as areas which are 'flat' where little or no flexion is taking place (see Fig. 5.28).

In some instances lordosis may be maintained in the lumbar spine even on full flexion, or flexion may be very limited, even without such lordosis. There may also be obvious overstretching of the upper back, as compensation for the relative tightness of the lower back.

Generally 'flat' areas of the spine indicate local shortening of the erector spinae group.

Can you observe 'flat', tense areas of the spine during either or both of these flexion exercises? Identify one or two such areas and palpate them lightly as your partner moves into flexion. Compare the feel of the tissues as they tighten, bind, compared with those areas which are flexible, where the curve is normal.

Also, if you identify flat areas, have your palpation partner lie prone and palpate lightly with your fingertips to assess the degree of hypertonicity and/or use some of the skin palpation methods discussed in Chapter 4 to evaluate other findings in the tense tissues (drag, for example, to locate trigger points) as compared with more normal ones.

Evaluate whether these tight muscles alongside the spine are areas of facilitation, by using Exercises 5.1–5.3 again. Record your findings.

EXERCISE 5.20: PALPATING FOR SHORTNESS OF UPPER TRAPEZIUS

Time suggested: A 3 minutes, B 2 minutes, C 5–7 minutes

5.20A

Your palpation partner is seated and you stand behind with one hand on the shoulder of the side to be tested and the other hand on the ipsilateral side of the head.

The neck is gently side-flexed, without allowing flexion, extension or rotation, to its 'easy' barrier, i.e. no force at all, while the shoulder of the tested side is stabilised from above (see Fig. 5.29).

The range is compared on each side and palpation (drag, for example) locates the shortened fibres.

If sitting is not possible then the same procedure is carried out in a supine position, with the ear being approximated to the shoulder during side-flexion.

5.20B

Your partner is seated and you stand behind with a hand resting over the muscle on the side to be assessed.

Your partner is asked to extend the arm at the shoulder joint, bringing the flexed arm/elbow backward. If the upper trapezius is stressed on that side, it will inappropriately activate during this movement. Since it is a postural muscle, shortness in it can then be assumed if it fires inappropriately.

5.20C

To test upper trapezius on the right side, your palpation partner should lie supine, initially with the neck fully (but not forcefully) rotated to the left. In order to evaluate the posterior fibres of upper trapezius, your left hand should support the upper neck/occipital area while your right hand, palm upward, rests so that the ulnar border lies against the right side of the neck. Your finger pads should be palpating the posterior fibres of upper trapezius, as you slowly side-flex it to the left, until you sense the first sign of 'bind' with your finger pads or resistance with your hand which is supporting and transporting the head.

You should now stabilise the head in this position of side-flexion and rotation with your right hand and cross your left hand over to cup the shoulder (see Fig. 5.30). With the cupped hand shoulder contact, assess the ease with which it can be depressed (moved caudally), while the head and neck are held firmly at their side-flexed and rotated barrier.

There should be an easy 'springiness' as you push the shoulder toward the feet, with a soft end-feel to the movement. Repeat this several times.

If when 'springing' the shoulder, there is a hard, wooden end-feel, those fibres of upper trapezius which are involved in the test are confirmed as shortened.

This same evaluation should be performed with the head fully rotated away from the side being assessed (posterior fibres), half turned away from the side being assessed (medial fibres), and slightly turned toward the side being assessed (anterior fibres), in order to respectively test for relative shortness, and functional efficiency, of the various subdivisions of the upper portion of trapezius.

continues

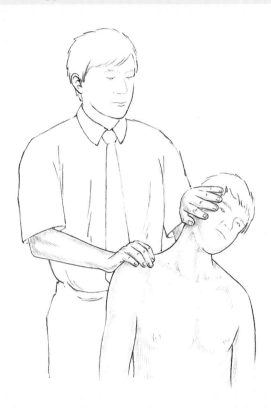

Fig. 5.29 Assessment of relative shortness of right side upper trapezius. The right shoulder is stabilised while the neck is side-bent to its first sign of resistance ('bind') without force. One side is compared to the other. Normal range is thought to be approximately 45°.

When introducing side-flexion when assessing medial and anterior fibres, the respective parts of the muscle should be palpated in a similar way to that described above, palm up or down according to comfort.

Can you identify the barriers of resistance simultaneously, with the transporting hand, and the contacts feeling for bind?

Do the different assessments in this exercise confirm each other? Which fibres are shortened based on these palpation tests?

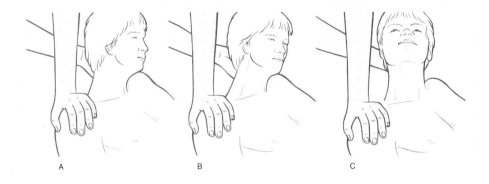

A   B   C

Fig. 5.30 Assessment of shortness in upper trapezius. The three head positions relate to posterior fibres (head fully rotated and side flexed); middle fibres (head half rotated and side-flexed); anterior fibres, side-flexed and turned slightly toward side being assessed.

Additional palpation exercises

Spend some time comparing the results of muscle tests, as described above with the finding you made when searching for trigger points and other reflex activity. Are muscles which house such points consistently short on testing? Usually or only sometimes?

Begin the final exercises in this chapter with you and your partner repeating the assessments of postural muscles as described above, noting on a chart those which are found to be shortened.

Results should then be compared with findings obtained after practising basic spinal NMT (or abdominal NMT) assessment, in which a note is kept on a chart of all areas, points, zones of soft tissue dysfunction (palpating as abnormal, indurated, contracted as well as sensitive). Also practise Nimmo's assessment sequence as described in Box 5.2.

Philip Greenman (1989) describes a pattern of palpation of muscle in the spinal region which is well worth carrying out, many times, until the tissues he asks you to feel for are indeed clearly noted. The following is a summary of part of his 'palpation prescription' for this region, which commences with superficial palpation, always an exercise worth repeating for we have done similar work before in Chapter 4.

EXERCISE 5.21: GREENMAN'S SPINAL 'PALPATION PRESCRIPTION'

Time suggested: A 7–10 minutes; B 7–10 minutes, C 15–20 minutes, D 15 minutes for each segment

5.21A
Sit or stand facing your seated partner's back and place your hands and fingers onto the upper portion of the scapulae, just overlaying the spines of these bones.

Palpate the skin for variations in temperature, tone, texture, thickness and elasticity, as you move your hands downwards over the shoulder blades.

At the starting position, move the hands slowly and sequentially in all directions, so that the skin moves on the subcutaneous fascia, and assess the degree of adherence between skin and fascia.

Gently lift the skin between thumb and index finger and perform skin rolling, moving medially and then laterally as well as superiorly, from whichever point you started palpating.

This elicits information as to the thickness and pliability of the skin as well as giving information about painful tissues.

Do this on both sides of the spine, symmetrically, and compare findings.

5.21B
Move your hands to a more central point and place the fingers of one hand so that they straddle the spine, one or two fingers on each side, close to the spine, between the shoulder blades.

Palpate the skin, moving it in various directions to assess the skin adherence. Compare the findings with those you assessed in tissue more lateral to the spine.

Now palpate through the skin in this region to the subcutaneous fascia, right down to the ligamentous structure (supraspinous) which lies

continues

between the segments, in the interspinous space. Compare its feel to the way it feels as it inserts into the spinous process. Palpate the spinous process and note the feel of bone, overlaid by skin and ligament.

Resting a finger on each of two or three interspaces at this level, have your partner slowly bend their head forward and backward. Spend some time doing this, gaining a sense of 'end-feel' of the ranges of motion involved.

5.21C

Now place the fingers of one hand on the soft tissues between the spine and the scapula on that side. Feel through the skin and subcutaneous fascia until you are aware of the fascia which overlays the first layer of muscle. Identify the direction in which the fibres of this muscle layer travel.

Have your partner draw the shoulder blade towards the spine, as you continue to palpate. This movement should highlight the horizontal fibres of the trapezius muscle which you are palpating.

Move your pressure deeper to the next layer of muscle on one side, the rhomboid, and try to feel for the oblique direction of its pull, from above downwards. As you palpate this with one hand, you can highlight the action of these fibres by having your partner draw the bent elbow (on the same side) downwards, against counterpressure offered by your free hand.

Going yet deeper, feel for a muscle which has a more fibrous, ropy texture, which runs vertically alongside the spine. Movement of your contact from side to side will help identify these fibres, which probably belong to the longissimus muscle, part of the erector spinae group. Move your palpating contact to the side of this ropy bundle, closer to the spine, and go more deeply in order to find evidence of a deeper layer of muscles, the rotatores and multifidi, which run from one segment to another providing fine control movement possibilities. Their direction of pull is obliquely from the spine outwards (as in the case of the rhomboids).

Greenman suggests that you try to identify any of the small muscles which are tender, more 'full and tense', and which are therefore involved in a degree of local dysfunction.

Moving to the outside of the longissimus muscle, palpate deeply into the fascial tissue. With the angle of your palpation being somewhat towards the spine, introduce a movement upwards and downwards, as you feel for the hollows and rises of the transverse processes and the interspaces between them.

5.21D

Review the assessment and palpation methods used in Chapter 4 and consider whether you could combine one such approach, say the 'skin drag' test, with, for example, Lief's NMT or the methods of Nimmo or Chapman.

Does skin 'drag' or reduced skin elasticity correlate with and help identification of the points described in Chapman's work or with trigger points as elicited by the Nimmo or Lief approaches?

continues

EXERCISE 5.21 *(Continued)*

Time suggested: A 7–10 minutes; B 7–10 minutes, C 15–20 minutes, D 15 minutes for each segment

Try also to combine skin assessment with the postural muscle tests, seeking localised areas of dysfunction in muscles which you have shown to be shortened. Having identified a short postural muscle, evaluate whether there are skin changes (drag, decreased elasticity, etc.) apparent near its origin and insertion, to a greater extent than in muscles which test as normal.

Are there more trigger points and/or localised areas of dysfunction in the soft tissues and corresponding skin changes in short postural muscles and/or their antagonists?

Try to find out the answer to these questions and reevaluate all the methods mentioned in this exercise, after you have treated such muscles with whatever method you consider appropriate.

Record your findings.

Palpation skill status

In this chapter on muscle palpation you have been exposed to a variety of approaches, all of which can be useful for uncovering evidence of functional integrity or dysfunctional adaptation, which adds to the knowledge gained in the previous chapter.

If you have successfully completed the exercises given in this chapter, you should now be comfortably able to evaluate for muscle shortness in appropriate (postural) muscles, as well as being able to identify localised changes in these.

If you have worked on the two segments of the last exercise (5.21) you will now have combined the use of the information residing in the skin with that which the muscles and other soft tissues have to offer, in respect of their structural changes.

As has been established, structure and function are intertwined to a degree that makes them inseparable in reality. Just as we can use structural analysis and palpation to predict what structural changes are likely, so can we evaluate function to guide us towards what structural changes are probable. This was made clear in the functional Exercises 5.13–5.15.

In the next chapter, the methods used are no longer looking for structural change alone but are concerned with the altered function which accompanies altered structure. Some of the methods are subtle, others less so. All are of proven value if you have the patience to develop the acuteness of touch needed to read the evidence which is waiting to be recognised.

REFERENCES

Arbuckle B 1977 Selected writings of Beryl Arbuckle. National Osteopathic Institute, Chicago, IL
Baldry P 1993 Acupuncture, trigger points and musculoskeletal pain. Churchill Livingstone, Edinburgh
Beal M 1983 Palpatory testing for somatic dysfunction in patients with cardiovascular disease. Journal of the American Osteopathic Association July
Becker R 1963 Diagnostic touch (part 1). Yearbook of the Academy of Applied Osteopathy, Newark, OH
Becker R 1964 Diagnostic touch (part 2). Yearbook of the Academy of Applied Osteopathy, Newark, OH
Becker R 1965 Diagnostic touch (part 3). Yearbook of the Academy of Applied Osteopathy, Newark, OH
Braggins S 2000 Back care: a clinical approach. Churchill Livingstone, Edinburgh
Chaitow L 1988 Soft tissue manipulation. Thorsons, Wellingborough
Chaitow L 1991 Soft tissue manipulation. Inner Traditions, Rochester, MA

Chaitow L 1996a Modern neuromuscular techniques. Churchill Livingstone, Edinburgh

Chaitow L 1996b Positional release techniques. Churchill Livingstone, Edinburgh

Chaitow L 2001 Muscle energy techniques. Churchill Livingstone, Edinburgh

Chaitow L 2002a Modern neuromuscular techniques, 2nd edn. Churchill Livingstone, Edinburgh

Chaitow L 2002b Positional release techniques, 2nd edn. Churchill Livingstone, Edinburgh

Chaitow L, DeLany J 2000 Clinical applications of neuromuscular technique (upper body). Churchill Livingstone, Edinburgh

Chaitow L, DeLany J 2002 Clinical applications of neuromuscular technique (lower body). Churchill Livingstone, Edinburgh

Cunxiny Y et al 1986 Creative effect and mechanism of acupoints Pishu and Weishu. Journal of Traditional Chinese Medicine 6(4)

Dvorak J, Dvorak V 1984 Manual medicine: diagnostics. Georg Thieme, New York

Erlinghauser R 1959 The circulation of CSF through the connective tissue system. Yearbook of the Academy of Applied Osteopathy, Newark, OH

Frymann V 1963 Palpation – its study in the workshop. Yearbook of the Academy of Applied Osteopathy, Newark, OH, pp 16–30

Goodridge J 1981 MET, definition, explanation, methods of procedure. Journal of the American Osteopathic Association 81(4):249

Greenman P 1989 Principles of manual medicine. Williams and Wilkins, Baltimore

Hoover H 1969 Method for teaching functional technique. Yearbook of the Academy of Applied Osteopathy, Newark, OH

Janda V 1978 Muscles, central nervous motor regulation, and back problems. In: Korr IM (ed) Neurobiologic mechanisms in manipulative therapy. Plenum, New York

Janda V 1982 Introduction to functional pathology of the motor system. Proceedings of the VII Commonwealth and International Conference on Sport. Physiotherapy in Sport 3:39

Janda V 1983 Muscle function testing. Butterworths, London

Janda V 1996 Evaluation of muscular imbalance. In: Liebenson C (ed) Rehabilitation of the spine. Williams and Wilkins, Baltimore

Jones L 1981 Strain/counterstrain. Academy of Applied Osteopathy, Colorado Springs

Kendall H, Kendall F, Boynton D 1952 Posture and pain. Williams and Wilkins, Baltimore

Korr I 1967 Axonal delivery of neuroplasmic components to muscle cells. Science 155:342–345

Korr I 1976 Proprioceptors and somatic dysfunction. Yearbook of the Academy of Applied Osteopathy, Newark, OH

Kuchera M et al 1990 Athletic functional demand and posture. Journal of the American Osteopathic Association 90(9): 843–844

Kuchera W 1997 Lumbar and abdominal region. In: Ward R (ed) Foundations for osteopathic medicine. Williams and Wilkins, Baltimore

Lewit K 1992 Manipulative therapy in rehabilitation of the locomotor system, 2nd edn. Butterworths, London

Lewit K 1999 Manipulative therapy in rehabilitation of the locomotor system, 3rd edn. Butterworths, London

Liebenson C 1996 Rehabilitation of the spine. Williams and Wilkins, Baltimore

Magoun H 1948 Osteopathic diagnosis and therapy for the general practitioner. Journal of the American Osteopathic Association December

McFarlane Tilley R 1961 Spinal stress palpation. Yearbook of the Academy of Applied Osteopathy, Newark, OH

McPartland J, Goodridge J 1997 Osteopathic examination of the cervical spine. Journal of Bodywork and Movement Therapies 1(3):173–178

Mense S, Simons D 2001 Muscle pain. Lippincott, Williams and Wilkins, Philadelphia

Murphy D 2000 Conservative management of cervical spine syndromes. McGraw-Hill, New York

Nimmo R 1966 Workshop. British College of Naturopathy and Osteopathy, London

Norris C 1998 Sports injuries, diagnosis and management, 2nd edn. Butterworths, London

Owens C 1963 An endocrine interpretation of Chapman's reflexes. Academy of Applied Osteopathy, Newark, OH

Patriquin D 1997 Chapman's reflexes. In: Ward R (ed) Foundations for osteopathic medicine. Williams and Wilkins, Baltimore

Rolf I 1962 Structural dynamics. British Academy of Osteopathy Yearbook, Newark, OH

Rosero H et al 1987 Journal of the American Osteopathic Association February

Selye H 1984 The stress of life. McGraw-Hill, New York

Simons D, Travell J, Simons L 1999 Myofascial pain and dysfunction: the trigger point manual, vol 1, upper half of body, 2nd edn. Williams and Wilkins, Baltimore

Smith F 1986 Inner bridges: a guide to energy movement and body structure. Humanics New Age, New York

Speransky AD 1944 A basis for the theory of medicine. International Publisher, New York

Thomson H, Francis D 1977 Abdominal wall tenderness: a useful sign in the acute abdomen. Lancet 1:1053

Travell J, Simons D 1992 Myofascial pain and dysfunction – the trigger point manual. Williams and Wilkins, Baltimore

Upledger J 1987 Craniosacral therapy. Eastland Press, Seattle

Wallace E, McPartland J, Jones J, Kuchera W, Buser B 1997 Lymphatic system. In: Ward R (ed) Foundations for osteopathic medicine. Williams and Wilkins, Baltimore

Walther D 1988 Applied kinesiology. SDC Systems, Pueblo, CA

Ward R (ed) 1997 Foundations for osteopathic medicine. Williams and Wilkins, Baltimore

SPECIAL TOPIC 6
Red, white and black reaction

Many researchers and clinicians have described an assortment of responses in the form of 'lines', variously coloured from red to white and even blue-black, after application of local skin-dragging friction, with a finger or probe.

In the early days of osteopathy in the 19th century, the phenomenon was already in use. McConnell (1899) states:

> I begin at the first dorsal and examine the spinal column down to the sacrum by placing my middle fingers over the spinous processes and standing directly back of the patient draw the flat surfaces of these two fingers over the spinous processes from the upper dorsal to the sacrum in such a manner that the spines of the vertebrae pass tightly between the two fingers; thus leaving a red streak where the cutaneous vessels press upon the spines of the vertebrae. In this manner slight deviations of the vertebrae laterally can be told with the greatest accuracy by observing the red line. When a vertebra or section of vertebrae are too posterior a heavy red streak is noticed and when a vertebra or section of vertebrae are too anterior the streak is not so noticeable.

Much more recently, Marshall Hoag (1969) writes as follows regarding examination of the spinal area using skin friction.

> With firm but moderate pressure the pads of the fingers are repeatedly rubbed over the surface of the skin, preferably with extensive longitudinal strokes along the paraspinal area. The blunt end of an instrument or of a pen may be used to apply friction, since the purpose is simply to detect colour change, but care must be taken to avoid abrading the skin. The appearance of less intense and rapidly fading colour in certain areas as compared with the general reaction is ascribed to increased vasoconstriction in that area, indicating a disturbance in autonomic reflex activity. The significance of this red reaction and other evidence of altered reflex activity in relation to (osteopathic) lesions has been examined in research. Others give significance to an increased degree of erythema or a prolonged lingering of the red line response.

On the same theme Upledger & Vredevoogd (1983) write of this phenomenon:

> Skin texture changes produced by a facilitated segment [localised areas of hyperirritability in the soft tissues involving neural sensitisation to longterm stress] are palpable as you lightly drag your fingers over the nearby paravertebral area of the back. I usually do skin drag evaluation moving from the top of the neck to the sacral area in one motion. Where your fingertips drag on the skin you will probably find a facilitated segment. After several repetitions, with increased force, the affected area will appear redder than nearby areas. This is the 'red reflex'. Muscles and connective tissues at this level will:
>
> 1. Have a 'shotty' feel (like buckshot under the skin);
> 2. Be more tender to palpation;
> 3. Be tight, and tend to restrict vertebral motion; and
> 4. Exhibit tenderness of the spinous processes when tapped by fingers or a rubber hammer.

De Jarnette (1934), the developer of sacrooccipital technique (SOT), wrote extensively on the subject of the 'red reaction', with some complex interpretations suggested in his classic text *Reflex pain*. De Jarnette initially made assessments of patients (partly based on blood pressure readings) into various categories, during which process he has them treated in order to alter the relative oxygenation levels which he believed to be the basis of these categories. None of these methods are pertinent to this survey of skin reactions, but are a necessary preamble to his descriptions, which would be confusing otherwise. In a 'Type 1' patient (one of De Jarnette's categories), who has received the appropriate preliminary attention as outlined ('carbon dioxide elimination technic') he suggested the following:

> Sit or stand immediately behind the patient facing the patient's back. Have the patient bend slightly forward. Be sure the light is even on the patient's back to avoid shadows. Place the index and middle fingers of your right hand upon the 7th cervical vertebra, having the two fingers about an inch [2.5 cm] lateral from the spine of the 7th cervical vertebra. Keep the fingers evenly spaced as you go down the spine, so each line is as straight as possible. For the 'Type 1' patient (normal BP after appropriate techniques) use a light touch. To produce an even pressure of both fingers on the back they may be fortified by placing the fingers of the left hand over them. As you go down the spine, your pressure will be just hard enough to cause the fingers to dent the skin.
>
> Now *draw your fingers down the spine very quickly* ending at the coccyx. Step back and watch the reaction. A red line will usually appear all the way down the spine. This soon starts to fade and the fading is what you must watch. The area that appears reddest *as this fading starts*, is the major [lesion] for this patient and should be marked with a skin pencil. You will often notice on this type of patient that the major area is much wider than any other area of your lines down the back. This is caused by tissue infiltration.

The 'Type 2' category patient will have slightly high blood pressure after De Jarnette's preliminary treatment. After adopting the same starting position he suggests:

> Making a firm pressure, draw fingers down the spine, with a fairly slow motion. You should be able to count to 15 while drawing the fingers from the 7th cervical to the coccyx, by counting steadily. With a good light on the back, the results should show a line which becomes red, some portions brighter and some very faintly coloured. Now watch the lines fade. The area which shows the whitest is marked as the major [lesions] for this is the most anaemic spinal muscle area. It will be paler than any portion of skin on the patient's body.

Moving next to the final category (patients with high blood pressure) De Jarnette asks that you adopt the same start position and then:

> Making heavy pressure, come down the spine slowly, counting 20 as you go from 7th cervical to coccyx. Now watch the reaction. The line that shows the Whitest is the major [lesion]. In this type the blood pressure is over 180 (systolic) the whitest area shows a waxy, pale colour and may persist for several minutes.

Korr (1970) described how this red reflex phenomenon corresponded well with areas of lowered electrical resistance, which themselves correspond accurately to regions of lowered pain threshold and areas of cutaneous and deep tenderness (termed 'segmentally related sympatheticotonia'). Korr was able to detect areas of intense vasoconstriction which corresponded well with dysfunction elicited by manual clinical examination. He cautions:

> You must not look for perfect correspondence between the skin resistance (or the red reflex) and the distribution of deeper pathologic disturbance, because an area of skin which is segmentally related to a particular muscle does not necessarily overlie that muscle. With the latissimus dorsi, for example, the myofascial

disturbance might be over the hip but the reflex manifestations would be in much higher dermatomes because this muscle has its innervation from the cervical part of the cord.

By use of a mechanical instrument which quantified the pressure applied at a constant speed, followed by measurement of the duration of the redness resulting from the action of the frictional stimulator on the skin, Korr could detect areas of intense vasoconstriction which corresponded well with dysfunction elicited by manual clinical examination.

It could be said that the opportunity to 'feel' the tissues was being ignored during all these 'strokes' and 'drawing' of the fingers down the spinal musculature and this thought was not lost on Morrison (1969), who describes his views as follows.

> Run your fingers longitudinally down alongside the dorsal and lumbar vertebrae (anywhere from the spinous processes extending laterally up to two inches [5 cm]) and stop at any spot of tissue which seems 'harder' or different from normal tissue. These thickened areas, stringy ligaments, bunched muscle bands, all represent indurated tissue; they are usually protective and indicate irritation and dysfunction. Once these indurated areas are palpated press down and almost always they will be sensitive, indicating a need for treatment.

Morrison used a technique for easing such contractions similar to that later described by Lawrence Jones, in his strain/counterstrain system (Jones 1981).

Osteopathic researchers Cox et al (1983) wrote regarding their work on identification of palpable musculoskeletal findings in coronary artery disease (see notes on facilitated segments in Chapter 5) and describe their use of the red reflex as part of their examination procedures (other methods included range of motion testing of spinal segments and ribs, assessment of local pain on palpation and altered soft tissue texture). In their work the most sensitive parameters, which were found to be significant predictors for coronary stenosis, were limitation in range of motion and altered soft tissue texture:

> 'Red reflex' cutaneous stimulation was applied digitally in both paraspinal areas [T4 and T9–11] simultaneously briskly stroking the skin in a caudad direction. Patients were divided arbitrarily into three groups.
> Grade 1 – erythema of the spinal tissues lasting less than 15 seconds after cutaneous stimulation.
> Grade 2 – erythema persisting for 15 to 30 seconds after stimulation.
> Grade 3 – erythema persisting longer than 30 seconds after stimulation.

In this context the Grade 3 – maintained erythema – is seen to represent the most dysfunctional response.

Newman-Turner (1984) describes the research of another osteopath/ naturopath, Keith Lamont, who first described the 'black line' phenomenon.

> It is a common observation of osteopaths who use a spinal meter, to detect the most active lesions, that pressure on either side of the spine with a hemispherical probe of approximately 0.5 cm diameter, will, in some patients, elicit a dark blue or black line. The pressure of the probe is usually very light since it is intended to register variations in skin resistance, but it has a pinching-off effect on the arterioles and venules of the capillary network beneath the skin. Local engorgement of the capillary bed with deoxygenated venous blood causes the appearance of the line which slowly fades as the circulation returns.

This is considered by some to relate to a nutrient deficit in those patients in whom this sign is seen. Newman-Turner suggests that Lamont, who first drew attention to the black line phenomenon, found that administration of vitamin E, bioflavonoid complex and homoeopathic ferrum phosphate corrected this deficiency.

Hruby et al (1997) describe the thinking regarding this phenomenon.

> Perform the red reflex test by firmly, but with light pressure, stroking two fingers on the skin over the paraspinal tissues in a cephalad to a caudad direction. The stroked areas briefly become erythematous and almost immediately return to their usual color. If the skin remains erythematous longer than a few seconds, it may indicate an acute somatic dysfunction in the area. As the dysfunction acquires chronic tissue changes, the tissues blanch rapidly after stroking and are dry and cool to palpation.

The reader is reminded that Hilton's Law confirms simultaneous innervation to the skin covering the articular insertion of the muscles, not necessarily the entire muscle. Hilton's Law states that the nerve supplying a joint also supplies the muscles which move the joint and the skin covering the articular insertion of those muscles.

Making sense of the red reaction

Clearly there is a good deal to learn from and about the simple procedure of stroking the paraspinal muscles. Whether or not De Jarnette's preliminary methods are validated does not alter the possible wisdom of his subsequent observations, employing variable pressures and looking at the fading of redness, rather than the initial red reaction itself, for evidence of altered function.

Similarly, Lamont's nutritional observations would need verification, something which does not alter the fact that some patients demonstrate this unusual 'black streak'. As with so much in palpation, there is little question over whether 'something' is being felt or observed. It is the interpretation of what the 'something' means that excites debate.

The observations of Upledger, Korr, Hoag, Hruby, Morrison and McConnell (and their co-workers) are readily applicable and should be tested against known dysfunction to assess the usefulness of these methods during assessment. The research of Cox et al indicates that one musculoskeletal assessment method alone is probably not sufficiently reliable to be diagnostic; however, when, for example, tissue texture, changes in range of motion, pain and the 'red reaction' are all used, the presence of several of these is a good indication of underlying dysfunction which may involve the process of facilitation. This supports the thoughts expressed in Chapter 1.

A simpler use for the reaction

A less complex use of the red reaction is to go back a century to McConnell's method, in order to highlight spinal deviations. By creating erythema paraspinally you can stand back and visualise the general contours of the spine as well as any local deviations in the pattern created by application of your firm digital strokes.

Question

How do you know whether your palpating fingers or thumbs are applying equal pressure bilaterally during such assessments or when palpating elsewhere bilaterally?

A useful guide to the uniformity of pressure can be obtained by comparing the relative blanching of your nailbeds: are they equally white, pink, red?

SPECIAL TOPIC EXERCISE: RED REFLEX ASSESSMENT

Time suggested: 20 minutes

Perform the various 'strokes' as described in the descriptions above. Run your fingers or probes firmly down the tissues close to and parallel to the spine. Observe the 'red reaction' as well as how it fades. Look for areas which become more irritated and those which become less irritated, when compared with surrounding tissues.

Having marked the ones which respond most dramatically and those which fade fastest, repalpate the tissues using some or all of the methods discussed in Chapters 4, 5, 6 and 9, in order to evaluate what it is you sense as being different about the tissues.

Do tissues which seem hypertonic respond to brisk stroking of this sort differently to normal or more flaccid tissues?

Do you note increased sensitivity in areas which redden or blanch when stroked in this way or is there little difference?

How does the degree of skin 'tightness' vary over these different areas?

What is the degree of skin adherence to underlying connective tissue (when skin rolling or lifting) in the different areas?

If you scan from off the body can you sense differences in temperature in these contrasting areas?

Is eliciting of the 'red reflex' likely to be of any clinical value to you?

REFERENCES

Cox J, Gorbis S, Dick L, Rogers J 1983 Palpable musculoskeletal findings in coronary artery disease (double blind study). Journal of the American Osteopathic Association 82(11): 832
De Jarnette B 1934 Reflex Pain. Nebraska
Hoag M 1969 Osteopathic medicine. McGraw-Hill, New York
Hruby R, Goodridge J, Jones J 1997 Thoracic region and rib cage. In: Ward R (ed) Foundations for osteopathic medicine. Williams and Wilkins, Baltimore
Jones L 1981 Strain/counterstrain. Academy of Applied Osteopathy, Colorado Springs
Korr I 1970 The physiological basis of osteopathic medicine. Postgraduate Institute of Osteopathic Medicine and Surgery, New York
McConnell C 1899 The practice of osteopathy. Kirksville, MO
Morrison M 1969 Lecture notes. London
Newman Turner R 1984 Naturopathic medicine. Thorsons, Wellingborough
Upledger J, Vredevoogd W 1983 Craniosacral therapy. Eastland Press, Seattle

Palpation of subtle movements (including circulation of CSF, energy and 'has tissue a memory?')

Evaluating movement

In seeking methods for evaluation of subtle movement in the body we can once again turn to Viola Frymann (1963) for an introduction, as she describes what we should expect as we begin to palpate muscular tissues for anything other than their mechanical status.

> If the hand is laid on a healthy muscle mass, of a resting limb, it is often possible, in the space of a few seconds, to 'tune in' to the inherent motion within. A state of rapport, of fluid continuity, between the examiner and the examined may be established, and a whole new realm of palpatory exploration lies ahead. The continuity of fluid within the body is never interrupted in health – intra and inter-cellular fluid, lymph, cerebrospinal fluid – which is in a constant state of rhythmic, fluctuant motion.

Frymann maintains that the vitality of tissue can be judged by the strength of such motions, with a wide variety of grades of tissue vitality being apparent. The example is given of the difference in the 'feel' noted when a previously paralysed and a presently paralysed limb are palpated. In the first a mere 'murmur' of motion will be felt, whereas in the latter there will be no detectable rhythmic motion at all. Frymann goes further and states that judgement can also be made as to the likelihood of improvement, based on information such as this.

EXERCISE 6.1: SIMULTANEOUS PALPATION OF INNERVATED AND DEINNERVATED TISSUES

Time suggested: 3–5 minutes

If you have access to someone with a totally or partially paralysed limb (a stroke victim perhaps?), Frymann (1963) suggests you start by simultaneously placing one hand on the spinal segment which supplies the principal innervation to the affected limb and the other on the affected limb itself. Having done this, pause for a few minutes, all the while concentrating on any 'activity' under your hands.

The spinal hand should begin to register a rhythm. The degree to which the ('rhythmically integrated') response is subsequently felt in the other hand as well may represent the ultimate/potential viability of the presently paralysed tissues.

Frymann calls this communication, which in normal tissue has a surging, rhythmic, nature, the 'vital fluid tide' within. Can you sense this?

If you do not have immediate access to someone with a disability involving total or partial paralysis of a limb, then palpate for rhythmic activity such as that described by Frymann in normal tissue, until the

continues

EXERCISE 6.1 *(Continued)*

'reading' of its presence becomes easy for you, and when a paralysed limb is accessible palpate this too, in order to register the profound difference.

What is the rhythmic 'fluid tide' which can be felt when we palpate, for example in Exercises 3.18, 3.19, 3.20?

It is necessary to come to an understanding of aspects of physiological function as it relates to this vital fluid tide, most notably how cerebrospinal fluid circulates, possibly throughout the whole body, as well as something of the trophic function of nerves.

Erlinghauser's research – cerebrospinal fluid circulation

For a deeper understanding of the concepts being discussed here, you are referred to an article by Ralph Erlinghauser (1959), as well as to Upledger & Vredevoogd (1983). The subject is further developed by Oschman (2001) in his evaluation of energy fluctuations and the topic of entrainment (see Chapter 3).

Erlinghauser starts his discussion with the news that research has demonstrated that collagen (connective tissue) has a tubular structure (Kennedy 1955, Wyckoff 1952), a discovery which, he believes, will revolutionise our understanding of human physiology. Cerebrospinal fluid (CSF) motion is considered by many cranial osteopaths to play a major part in controlling a vital 'semiclosed' hydraulic system. This is bounded by the cranial vaults themselves and the dural membranes which, together, form the semiclosed aspects of the unit.

CSF enters and leaves this hydraulic system via the choroid plexuses and the arachnoid villi. As well as giving shape and stability (and, some believe, motion) to this system, the largely incompressible CSF also fluctuates through the tubular collagen fibrils of the connective tissues throughout the body. CSF is seen to act as a transport medium between the subarachnoid space and cells of the body. Additionally, as Oschman (2001) points out, CSF (as well as blood and lymph) is an excellent conductor of electricity and probably forms pathways via which electromagnetic impulses are channelled throughout the body.

> Oscillations of the brain's direct current field, the brain waves, are not confined to the brain. Instead, they propagate through the circulatory system, which is a good conductor, and along the peripheral nerves, following the perineural system, which reaches into every part of the body that is innervated. Similarly, oscillations of the heart's electrical activity are not confined to the heart muscle, but are propagated through the vascular system, perivascular connective tissue, and living matrix to all parts of the body.

Erlinghauser's discovery of collagen's tubular structure indicates that, far from connective tissue being merely structurally supportive (as it anatomically connects epithelial, muscular and nervous tissues), it can also be assumed to be linked to these tissues histologically, biochemically, physiologically, energetically and, of course, pathologically, when dysfunction/disease is present.

Connective tissue, with its hollow, tubular fibril structure, is continuous throughout the body, from the fascia of the skull to that of the feet. It provides fascial planes, envelopes, reflections and spaces, as well as ligaments and tendons, giving protection, cohesion, form, shape and support to the circulatory, lymphatic and nervous systems, which it separates, shapes and binds.

In 1939, WG Sutherland (1948), having established that the cranial bones had a constant rhythmic physiological range of motion, postulated that CSF fluctuation provided the mechanism which moved these. While the CSF theory is not fully

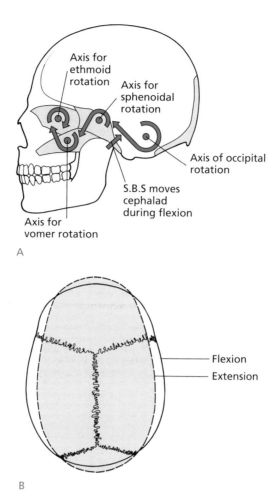

Fig. 6.1A Schematic representation of cranial motion. During flexion, the occiput is thought to move anterosuperior, which causes the sphenoid to rise at its synchondrosis. Simultaneous movement occurs in the frontal, facial and nasal bones as indicated. The extension phase of this motion involves a return to a neutral position. (**B**) The flexion phase of cranial motion (inhalation phase) causes the skull, as a whole, to widen and flatten.

accepted by cranial therapists, subsequent studies have certainly confirmed that, although sutures provide a strong bond between cranial bones, they do allow movement (Chaitow 1999). Other workers have considered that such motion as is observed relates to variations in venous, arterial and respiratory pressures, and these do undoubtedly have the potential for such an influence, (see Fig. 6.1).

It is also considered that there exist within the brain cells which provide a further rhythmic pulsation which influences fluid motion (the oligodendroglia). Pulsations of between 6 and 12 per minute are now considered to be the norm in good health, for what has been termed the 'primary respiratory mechanism' in cranial osteopathy. These rhythms are unrelated to normal respiration or heart rate and are seen to operate in all mammals. Research indicates that oxygen reaches fine neural structures at this rate (8–12 waves per minute) and that administration of carbon dioxide (30%) stops the waves in humans. In animal studies, the administration to anaesthetised dogs of high concentrations of carbon dioxide has been shown to lead to a precipitous rise in CSF pressure. In the rhythmical coiling and uncoiling of the oligodendroglial cells, which possibly provide part of the pulsating impetus for CSF fluctuation, we may have one explanation for its motive power through the channels which exist within connective tissue.

Erlinghauser provides ample research validation for this concept (much simplified in this account) of the circulation of CSF, from the subarachnoid spaces via tubular collagen fibrils to the intercellular spaces, where it combines with tissue fluids, being in turn reabsorbed by the end-lymph vessels into the lymph system and thence to the venous system. This leads, naturally enough, to the conclusion that any derangement of the connective tissue system must result in limitations to the physiological flow of CSF within the collagen fibrils, with negative consequences to cellular health.

If we want to obtain palpatory evidence of dysfunction affecting the musculoskeletal system (which will always involve connective tissue), the ability of the palpator to 'read' the rhythmic pulsation of CSF becomes very important indeed. This is the 'vital fluid' which Frymann referred to above.

Whatever moves CSF, what matters in our palpation studies is the fact that fluid fluctuations occur, that they can be palpated and they have significance. Upledger (1983) summarises the cranial (and other osseous and soft tissue) motions which result from, or which take part in, the rhythmic motion of CSF. Recall that this has a rhythm of 6–12 cycles per minute under normal circumstances. Primary respiratory flexion is the term applied to the extreme range of motion occurring during each of these cycles, at which time the head becomes wider transversely and shorter in its anteroposterior dimension (see Fig. 6.1). At the same time, the entire body externally rotates and widens. There is then a brief pause before the body returns to the starting position (termed cranial extension) during which time the head narrows and elongates, as the rest of the body goes into internal rotation. All these motions are very slight indeed (measurable in microns) but once you learn of their existence, palpation of them during the approximately 6–8 seconds of a full cycle can be learned fairly quickly.

Upledger (1983) says:

> Once you tune into these motions, you can perceive your own body doing flexion-extension cycles as you stand or walk. After a time you will learn to tune yourself in and out of your own physiological body motion as well.

The craniosacral connection

One other anatomical link needs to be explained regarding this concept – the cranial link to the sacrum. The connection between the occiput and the sacrum involves the dural membrane, which is itself continuous with the meningeal membranes. If the occiput moves (minutely) anteriorly as the flexion phase of the cranial respiratory cycle commences, it appears to create a synchronous movement at the sacral base (see Fig. 6.2), which moves posteriorly during this phase (taking the sacral apex and coccyx anteriorly).

Remarkable video evidence of this synchrony of motion has been made as a result of the clinical and research work of Dr Marc Pick (2001), screened at a conference in London (see Fig. 6.2). What should we be trying to learn from our palpation of these rhythms and cycles? Upledger summarises:

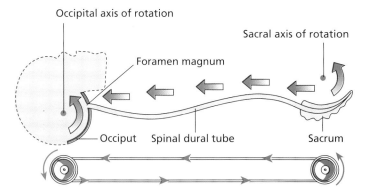

Fig. 6.2 Schematic representation of synchrony of motion between the sacrum and the occiput.

From the diagnostic, prognostic and therapeutic points of view, we are interested in a qualitative estimate of the strength of the inherent energy which is driving the physiological motion, the symmetry of the body motion response (both of the craniosacral system and of the extrinsic body connective tissues), and in the range and quality of each cyclical motion. Is it fighting against a resistance barrier?

Not only is there useful information available when palpating the cranial and sacral components of this complex but it is possible to feel the cycle in any tissues of the body, even in patients who are in a vegetative state.

Palpation hint

It is suggested that in all early exercises in which cranial motion or craniosacral rhythms are being assessed, you should think in terms of a slight 'surging' sensation, sometimes described as feeling 'as though the tide is coming in' or a feeling of 'fullness' under the palpating hand, rather than expecting to feel movement of a grosser nature. After a few seconds this 'surge' will be felt to recede; the tide goes out again. This is a subtle sensation but once you have tuned into it, it is unmistakable and very real indeed.

EXERCISE 6.2: PALPATION OF SYNCHRONY BETWEEN OCCIPUT AND SACRUM

Time suggested: approximately 7 minutes for each of Exercises 3.18, 3.19, 3.20, which should be repeated, plus 5–8 minutes for Exercise 6.2

Go back to Chapter 3 and repeat Exercises 3.18, 3.19, 3.20, which focused your attention on cranial and sacral rhythms. Follow these with this exercise.

Your partner lies on her side, pillow under the head in order to avoid any side bending of the neck. You are seated behind and place one hand on the occiput (fingers going over the crown) and the other on the sacrum, fingers towards the coccyx.

Take some minutes to 'tune in to' the motions of the occiput and the sacrum. Are they synchronous?

When you have satisfied yourself (5 minutes should be ample), have the model remove the pillow so that the neck is side bent (Fig. 6.3). Repalpate and compare the results.

Can you feel the synchronous motions under your hands? What changes occur when the neck is not supported on the cushion?

continues

EXERCISE 6.2 *(Continued)*

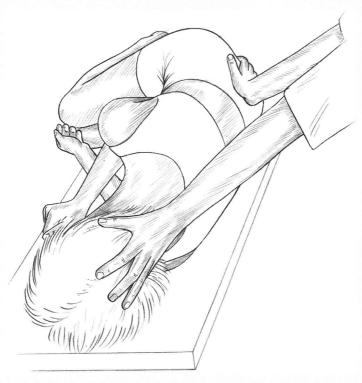

Fig. 6.3 Palpation for the synchrony of motion between the sacrum and the occiput.

EXERCISE 6.3: PALPATING CRANIAL MOTION FROM THE LEGS

Time suggested: 3–5 minutes

Have your palpation partner lie supine. You stand at the foot of the table, cradling one foot (heel) in each hand. Close your eyes and feel for external rotation of the leg during the flexion phase of the craniosacral cycle and internal rotation as it returns to neutral, during the extension phase (see Fig. 6.4). Does holding the breath change this?

Once you have become keenly aware of this motion, compare the ease of motion in the intrinsic rotation of the two legs. Does there seem to be an easier feel to the external or the internal rotation, symmetrically or in one leg or the other?

continues

EXERCISE 6.3 *(Continued)*

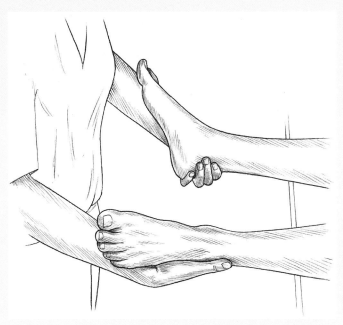

Fig. 6.4   Palpating craniosacral rhythmic motion via the feet.

EXERCISE 6.4: SPHENOIDAL DECOMPRESSION 'LAYER' PALPATION

Time suggested: 5–7 minutes

In this palpation you will attempt to evaluate sensations which partly involve mechanical/structural cranial features, as well as more subtle sensations. The patient's head is cradled in your hands so that the fingers enfold the occiput and the thumbs rest lightly on the great wings of the sphenoid (see Figure 3.2, p. 66).

First take out all the skin slack under your thumbs so that you have a firm purchase over the wings themselves, not on the supraorbital ridges or the orbital portions of the zygomae. Milne (1995) suggests $1/5$ of an ounce contact pressure, which is approximately 5.5 grams, much the same as recommended by Upledger & Vredevoogd (1983).

By lightly drawing your thumbs toward your hands, the sphenoid is 'crowded toward the occiput'. This crowding is held for several seconds, after which the thumbs should alter their direction of effort, as they are lightly drawn directly toward the ceiling, so (theoretically) decompressing the sphenobasilar junction and applying traction to the tentorium cerebelli (one of the reciprocal tension membranes within the skull), as the weight of the cranium drags onto your palms and fingers.

Milne (1995) suggests that it is possible to distinguish six levels of tissue separation, from first contact to final completion, during this exquisite palpation exercise.

1. Skin, scalp and fascia
2. Slow release of the occipitofrontalis and temporalis muscles (mainly)
3. Sutural separation ('akin to prising apart a magnet from a piece of metal')
4. Dural release (like 'elastic bands reluctantly giving way')

continues

5. Freeing of the cerebrospinal fluid circulation ('the whole head suddenly feels oceanic, tidal, expansive. This is the domain of optimized cerebrospinal fluid')
6. Finally energetic release ('a tactile sensation of chemical electrical fire unrolling and spreading outwards in waves under your fingers')

In this poetic language we can sense the nature of the debate between those who wish to understand what is happening in orthopaedic terms and those who embrace 'fluid/electric' and energetic concepts.

Creating a still point

Upledger's writings are a treasure house of information for anyone who wishes to add craniosacral work to their repertoire. Instruction in workshop or seminar settings is, however, essential before this is applied therapeutically.

It is both possible and desirable during palpatory training for the student to learn to briefly interrupt the cranial cycles, a process known as inducing a 'still' point. This can be done from many places in the body, for example from the feet, as in Exercise 6.3, or from the sacrum or occiput.

What is required is that the palpating hands follow the palpated part as it goes to the limit of the flexion or extension phase and to then 'lock' the part(s) at this limit of motion, not by applying pressure but by means of restraining the tendency to go into the next phase of the cycle, the return to neutral. This attempt to halt normal motion is repeated after subsequent cycles, until the rhythm stops completely, for some seconds or even minutes This is the 'still' point (see Exercise 6.5).

After a while, the palpating (restraining) hand(s) will begin to sense the movement trying to start again. The normal motion is then allowed and a general improvement is usually noted in the amplitude and symmetry of the motion.

Time suggested: 10–12 minutes

To start the exercise in establishing a 'still' point, go back to Exercise 5.3. When you have established that you can clearly sense a rhythm of external and internal rotation of the legs, during the flexion and extension phases of the craniosacral movement cycle, start to follow the external rotation while preventing any return to internal rotation of the legs, when this phase is perceived.

Do not forcibly rotate the legs, simply go with the external rotation each time it occurs, taking up additional slack to its limit, and then prevent any return to the neutral position.

After a number of cycles (Upledger says anywhere from five to 20 repetitions), during which slight increases in external rotation will be achieved, the impulses should cease.

continues

EXERCISE 6.4 (Continued)

There may be sensations of tremor, slight shuddering or pulling noted through your contact hands, possibly arising from elsewhere in the system (as the cranial impulses try to deal with the restriction), but eventually this too should cease and the 'still' point will have been reached.

During this phase the person acting as your model will relax deeply, breathing may alter and corrections may occur spontaneously within the musculoskeletal system.

CAUTION: The 'still' point may easily be initiated via cranial and sacral structures but practising of this approach on such structures is not recommended without guidance and training, as it is all too easy to traumatise the craniosacral mechanisms. Working on the same mechanism from the feet is safe.

DISCUSSION REGARDING EXERCISES 6.1–6.5

From a palpation point of view this is as far as we can go with our exercises in assessment and manipulation of cranial fluid fluctuations and rhythms.

By practising the exercises as described, you should have become sensitive to the subtle, yet powerful phenomenon which has been described as the primary respiratory mechanism and which forms a major information source and therapeutic tool in cranial manipulation.

Just how this is integrated into your work depends on the degree of interest this avenue excites in you and how much cranial study/training you undertake. The heightened awareness of subtle rhythms which these palpation exercises should have produced is, however, of value whether or not your work ultimately involves cranial manipulative methods.

Therapeutically this has the effect of enhancing fluid motion, restoring flexibility and reducing congestion.

Energy

The ideas of a number of eminent clinicians and researchers now take us from CSF fluctuations and cranial rhythms to an area which can best be described as the palpation of energy flow. This is a topic which many find difficult to deal with, either intellectually or practically. The best advice the author can give is that you temporarily suspend disbelief and attempt the various exercises outlined below, based on the work of Becker, Smith, Oschman and Upledger, amongst others, and see what you feel. Whether or not you accept the explanations which these respected researchers and clinicians give for 'their' approach to reading and manipulating what they conceive as energy fluctuations in the body is quite another matter.

If you have patience, you will undoubtedly feel movements and rhythms as you follow the exercises given below and for the purpose of learning to 'feel', you are asked to accept that these represent, in one form or another, 'energy'. In Chapter 11 we will be looking at even more subtle energy manifestations, as used in methods such as 'therapeutic touch', and the discussion below should be kept in mind as that chapter is studied, for we are entering an area which is ill-defined, where function and concepts of energy interactions are mixed and blurred.

That something palpable exists which is called energy by numerous researchers and practitioners is not in question. What remains controversial is its nature and function.

Before exploring the work of clinicians, a major researcher into energy phenomena offers a glimpse of what may be happening as we enter this twilight zone of current understanding. Oschman (2001) has researched this topic deeply and these are some of his observations.

> Over half a century ago Burr (1957, 1972) and his colleagues published evidence that early stages of pathology, including cancer, can be diagnosed as disturbances in the body's electrical field and that reestablishing a normal field will halt the progress of disease.
>
> In 1962 Baule & McFee (1963) used a pair of 2 million-turn coils on the chest to pick up the magnetic field produced by the electrical activity of the heart muscle.
>
> Also in 1962 Josephson (1965) developed the concept of quantum tunnelling which found many important applications, including the development of a magnetometer of unprecedented sensitivity, known as the SQUID (Superconducting Quantum Interference Device).
>
> By 1967 the SQUID was able to record the heart's biomagnetic field clearly (Cohen 1967). Magnetocardiograms produced in this way were clearer than electrocardiograms, because electrical fields are distorted as they pass through the various layers of tissue between the source and the skin surface, however these tissues are transparent to magnetic fields.
>
> By 1972 the biomagnetic field of the brain could be recorded (magnetoencephalogram). The field of the brain has been found to be hundreds of times weaker than the heart's field (Cohen 1972).
>
> In the 1970s Bassett and colleagues developed pulsing electromagnetic field therapy (PEMF) that stimulates repair of fracture non-unions. By 1979 the FDA approved this method and by 1995 more than 300,000 non-union fractures, world wide, had been treated this way. The PEMF method has since been modified for treating soft tissues, such as nerves, ligaments, skin, and capillaries (Bassett 1978, MacGinitie 1995).
>
> Using the SQUID magnetometer, Zimmerman (1990) has been able to demonstrate that a signal can be measured emanating from the hands of practitioners using Therapeutic Touch, as well as non-practitioners, in the range of 7–8 Hz. Similar studies in Japan showed the hands of martial arts practitioners (QiGong, yoga, etc.) emitting pulsed biomagnetic pulses centred around 8–10 Hz, precisely the range used by biomedical researchers to 'jump-start' the healing of soft and hard tissues (Seto et al 1992).

You must make of this information what you will; however, the evidence is that forms of electromagnetic energy emerge from the human hand which, when generated by machines, have a healing potential. And as the SQUID evidence shows, large, measureable electromagnetic energy fields exist around the heart (and other organs) and particularly the brain. Whether we can sense, feel, palpate these

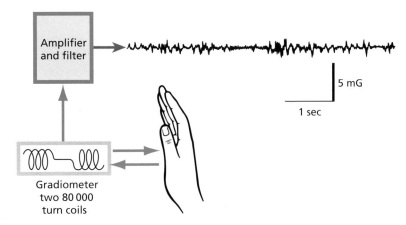

Fig. 6.5   Biomagnetic field measurement during 'chi emission' from the hand of a female subject in Tokyo. The double-coil magnetometer recorded a pulsating magnetic field that averaged 2 mGauss, peak to peak, with frequency of 8–10 Hz (after Seto et al 1992, with permission from Oschman 2001).

energies and whether we can consciously activate the forces which our hands emit is a matter for debate. (Palpation without touch will be evaluated in Chapter 11.)

Some of the ideas of different practitioners outlined below seem clearly to impinge on this area of energy medicine.

Layers of energy?

Dr Fritz Smith (1986) outlines his model of energy patterns within and around the body. Smith suggests that there is a non-differentiated field which pervades the body, which extends some distance beyond the limits of the physical body. He suggests that the currents which move within us are organised into:

1. A deep layer which flows through the skeletal system;
2. A middle layer which flows through the soft tissues (neurovascular bundles, fascia, muscle cleavages, and so on) as described in Traditional Chinese Medicine, and;
3. A superficial layer which is found just below the skin.
   These energy patterns are capable of disruption if the physical medium through which they pass (bone, soft tissue, skin) is traumatised or stressed, and the non-differentiated field may carry 'imprints' of imbalances caused by physical, toxic or emotional insults and traumas, especially if these have not been absorbed by specific tissues or systems.

Energy cysts and chakras

Before examining the work of Smith and of Rollin Becker in relation to such energy patterns, we will also need to become familiar with Upledger's concept of the 'energy cyst' and in order to do so we need to look at the chakra system, as described in Ayurvedic medicine. One of the palpable phenomena of the energy system is said to be the chakras, or energy centres, which are situated at specific sites on the body and which can be palpated on the surface or just off the surface. It is not necessary to accept the existence of chakras as such in order to palpate them, as they can simply be conceived as areas where circulating energy is more organised, or dense, or where neurological activity creates increased rhythmic patterns of subtle movement. The original concept of chakras was Ayurvedic (Indian), as was the word *prana* (energy), used to describe the vital 'substance' with which they are associated. The chakras are described as involving a clockwise circulation of energy (prana, chi) at seven specific sites, said to range in size from about 3 to 15 cm in diameter.

1. The root chakra is palpated just above the pubis, Upledger suggests, with one hand under the sacrum and the other resting on the lower abdomen. It is said to relate to sexual function.

2. The navel chakra is best palpated similarly, one hand under the lumbar spine, the other just below the navel (no hand pressure, just a touch). This is said to relate to emotions and sensitivity.

3. The spleen chakra is best palpated, says Upledger, with one hand over the lumbodorsal junction and the other over the epigastrium and is said to relate to energy assimilation and immunity.

4. The heart chakra requires one hand under the midthoracic spine and the other touching the central sternal area and is said to relate to emotions connected with love as well as 'hurt' feelings.

5. The throat chakra should be palpated with one hand behind the neck and the other over the centre of the throat. It may be felt as two centres of spinning energy and is said to relate to personal communication and relationships.

6. The brow chakra may be palpated with a hand under the occiput and three fingers over the glabella. It has an intense energy 'feel' relating, it is said, to intuitive perception.

7. The crown chakra is palpated at the crown of the head where it may be felt as an energy outflow rather than a spinning energy centre, related, it is said, to the pineal gland and to spiritual factors.

EXERCISE 6.6: CHAKRA PALPATION

Time suggested: 2 minutes per chakra centre

Your palpation partner should be supine (or seated). Place one hand beneath (behind) and one above (in front of) the chakra centre as described above (see also p 347, Fig. 10.3), resting your hands on the tissues.

As you palpate the chakras, do you sense any surge, vibration, churning, fluctuation of motion under your hands?

This is an exercise to repeat after completing some of the work suggested in the exercises below, if the chakra concept interests you.

Restricted energy flow: the Varma and Upledger models

Both TCM and Ayurvedic medicine hold that there are channels over the surface of the body, and within it, which are conduits for the flow of energy. If these are blocked or altered, the result is dysfunction or disease.

It may be useful to consider a similarity in the ideas of different clinicians, separated by time and culture, whose concepts were very close, if not identical. Stanley Lief, the developer of neuromuscular technique (see Chapter 5) was greatly influenced by Dr Dewanchand Varma, an Ayurvedic practitioner working in Paris in the early 1930s, whose method of treatment of energy imbalances utilised an early form of NMT, which he called 'pranotherapy'.

Varma (1935) discussed the ways in which 'electromagnetic currents' derived from the atmosphere (at the chakras) were capable of becoming obstructed 'by certain adhesions, in which the muscular fibres harden together so that the nervous currents can no longer pass through them'. Varma mentions changes in the skin when such obstructions occur, saying:

> If the skin becomes attached to the underlying muscle, the current cannot pass, the part loses its sensibility.

This is remarkably close to Lewit's description of hyperalgesic skin zones (see Chapter 4).

Varma's pranotherapy method, a form of manual soft tissue manipulation designed to release these palpable obstructions, was incorporated by Lief into what became NMT (see Chapter 5). But how were the obstructions and adhesions dealt with?

Varma suggested a two-stage treatment which, as in NMT, is actually an assessment during which treatment can be imparted. The first part of the assessment/treatment involved the tissues being prepared by rubbing with oil. The actual manipulation of the tissues was performed by first 'separating' skin from underlying tissue, followed by a gentle 'separation' of the muscle fibres, a process which required:

> . . . highly sensitive fingers able to distinguish between thick and thin fibres, and
> . . . highly developed consciousness and sensitivity, attained by hours of patient daily practice on the living body.

While these are descriptions of some interest, they fail to describe adequately what Varma actually did to the tissues.

My late uncle, Boris Chaitow (the co-developer of NMT with his cousin Stanley Lief), has commented on Varma's methods, saying that the most valuable essential which he derived from Varma came as a result of having treatment from him, many times (Chaitow 1983, personal communication). It was during one of these sessions that the 'variable pressure' factor become apparent, something which Chaitow believed to be invaluable in both assessment and treatment. This subtle factor, which allows the palpating hand/digit to 'meet the tissues', not overwhelm them, is a factor which will be seen again when we come to examine Fritz Smith's research work, later in this chapter.

John Upledger (1987) has described how his concept of an 'energy cyst' developed as he worked with biophysicists, psychologists, biochemists, neurophysiologists and others at the Michigan State University College of Osteo-pathic Medicine:

> The energy cyst is a construct of our imagination, which may have objective reality. We believe that it manifests as an obstruction to the efficient conduction of electricity through the body tissues (primarily fascia), where it resides, acts as an irritant contributing to the development of the facilitated segment [see Chapter 5] and as a localised irritable focus.

Varma had hypothesised his 'obstructions' to energy (prana) flow over 60 years before Upledger's development of the 'energy cyst' theory, which is quite remarkably similar. (There is no suggestion whatever that Upledger or his fellow workers had, or have, any knowledge of Varma and his work, which quite simply vanished, almost without trace, during the Second World War, leaving behind Lief's NMT.)

Upledger believes that the 'cyst' interrupts the flow of chi, the Chinese term for energy, and that, by palpation, these obstructions can be readily located. They can result, says Upledger (1987), from trauma, infection, physiological dysfunction (see commentary in Chapter 5 as to how soft tissue changes occur and progress) mental or emotional problems or through disturbance of the chakras. What do 'energy cysts' feel like? 'The cyst is hotter, more energetic, less organised and less functional than surrounding tissues' (Upledger 1987).

How does Upledger pinpoint a cyst? He uses a method which he terms interference arcing, in which he 'feels' for waves, or arcs of energy, relating to such dysfunctional centres. The cysts seem to generate interference waves which can be sensed (usually pulsating at a much faster rate than normal tissue) superimposed on the normal rhythms of tissue. If these waves can be imagined as being like ripples on a pond surface, after a pebble has disturbed the surface, it is possible to visualise that the palpating hands could 'zero in' on the centre of the wave pattern, to locate the source, the cyst. It would not matter from which direction, in relation to the cyst, the hands were coming in their palpation, for the centre would remain constant, as would the wave pattern.

Note: It may prove useful to compare the image of an energy cyst, as pictured by Upledger, with that of the 'eye' of the disturbance, which Becker describes in his work later in this chapter.

EXERCISE 6.7: PALPATING FOR AN 'ENERGY CYST'

Time suggested: 10–15 minutes

Your palpation partner should be lying prone or supine.

Palpate for 'energy cysts/arcs' in an area of soft tissue dysfunction, previously identified using the methods of Lewit, Lief or Nimmo (i.e. use a trigger point or other area of reflex activity as your starting point).

Place your finger(s)/hand(s) in touch with the surface being palpated, without force, waiting for a sense of rhythmic patterns present in the tissues.

Try to determine from which direction waves are being sensed.

Reposition your hands whenever you wish, in order to more clearly localise the focal centre of any wave-like patterns you may be picking up.

Can you sense the waves? Can you localise the centre of an area of disturbance?

If you find this particular exercise difficult, in that the patterns being sought seem hard to identify, the work of Smith, as described below, may help.

A brief introduction to zero balancing

Smith (1986) has explained his concepts and methods, which he named 'zero balancing'. He has clarified this as representing a 'guide to energy movement and body structure'.

He describes the following realisation, after 10 years of study of both orthodox and traditional (mainly Oriental) medical methods:

> During this process I came to recognise a specific area in a person where movement and structure are in juxtaposition, similar to the situation in a sailboat where the wind (movement) and the sail (structure) meet. From the explanation of the interface, in 1973, I formulated the structural acupressure system of Zero Balancing, to evaluate and balance the relationship between energy and structure.

Smith has examined the relationship between ancient energy concepts and modern medicine, Eastern esoteric anatomy and Western human anatomy, subjective inner experiences and objective observation. This approach is of considerable value and importance to those practitioners who struggle to align the apparent contradictions faced when comparing the variables in theory and methodology which exist between Western and Eastern medicine.

Smith examines what he terms 'the foundations for the energetic bridge' and looks at, among other areas, 'foundation joints'.

These, he says, are the:

- cranial bones of the skull
- sacroiliac articulations
- intercarpal articulations of the hand
- pubic symphysis
- intertarsal articulations of the foot.

These, he maintains, transmit and balance the energetic forces of the body, rather than being merely involved in movement and locomotion. They have in common small ranges of motion and little or no voluntary movement potential. In all cases, movement in these structures occurs in response to forces acting upon them, rather than being initiated by the part itself.

Therefore, if there is an imbalance or altered function in any of these joints, the body is obliged to compensate for the problem, rather than being able to resolve the situation through adaptation. Such compensation can be widespread and will often involve other associated structures, commonly becoming 'locked into' the body, limiting its ability to function normally. Smith believes that these joints have the closest relationship with the subtle (energy) body and any limitation in them, he suggests, can be seen as a direct read-out of the energetic component of the body.

He reminds us of the basic law of physics (Hooke's Law) which states that the effect of stress on any mechanism will spread until it is absorbed or until the mechanism breaks down. What Smith is pointing to is the fact that stresses will spread into these 'foundation areas' and that, because they have no power of voluntary motion, they will absorb the strains until these become locked into them or until there is a restoration of normality by outside forces. Smith further identifies what he terms 'semi-foundation' joints, such as the:

- intervertebral articulations
- rib joints (costovertebral, costochondral, costotransversus)
- clavicular articulations with the first rib and sternum.

He describes a variety of assessment methods capable of identifying reductions in the normal energy flow, in tissues associated with distressed foundation and semi-foundation joints, and describes methods which he uses to restore normal function, when reduced energy flow is perceived. He makes much of the usefulness in assessment of the ability to identify 'end of motion range' in joint play (discussed in Special topic 9, relating to joint play and end-feel).

Smith's 'essential touch' palpation

Smith's work, therefore, seems to be a bridge between the gross methods of Western physiological methodology and the apparently abstract concepts of 'energy' medicine. He explains the way he makes contact with the patient. He calls this 'essential touch', saying, quite rightly, that it is common in bodywork to be touched only on the physical level, not to have a significant energetic interchange take place. The connection which he wants to achieve transcends the physical touching and involves an instinctive, intuitive, yet conscious action on the part of the aware therapist.

What should we feel when this is achieved? Smith describes it thus:

> There are a number of sensations, mostly involving the feeling of movement or aliveness, which let us know we are engaging an energy field. We may perceive a fine vibration in the other person's body, or in the aura, a feeling we are making contact with a low voltage current. This may be described as tingling, buzzing, a chill sensation, 'goose bumps', as well as a subtle sensation that some people describe as 'vibration'. We may also perceive a grosser feeling of movement as though the person's body, or our own, were expanding or contracting, even though we see no physical change.

This is not dissimilar to Frymann's description early in this chapter. Smith uses the concept of a fulcrum in order to establish his contact, as do other workers in this field, notably Becker and Lief, although in each case the descriptions of their individual fulcrums are somewhat different. A fulcrum is defined, says Smith, as a balance point, a position, element or agency through, around or by means of which vital powers are exercised.

> The simplest fulcrum is created by the direct pressure of one or more fingers into the body, to form a firm support, around which the body can orient.

The fulcrum needs to be 'deep' enough into the body, so that the physical slack of the tissue is taken up; this is the point at which any further pressure meets with resistance in the tissue beneath the fingers. Getting 'in touch' with the person's energy field is thus achieved by taking up slack from tissues, so that any additional movement on your part will be translated directly into the person's experience.

Compare the similarity between this description and the request, by Lief and Boris Chaitow, that digital or hand pressure, being applied in use of NMT, should be 'variable', matching that of the tissues it is meeting.

Note: Smith insists that there should be frequent breaks (he calls these 'disconnects') from the patient when energy exercises (or therapy) are being performed. A loss of sensitivity (which he calls 'accommodation') otherwise takes place, as well as a draining of the therapist's vital reserves.

EXERCISE 6.8: SMITH'S BALLOON AND RUBBER BAND PALPATIONS

Time suggested: 3–4 minutes

Smith suggests we learn to practise this approach using a water-filled balloon, 25 cm or so in diameter. Place this on a table and slip your fingers under it. Raise your fingers slowly and be sensitive to the pressure on your finger tips.

As the fingers are raised, slack is taken out of your own tissues as well as the slack of the balloon.

As you increase pressure there will come a moment when you make 'connect' with the mass of water in the balloon and, at that moment, the fingertips are acting as a fulcrum for the balloon. At any fulcrum or balance point, there is solid contact with the material. In this instance the mass orients around the finger and any further pressure will affect the energy.

When you are performing this exercise on the partially water-filled balloon, can you sense the moment when your contact stops removing slack and becomes a fulcrum?

continues

EXERCISE 6.8 *(Continued)*

Other ways of creating a fulcrum, apart from direct pressure with finger or hand, can involve stretching, twisting, bending or sliding contacts. For example, Smith suggests you take a rubber band and stretch it, taking out the slack. At that point he likens what you have done to 'making contact' in the patient situation. Any further movement or stretch will involve the rubber itself.

EXERCISE 6.9: PALPATION USING HALF-MOON VECTOR

Time suggested: 10–15 minutes

Your palpation partner should lie prone.

With the experiences of the rubber band and the balloon fresh in your mind, make contact by placing a hand onto soft tissues and lightly pull the hand towards yourself and when the slack has been removed in that direction, slightly 'lift' your hand from the tissues, without actually losing contact.

Smith describes this as a 'half-moon' vector, since it combines both lifting and pulling motions which translate into a curved pull, which is the key to what he seeks.

Once you have taken out the physical slack and established an interface (fulcrum) with the tissues, any additional movement on your part will be felt by the person being touched and any movement in the person's body (even very subtle ones) should be perceived by you.

At this point you are in touch at the energy level. Can you feel it? Stay with the contact for some time and assess what you feel.

Record your description of the sensations you are feeling.

Fine-tuning

It is with such a contact (half-moon vector), Smith states, that you should feel vibrations and currents and by adding more movement yourself, you can judge how the tissue (or the patient as a whole) responds.

To fine-tune the fulcrum contact he asks himself 'How does this feel to the patient?' or 'How would this feel if it were done to me?'. The response helps him decide whether to pull harder or more gently, to twist more or less. He also asks the patient how it feels to them, suggesting that with a straight pressure fulcrum a 'nice hurt' is what is desirable.

Personal note

Long before I was aware of Smith's work (but possibly after reading Becker's ideas) I came to use a contact which achieves very similar results, in a diagnostic sense, to that described by Smith. I would make a hand contact, mainly involving the palmar surface, with fingers lightly touching but not usually involved. I tried to think of the palm as though I were applying a suction pad to glass, lifting and slightly turning the cupped contact until there is a feel of 'suction' between my hand and the patient. The writhing, pulsating or flickering sensations of the energy field are noticed almost immediately.

Try this and see what you feel. Compare it to the 'half-moon vector' exercise above. Is it the same?

Smith suggests the following exercises to help in assessment of bone status.

EXERCISE 6.10: PALPATING AN ENERGY INTERFACE IN THE FOREARM

Time suggested: 7–10 minutes

1 Take hold of your palpation partner's forearm, above the wrist and below the elbow. Take out the slack by 'pulling' your hands apart, until the point is reached where you have created a fulcrum.

2 After taking up the slack of the physical body, and the soft tissues, by pulling your hands apart (see Special topic 8 notes on end-feel), the resistance of the bone itself will be encountered. Any additional movement, from this interface position, will be felt by both the person being palpated and yourself.

Now gently put a bend or 'bow' into the arm. Try making this 'bowing' motion in one direction, just as far as the tissues will allow, and then gently release the tension, before making a bowing motion in the opposite direction (see Fig. 6.6).

Try this several times, once with your eyes open and once with eyes closed. Repeat the exercise on the person's other forearm, and compare the findings. Record your findings.

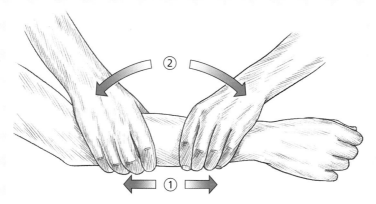

Fig. 6.6   Smith's palpation exercise to assess the interface between the physical and the 'energetic' structures of the arm.

See 'Interpretation' notes below, on Smith's explanation of the meaning of what may be felt during these exercises.

How much force?

Caution: I suggest, when you are trying to introduce twisting or bowing or any other direction of motion to bony structures or soft tissues, that you do not try to produce this effect by means of force from your hands alone.

Having made the initial contact and allowed time for a melding of the contours of your hands with the tissues, use your arms to take out the slack or to introduce a direction of motion. Indeed, consider the hands in this situation to be the contact only, with the motive force coming from the shoulders and arms. Consider – if you were trying to use a spanner to free a tight nut, say, you would not use the strength of the hands alone but would introduce the effort through the whole arm. In a far more subtle manner, the motion or direction of effort in this sort of exercise is best achieved by very fine, whole-arm movements rather than just the hands trying to achieve the desired objective. Anyone who has performed work on the cranium (after suitable instruction) will know that motion in the skull can be palpated, or introduced, in a similar manner, far more effectively and with less chance of injury if leverage is applied by subtle use of arm muscles to guide the hand, rather than letting the hands act alone.

Interpretation of Exercise 6.10

Smith states clearly that this is not an exercise in judging whether things are 'good or bad', but is designed to help you to become sensitive to motions and energies not previously registered.

Smith states that, if the arm is normal, not injured, it may bow more easily in one direction than the other; a bow in one direction may feel obstructed or it may suggest a twisting distortion or have the feel of a steel bar or be more rubbery. Great variations exist and it is up to each of us to establish what 'normal' feels like; to become aware of what is acceptable and what needs working on.

He then suggests a similar exercise involving the long bones of the lower leg, which are probably a better testing ground for practice than the forearm, which has a natural rotational tendency anyway and so can confuse assessment.

EXERCISE 6.11: PALPATING AN ENERGY INTERFACE IN THE LOWER LEG

Time suggested: 2–4 minutes

Place one hand just above the ankle and the other below the knee of one leg. Take up slack in the soft tissue (pull hands apart) and gently twist with your hands going in opposite directions, feeling the bony resistance, as if gently wringing a sweater.

Repeat this in the other direction.

What do you feel?

Smith says:

> Because the bones are denser in the leg than the forearm, and because the muscles are heavier, it takes a moment longer to perceive the energy currents interacting in the twisting motion. It is an exaggeration to say that energy on this level moves with the speed of molasses, but the principle is true.

Repetition and comparison

As with most exercises in this text, these previous two exercises should be performed on several people, within a short space of time, making comparisons easier. By sharing experiences with others it is possible to validate the subtle perceptions derived from these palpation experiences.

If it is possible to palpate limbs which have previously been fractured and which have healed, energy variations may become very instructive. Smith tells us that:

> Energy fields across a fracture may feel heavy and dense, have low vitality, or be disorganised and chaotic. These qualities relate to the process of reconnecting or bridging the energy fields across the damaged bone.

Can the palpated patterns be altered? Yes, says Smith. He takes a forearm, for example, which has an old fracture, grasping it as in Exercise 6.10. He takes out the slack by stretching apart his hands:

> Holding this, I might add a further stretching force, and then, in addition, a bowing or twisting force. I hold this configuration, being sensitive to the resilience of the bone, for a brief period, possibly 15 to 20 seconds, and then gently release.

On reevaluation he would expect a lessening of the asymmetry of the original force fields, a greater freedom of energetic movement through the long bone. He says that he allows three such attempts in order to create the greatest degree of 'shift' at any one session.

Soft tissue palpation using Smith's methods

Where energy motion in soft tissues is concerned, Smith tells us that a difficulty arises, since taking out the slack in pliable tissues is far less easily accomplished, making the reading of energy currents and movements in soft tissues more difficult. He suggests that a good way to start is to make two energetic contacts with the fingers and to 'read' the current as if flows from one point to the other.

EXERCISE 6.12: TWO-FINGER ENERGY PALPATION

Time suggested: 3–4 minutes

Make skin contact with one finger pad on soft tissue below someone's elbow. Place a finger of the other hand at wrist level.

Does a sense of linkage between these contacts appear? This may be noted as a pulsation, subtle movement, a 'buzzing' or just a sense of 'connectedness'.

Both the time taken for this connection to happen and the strength and quality of the sensation should be noted and recorded.

Repeat this in different sites.

See Smith's thoughts, below, which introduce Traditional Chinese Medicine concepts into the discussion as to what may be happening.

The link with Traditional Chinese Medicine (TCM)

Smith debates whether the right hand receives such impulses or sends them and states his conclusion that the practitioner's thoughts determine the direction of flow. Upledger (1987) concurs. Let both hands be neutral, is his advice and allow the patient's body to organise itself around your two contact 'poles', allowing these to be organisational fulcrums, rather than predetermining the direction in which you want flow to take place.

Smith suggests that TCM has long used just such energy readings, most obviously during pulse diagnosis, and that once you have convinced yourself that you can indeed feel energy flows, it is time to start understanding the subtle ways in which you can use this information in evaluating the state of the patient. Therapy using these energy flows is only a small step beyond the palpation stage (see Special topic 11).

Smith states that evaluation of the superficial level of internal energy flow (known as protective chi in TCM) is best achieved using your hands just above the body surface, as in 'therapeutic touch' (Chapter 11), as well as scanning/palpating the skin texture and temperature (Chapter 4).

Beyond the energy fields which are related to the superficial soft tissues and bones lies an energy field which he terms 'background' energy, on which can be 'imprinted' past trauma – chemical, emotional and psychic, as well as physical. This brings us close to Becker's concepts involving tissue 'memory' which we will examine next.

There is also an interesting resemblance between craniosacral still point concepts and something Smith describes in energy work.

EXERCISE 6.13: PALPATION OF THE ENERGY BODY

Time suggested: 5–7 minutes

Your palpation partner lies supine with feet extended slightly over the end of the table. You stand at the foot of the table and with each hand grasp just above the ankle (as in Fig. 6.4). Introduce traction until all the soft tissue slack has been removed.

Sense the connection with the energy field of the patient. Does this seem to 'elongate' and eventually try to contract? If so, slowly release the tension in your traction, as though it were an elastic band.

What do you think was happening during this palpation exercise?

Explanation: manipulating energy?

Once he has established the fulcrum between himself and the patient (as in Exercises 6.10, 6.11 and 6.13), a number of sensations are possible, Smith declares. As he holds traction, for example in Exercise 6.13, he states that he may sense that the patient's energy body is elongating, 'stretching' or 'flowing' into his hands, a process which at some point will stop.

If following this there is not a feeling of contraction, as though the energy body is returning to its previous state, but rather of a stillness, a resting in the 'elongated' state, Smith would gradually release the traction and rest the patient's legs on the table. The patient might then remain in a very deep relaxed state for some moments, before returning to normal (he watches eye movements, the patient's colour and breathing pattern to assess states of consciousness).

However, if, for therapeutic reasons, Smith wishes to anchor the energy field as it tries to contract again, he can do so by maintaining traction. This is very similar to the idea of holding the still point (see Exercise 6.5) as the body tries to normalise ('organise' or 'unwind') itself around that fulcrum, in cranio-sacral methodology or functional technique in osteopathy (see Chapter 8). If, however, he decided to go with the retraction rather than anchoring it, this would be 'like letting a stretched rubber band slowly go back to its slack position'.

Were you aware of any of these sensations during Exercise 6.13?

DISCUSSION REGARDING EXERCISES 6.6–6.13

In this series of palpation exercises you have been trying to evaluate the presence or otherwise of fluctuating movements which seem to be housed in the soft and hard tissues of the body. The explanations regarding the existence of chakras, and of Smith's and Upledger's concepts of palpable energies, are irrelevant to the reality that 'something' can be palpated. What 'it' is, what it means and how it can be used diagnostically, prognostically and therapeutically must remain a matter for you and your particular understanding of the body, your belief system and approach to health enhancement.

The very fact of being able to sense subtle motions is, at this stage, adequate reward for the time and effort you have put into these exercises thus far. If, on the other hand, you cannot feel what has been described then repetition and quiet application of the methods outlined thus far in this section is essential, before moving on to the remaining exercises in this chapter.

Reading the history of trauma

Smith (1986) suggests that we try to distinguish between palpable energy fields which lie beyond the surface of the body, which may reflect present states of health in body and mind (these vibrations not being 'imprinted' on the energy field), and those patterns of energy related to forceful trauma or stimulus of a physical, chemical, emotional or psychic nature.

These latter imbalances exist, he says, as freestanding energy waveforms, abnormal currents, vortices or an excess or deficiency of energy within the field. These 'imprinted' changes are, he suggests, likely to develop in response to trauma of a physical nature, interacting with emotional trauma or when a highly aroused or depressed state existed at the time of trauma.

This combination of interacting stress factors disrupts the subtle body. Smith uses the metaphor of 'wrinkled clothing' to describe these changes in the subtle energy fields around us; they may disappear on their own or may require help to 'iron them out'.

Assessment of such changes involves two tasks.

1. First, we need to quiet the physical body so that we can feel the deeper energy patterns.
2. Second, we have to 'take up the slack', a common theme in Smith's work.

We have already noted (Exercise 6.13) that we can achieve this reduction in slack by means of a traction fulcrum, through the legs. Alternatively, for example, we could use a compression fulcrum through the shoulders. Describing the latter he says:

> I sit at the head of the table, rest my hands firmly and comfortably over the person's shoulders, and gently press down towards the feet, compressing the body to the point of energetic contact. As I gently push . . . the body will move beneath my hands until it reaches its compression limit for the amount of pressure I am applying. In doing this I have taken up the slack. Having engaged the physical body fully, I add slight pressure, which establishes the connection with the energy fields. When I have made good contact with this I just hold the pressure. If there are abnormal waves in that area, I am able to feel the sensations from the person's body in my hands.

EXERCISE 6.14: PALPATION OF ENERGY BODY VIA THE SHOULDERS

Time suggested: 5 minutes (reducing to 30 seconds with experience)

Sit at the head of the table, with your partner supine, and place your hands over the shoulders. Press toward the feet, taking out slack by compression. When this is achieved add just a little more pressure to 'engage the energy fields', as Smith describes it in the quoted text above. Take your time and see what you (and your partner) feel.

Naturally this requires practice to do well, so practise over and over again. Having taken out the slack and applied additional force (slight), allow yourself to be passive when waiting to sense subtle sensations.

Smith states that this particular evaluation takes him anything from 10 to 30 seconds. This is what you should aim for once you are comfortable with the concepts and your palpatory skills in this area are 'literate'.

Balancing energy

How does Smith balance any abnormal energy waves he perceives? He could, he says:

- override an abnormal pattern with a stronger, clearer energy field
- introduce a force field which matches the aberrant pattern and by holding it allow the original field to diminish and vanish
- make an 'essential connection' with the aberrant pattern and anchor this as the body tries to pull away.

Whichever he chooses, immediate reevaluation will often show that the aberration is still present. However, reassessment some days, or even weeks, later may show that it has normalised. This is not dissimilar to many manual treatment results, in which changes at the time of treatment may be apparent but minor, with the majority of change taking place later, as homeostatic mechanisms accomplish their self-regulating tasks.

Example

Smith illustrates his ideas with clinical examples. In one instance he examined a patient who had been in pain since an automobile accident over a year before, in which no significant injury had occurred apart from bruising. Smith was unable to find any cause for the pain until he noted a strong twisting force in the energy field, from the right side of the chest to the left abdomen. This represented the twisting force exerted at the time of the accident.

He used traction on the legs to 'engage' this force field (an alternative to the method mentioned above, of pushing down through the shoulders to engage it) and exerted a slightly stronger force field through his body, noting:

. . . a sensation of a rebounding effect along the energy imprint itself. By anchoring the new field I allowed the rebound to subside.

A gradual release, initially of the energy body and then the physical body, and a subsequent resting of the legs on the table left the patient with a sense of well-being and quietness. Two days later, on examination, he was free of pain and there were no twisting currents to be found. A number of zero-balancing sessions may be needed if greater degrees of imprinting of forces exist.

Horses and camels

In palpating areas of trauma, Smith (1986) tells us something of variations in patterns we may expect to palpate, depending upon the type of trauma a patient has experienced, specifically detailing ancient Chinese distinctions between 'horse kick injury' and 'camel kick injury'.

The first, involving hard hooves, results in local physical trauma, severe at the onset, with healing after days or weeks.

The second, involving softer camel hooves, results in mild initial reaction with increasing symptoms as time passes, as the injury 'moves deeper'. It is as though the 'soft' injury fails to stimulate defence mechanisms and therefore disperses through the body/mind/energy fields of the person, with subsequent symptoms emerging.

Focus

Smith makes an important statement when he says:

> Energetic connections can be lost if our thoughts drift or we are focused elsewhere. Energy follows thought.

Upledger makes very similar pronouncements, as do most workers in the 'energy field', and this is something the beginner may find useful. When results don't come, ask yourself where your attention was.

Tissue memory

Upledger (1987) reports evidence showing that decerebrate laboratory rats are able to solve food-orientated maze problems, indicating a 'memory' and decision-making facility within the spinal cord. He also reports studies indicating a degree of decision making taking place in the hands of a musician without CNS input. He suggests:

> Perhaps these powers develop in these peripheral locations, in response to a person's need to develop certain skills.

Upledger employs techniques such as somatoemotional release in which emotional 'scars' are dealt with and he, along with Smith (see above), holds to the concept that palpable changes occur in the energy fields of the body related to physical, chemical and emotional trauma.

Is this physiologically possible? Professor Irvin Korr, a physiologist of international stature, enters this controversial arena, albeit on a neurological rather than an energy level. In an article entitled 'Somatic dysfunction, osteopathic manipulative treatment and the nervous system', Korr (1986) states:

> Spinal reflexes can be conditioned by repetition or prolongation of given stimulus. According to the hypothesis, like the brain, the cord can learn and remember new behaviour patterns. Whether the (memory) once recorded, needs reinforcement by some kind of afferent stimulation is an open question.

On the influence of somatic changes on the mind he says:

> Clinical experience indicates that somatic dysfunction (and manipulation) are powerful influences on brain function and on the perceptions and even the personality of the patient. This experience . . . raises many fundamental questions and exciting clinical implications.

So Korr seems to be supporting the ideas of a 'memory' independent of the brain as well as of tissue changes (from whatever cause) having a continual impact on 'perceptions and personality' factors.

To conclude this survey of opinions, let us look at what Hans Selye, the premier researcher into stress, said on the subject (Selye 1976).

> The lasting bodily changes (in structure or chemical composition) which underlie effective adaptation, or the collapse of it, are after-effects of stress; they represent tissue-memories which affect our future somatic behaviour during similar stressful situations. They can be stored.

Speransky (1944), the great Russian researcher, not only hypothesised such a state of affairs, he also proved it and showed how to reverse it. He stated:

> Chemical and infectual trauma of nerve structures result in nervous dystrophy, this, in turn, gives the impulses for the development in the tissue of other pathological change, including those of an inflammatory character. Their disposition at the periphery can be predicted by us in advance, and their boundaries remain unchanged often throughout long periods.

Rollin Becker (see below) reports that Speransky changed these imprinted messages by 'manually flushing or washing the CNS with the animal's or human's own CSF, and the disabled condition in the peripheral tissues normalised' (Becker 1963).

Becker himself declares:

> Memory reactions occur within the CNS system in all traumatic cases . . . An area of the body that has been seriously hurt is going to send thousands of sensory messages into the spinal cord segments, and brain areas, that supply that part of the body. If the injury is severe, or long lasting, these messages will be imprinted into the nervous system similar to imprinting a message on a tape recorder.

Thus the tissues and the nervous system 'remember' the injury and its pattern of dysfunction long after healing has occurred. It becomes 'facilitated' to that pattern long after the trauma.

Finding the eye of the hurricane, the still point, is the formula which Smith, Upledger and Becker advocate, if we are to quieten those aberrant patterns of energy which exist after trauma or misuse.

The brilliant research of Bjorn Nordenstrom is outlined below. This former Chief of Diagnostic Radiation at the famed Karolinska Institute in Stockholm has shown that there exists a previously unsuspected energy system, which could help to explain the work of researchers such as Smith and Becker.

However, before examining his research results we should investigate the dedicated studies and palpatory techniques of Rollin Becker (1963, 1964a,b, 1965) and Alan Becker (1973).

Becker's diagnostic touch

According to Rollin Becker, when a practitioner is first faced by any patient:

> The patient is intelligently guessing as to the diagnosis, the physician is scientifically guessing as to the diagnosis, but the patient's body knows the problem, and is outpicturing it in the tissues.

Learning to read what the body has to say is the necessary task of diagnosis and much of this depends upon palpation:

> The first step in developing depth of feel and touch is to re-evaluate the patient from the standpoint, just what does the patient's body want to tell you? Having set aside the patient's opinions and your initial diagnosis:
>
>> Place your hands and fingers on the patient in the area of his complaint or complaints. Let the feel of the tissues from the inner core of their depths come through to your touch and read, and 'listen' to their story. To get this story it is

necessary to know something about potency . . . and something about the fulcrum.

'Potency' and 'fulcrum' are two areas which we must examine closely as we learn of Becker's remarkable palpatory method.

Potency tells us the degree, the power of strength, of whatever is being discussed; it also, Becker reminds us, speaks to the ability to control or influence something. The diagnostic tool which Becker will teach us to use, as we learn to read and understand potency, is the fulcrum, in which the fingers and hands create a condition in which potency becomes apparent.

Becker asks us to acknowledge that:

> At the very core of total health there is a potency within the human body manifesting itself in health. At the core of every traumatic or disease condition within the human body is a potency manifesting its interrelationship with the body in trauma and disease. It is up to us to learn to feel this potency.

He likens this concept to the eye of a hurricane, which carries the potency, or power, of the whole storm. In just this way, within each trauma or disease pattern there is an 'eye', 'within or without the patient', which carries in itself the potency to manifest the condition. This eye is a point of stillness, the existence of which he asks you to accept, as you take the time to develop a sense of touch which can perceive it.

The *fulcrum* is a support, or point of support, on which a lever turns in raising or moving something, therefore being a means of exerting pressure or influence.

Lief used the term 'fulcrum' to describe the still resting state of the fingers as the thumb moved towards them in its searching mode in NMT methodology. Smith uses the term 'fulcrum' to describe a 'balance' point via which the therapist 'gets in touch' with the energy body. It is established once the 'slack has been taken out' of the tissues and an interface created. Becker suggests that his fulcrum should be understood as a 'still-leverage' junction, which may be shifted from place to place, all the while retaining its leverage function. The would-be palpator achieves this by placing her hand(s) near the site complained of by the patient. A fulcrum is then established using the elbow, forearm, crossed legs or other convenient area as a supporting point (the fulcrum), allowing the contacting fingers/hand(s) to be gently yet firmly moulded to the tissues. The fulcrum provides the working point, free to move if needed, yet stable as the palpation proceeds.

Example of Becker's fulcrum

An example is given in which a supine patient with a low back problem is to be examined. The practitioner sits beside the patient, placing a hand under the sacrum, fingers extended cephalad and the elbow of that hand supported either on the table or on the practitioner's own knees. 'By leaning comfortably on his/her elbow, the physician establishes a fulcrum from which to read the changes taking place in the back.'

It is the elbow which is the fulcrum. By applying increased pressure at the fulcrum, causing a slight degree of compression at the sacrum, the practitioner will 'initiate a kinetic energy that will allow the structure-function of the stress area to begin its pattern to be reflected back to his/her touch' (Becker 1963).

If the other hand were similarly placed under the low back, the fulcrum could be the edge of the table, against which the forearm rests (or the elbow could rest on the knee). Either or both fulcrums may be employed, to feel 'the tug of the tissues deep within'. The practitioner will also become aware, says Becker, of 'a quiet point, a still-point, an area of stillness within the stress pattern, that is the

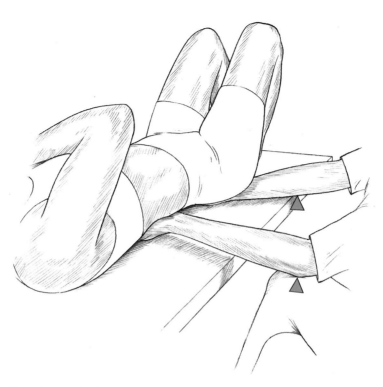

Fig. 6.7   Low back palpation. Hands under sacrum and low back apply no pressure – contact only. Forearm resting on the edge of the table acts as Becker's fulcrum. Increased pressure downwards at the fulcrum enhances the palpator's awareness of tissue status.

EXERCISE 6.15: PALPATION USING BECKER'S FULCRUM

Time suggested: 5 minutes

Palpate a sacrum using Becker's fulcrum, as described above.

Compare this with the sensations noted when using Upledger's sacral assessment, in Exercise 6.2, Figure 6.3.

Also compare these results with those you will obtain when you perform Exercise 6.17, later in this chapter.

point of potency of that particular strain' (see Fig. 6.7). Becker makes it clear that he is discussing the kinetics of the energy fields that make up the stress pattern and not anatomical/physiological units of tissue, when he describes the point of potency.

What are we palpating?

What is the form of energy being assessed here? Becker does not know and says we do not need to know, any more than we need to know the nature of electricity before being able to use it safely. This thought has been deeply satisfying to those practitioners, aware of the effectiveness of these ideas and methods, who are unable to accept the Upledger/Smith/chakra/acupuncture models of 'energy'.

Is there any other model? We have seen that Oschman's perspective (earlier in this chapter) offers explanations which emerge from the world of quantum physics. It would be appropriate at this point to bring in Nordenstrom's research results, since they may answer the question as to what the form of energy being palpated represents. Nordenstrom, formerly chair of the Karolinska Nobel Assembly, which selects Nobel prize winners in medicine, is hardly a rebel or maverick. His discoveries are, however, revolutionary. He described his results in his book *Biologically closed electric circuits* (Nordenstrom 1983). It was when using a small spot X-ray technique, in order to define breast and lung tumours, that he first noted an unusual zone around some tumours. He called this a 'corona' and decided to investigate the phenomenon, as there was no histological evidence of change in these tissues. By inserting fine needles into these tissues he demonstrated an electrical flow. He continued his research on humans and animals, alive and dead, before developing a series of principles.

The first was that energy conversion in tissues over a biologically closed electric circuit can be defined as a fluctuation in electrical potential in a limited area, resulting from injury, tumour and healing. He found that there was an electrical flow in tissues which followed selected pathways and that large blood vessels function as insulated electricity conducting cables (as described by Oschman earlier in this chapter). He also demonstrated that biologically closed electric circuits produce magnetic changes around an area which can be measured from a distance.

Nordenstrom also discovered that biological factors which cause cancer, of a chemical or physical nature, have the ability to polarise tissues and that therefore 'inactivated biologically closed electric circuits' may represent a common factor in carcinogenesis. He was able to show that there exist differences in electrical potential, over an area of a few millimetres, around injured (or malignant) tissues.

Is this electricity the energy Smith and Becker are feeling? Are polarisations and fluctuations what is being palpated in an energy cyst? What Nordenstrom has proved is that there is another circulation in the body, that of electricity (or energy), and that it changes measurably in response to disease or injury. It can be assessed by machine and probably, therefore, by palpation. Reviewing this book, Martyn Richardson (1988) states:

> I had a chemistry professor in college who demonstrated that the molecule consisted of atoms, which consisted of electrons, protons and neutrons, which were not 'solid matter' but electric charges. Therefore everything was nothing – except a collection of electric charges.

Clyde Ford (1989) explains a different energy research study which evolved from the simple observation of a chiropractor, I.N. Toftness, that skin drag occurred on palpation of 'problem areas' (see Chapter 4 for a reminder of skin drag palpation). Toftness's research showed that microwave emissions emanating from the body could be measured, that these varied in relation to areas of excess or diminished activity and also that they changed after sustained light pressure was applied to such areas.

> Toftness used light pressure to manipulate the body and had a wealth of clinical studies to document the effectiveness of this method. To this he now added the ability to objectively monitor the human electromagnetic field and demonstrate its relationship to the physical condition of the human body. Typically, the radiometer detected abnormally high, or abnormally low, microwave readings, in problem areas of the body. After sustained light pressure, these peaks and valleys normalised – the high readings were reduced, and the low readings raised. Monitoring the electromagnetic field produced by the body is a unique form of diagnosis because it is truly non-invasive.

Clearly, this 'electromagnetic' or microwave transmission from body tissues is a strong contender for what Smith and Becker (and the others we have discussed) are palpating when they speak of 'energy'. Whatever Becker is palpating, it seems to be significant and worthy of our learning to do the same.

How long does it take to make an assessment using Becker's methods? Less than 10 minutes is necessary to identify the focal point of potency, he says, and with practice it becomes possible to date old strains (are they weeks, months or years old?) and to tell the difference between the energy patterns of these and those found with new strains. The following exercise, which Rollin Becker describes (1963, 1964a), is well worth attempting several times until the principles he is teaching become clear.

EXERCISE 6.16: PALPATING FOR TISSUE STATUS FROM THE KNEE

Time suggested: 5–7 minutes for each stage

Stage 1: First sit facing a patient/model who is seated on the edge of a treatment table. Place your hands around the knee, fingers interlocked in the popliteal space. Try to sense as much as you can about the knee, applying a compression force towards the hip to see what you can tell about that area. You may get some information, but not much.

Stage 2: Now adopt the same contact with the knee but this time rest your own elbows on your knees as you do so. Apply the same compression towards the hips and assess what you feel, using the fulcrum points.

Becker describes what you might feel this time.

> Feel how the innate natural forces within the thigh and pelvis want to turn the acetabulum either into an internal rotation or an external rotation position. Note the quality and quantity of that turning. Note that if you lean lightly on your elbow fulcrum points you get a more superficial reading from the tissues under your hands even though your hands and interlaced fingers remain light in their control.

Note that when you then lean more firmly onto your elbow fulcrum points, you get a deeper and deeper impression from the tissues under examination.

The depth of perception is dependent on the firmness of the fulcrum contacts, not on the firmness of the examining finger contacts. If there exists a deep strain in the tissues, it is the fulcrum pressure which needs to be increased in order to reach these tissues and their patterns of dysfunction.

This can be done anywhere on the body surface by the simple expedient of creating a contact under the tissues to be examined, establishing a fulcrum point and 'turning in' to the information waiting to be uncovered.

There are two important riders to this, though, says Becker.

● You must know your anatomy and physiology in order to make sense of the information.
● You must divorce yourself from any sense of 'doing'. Just let the story come through. The fulcrum points are listening posts only.

And yet this is not quite the case. For Becker does suggest the introduction of a slight compression force, or traction, not in order to actively test the tissues but to 'activate already existing forces within the patient's body'.

The example of the pressure towards the acetabulum, in the previous exercise, is useful for, having applied this, it would be the innate tendency of the tissues to externally and internally rotate, which would then be palpated.

Becker is asking for contact with the 'interface', which Smith described, and the 'still point', which Upledger described, in different terms perhaps but in essence in much the same manner.

What he adds is the concept of being able to gain deeper perception of, and access to, tissue (or energy) states by means of the fulcrum.

Becker calls this diagnostic touch:

> It is a form of palpation that one might call an alert observational type of awareness for the functions and dysfunctions from within the patient, utilising the motive deep energy, deep within the tissues themselves. It is not the patient voluntarily turning the acetabulum but his tissues within the acetabulum turning it for you to observe.

What should you feel as the body's forces play around the fulcrum? To the outside observer watching our work, our hands are apparently lying quietly on the patient but the motion, the mobility, the motility we sense from within the patient is considerable, depending on the problem. There is a deliberate pattern that the tissues go through in demonstrating the strain that is within them. Kinetic energy-wise, they work their way through to a point at which all sense of motion or mobility seems to cease. This is the point of stillness. Even though it is still, it is endowed with biodynamic power.

The 'potency within the strain' and 'interference waves'

This then is the point of potency within the strain pattern, the still point in this functioning unit, which changes as the contact is held, following which a new pattern emerges and is felt. Normality has been encouraged or achieved. Upledger describes the 'interference waves' which result from restriction lesions or trauma. These waves superimpose on normal physiological body motions. Once you identify where the interference waves are coming from, the source of the problem is found.

Symmetrical placement (gently) of your hands on the head, thoracic inlet, inferior costal margins, pelvis, thighs and feet of the patient allows your hands to perceive the arcs or inherent wave patterns. If these are symmetrical all is well. If the arcs are asymmetrical, then you are asked to visualise the radii of these arcs and to determine where they interact. That will be the location of the lesion (restriction or trauma). You need to place your hands on as many sites as necessary to pick up the information required to make this assessment. It is as if there were an infinite number of concentric globes around the lesion, each vibrating and describing arcs. Where is the centre of all the concentric globes? The closer you get, the smaller are the arcs. Hands may be placed, one on the anterior, one on the posterior surface of the body; both hands may receive the impression of arcs, which you should evaluate in order to find a point of intersection. This gives the depth of the lesion. This is Upledger's way of finding 'the eye of the hurricane'. When you have performed a number of Becker's exercises (below) and you come to Exercise 6.20, compare the methods of Upledger and Becker (as well as Smith). One of these may well suit you better than the others, something you can only discover by trying them all. (See also Chapter 12, Figs 12.1, 12.2.)

Becker's exercises

Rollin Becker gives a series of examples in which he palpates different body regions and describes his contact and fulcrum points. It is suggested that all of these be used in any sequence, on appropriate palpation partners, selecting, if possible, areas where there is or has been dysfunction or pathology, so that variations in what is perceived can be observed and learned from.

Take as much time as possible.

EXERCISE 6.17: PELVIC PALPATION USING BECKER'S FULCRUM

Time suggested: 5–7 minutes

To assess the sacrum and pelvis (see Fig. 6.8) have your palpation partner supine, knees flexed. Sit on a stool of appropriate height, on your partner's right side facing the head, and place your right hand under the sacrum, fingertips on spinous processes of the fifth lumbar vertebra. Your right elbow rests on the table as the fulcrum.

Your left hand and arm bridge the anterior superior spines of the ilium, so that either the left hand on the left ASIS or the left elbow on the right ASIS can act as fulcrums if pressure is applied through them.

You may alternate the use of one or the other ASIS as a fulcrum point, in examining the opposite ilium in its functioning relationship with the sacrum.

The pelvis and its relationships with the sacrum, lumbar spine and hips below can all now be assessed. It is particularly useful for assessment of sacral involvement in whiplash injuries.

Compare the results of this exercise with those derived from Exercises 6.2 and 6.15.

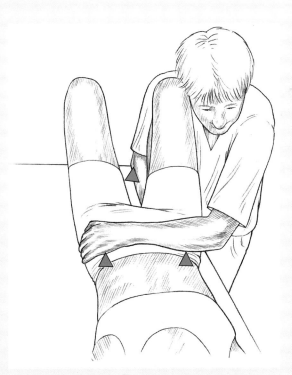

Fig. 6.8 Palpation of sacrum and pelvis. Becker's fulcrum points are the right elbow on the table and contacts on the anterior iliac spines with the left hand/arm.

EXERCISE 6.18: PALPATING THE LOWER THORAX USING BECKER'S FULCRUM

Time suggested: 5–7 minutes

To assess the rib cage, you should sit to the side of the supine patient, your caudad hand lying under the rib cage, with fingertips resting just short of the spinous processes. The fulcrum point is on your crossed knees.

The other hand rests on the anterior ends of the same ribs, the fulcrum point being the forearm which rests on the patient's ASIS (see Fig. 6.9).

A slight compression at the fulcrum points initiates motion at the heads of the ribs being examined, allowing strains to be evaluated and treated.

The entire rib cage can be assessed, the hands changing position as needed.

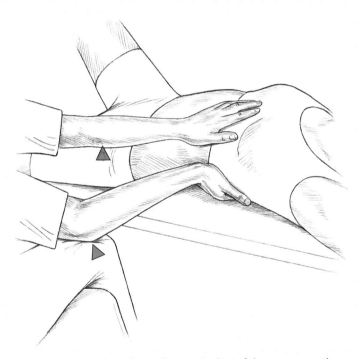

Fig. 6.9   Palpation of the rib cage. Becker's fulcrums are on the practitioner's crossed knees and the patient's ASIS (left).

EXERCISE 6.19: PALPATION OF THE CERVICAL SPINE USING BECKER'S FULCRUM

Time suggested: 5–7 minutes

Sit at the head of your supine palpation partner, with your hands bilaterally bridging the entire cervical region, from the base of the skull (hypothenar eminence contacts here) to the upper thorax, where the fingertips lie (see Fig. 6.10). The fulcrum points are the forearms, which rest on the table.

General assessment is possible of tissue status using these contacts. Individual segments can be localised by finger contact.

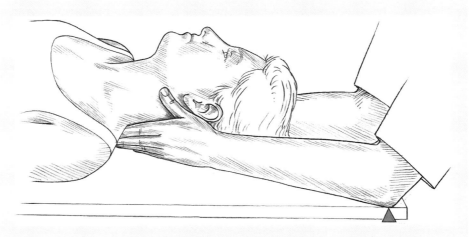

Fig. 6.10   Palpation of cervical spine. Becker's fulcrums are forearm and elbow contacts on the table.

The 'other' Becker's views

There are two Dr Beckers and we have so far been involved with the work of Rollin Becker.

Alan Becker (1973) discusses ingrained patterns which we all carry, in much the same way as computers which have been programmed, whether these allow normal or abnormal function. In assessment and treatment he carries Rollin Becker's 'diagnostic touch' concepts further, stating:

> I make contact with the involved tissues and apply enough pressure to get the patient's attention and to initiate the automatic response. Then I ask the patient to close his eyes and look at my fingers, to be aware of what is happening to his body. By this means I persuade him to take conscious control of the program and re-evaluate his standards of normal, acceptable and tolerable data. Then as I lead the structures towards increased ease and balance, the patient senses the changes and tends either to install new action programs which include the new data or to re-establish the ones which were in effect before abnormal data was encouraged.

In discussing a whiplash injury he illustrates this, saying:

> The problem is complicated by the fact that the body has been subjected to forces that entered it in a direction that crosses the normal direction of movement. Such forces tend to produce wavelike movement within the fluid cells of the body, and the inertia of the body, which is trying to continue whatever programs are in action at the time, causes a counterwave directed towards the point of impact.

These two forces, according to Alan Becker, set up a wave-like pattern, a ridge of energy, a built-in distortion around which the defensive patterns are built. These have to be removed by dissipation of the energy rather than by force. Only then, Becker insists, can new, more appropriate patterns be established by the patient. The resistance of built-in patterns, whether these relate to habit or to injury, is something the palpating practitioner should be acutely aware of, for this is a key feature of the territory being explored.

We are now entering the area of structural reintegration, postural reeducation, Alexander technique, Feldenkrais's work, somatics (Thomas Hanna) and other methods which require a relearning of how we use ourselves.

Alan Becker's contribution seems to be that he calls on a conscious awareness from the patient, as methods such as those of Rollin Becker are applied, in order to have them become aware of the changes which are taking place and to have them support and encourage these.

EXERCISE 6.20: COMBINED PALPATION OF TISSUE CHARACTERISTICS

Time suggested: open ended depending upon your selection of options, but at least 30 minutes if possible

Choose an area of dysfunction on your palpation partner and prepare to palpate, incorporating, sequentially or at the same time, the concepts of Smith and Rollin Becker, as you palpate the intrinsic expressions of function in various areas of your patient/partner.

Move from the methods of Smith (using a half-moon vector) to those of Becker (using the fulcrum) and back again. Which gives you the most information? Do the methods confirm each other's findings? Which do you feel more comfortable with?

Do you now agree that tissue has a memory?

Are these exercises likely to be of value in a clinical setting?

DISCUSSION REGARDING EXERCISES IN THIS CHAPTER

Where have we come to by performing the exercises in this chapter? Have we simply acquired a series of experiences which we find hard to use or find relevance for? Or have the subtle skills which these exercises have encouraged a practical value?

Consider the words of one of the leading American osteopathic clinicians and academics, Philip Greenman (1989), who, when discussing myofascial release technique, a subtle yet extremely clinical tool, states:

> This [myofascial release] is directed towards a biomechanical effect and a neurophysiological effect. Ward has coined a mnemonic: POE(T2). POE stands for point of entry into the musculoskeletal system. Entry may be from the lower extremity, the upper extremity, through the thoracic cage, through the abdomen, or from the cranial cervical junction. The two 'Ts' stand for traction and twist. In most of the techniques, traction produces stretch along the long axis of the myofascial elements that are shortened and tightened. The stretch should always be applied in the long axis rather than transversely across myofascial elements. Introduction of a twisting force provides the opportunity to localise the traction, not only at the point of contact with the patient but also at points some distance away.

continues

DISCUSSION REGARDING EXERCISES IN THIS CHAPTER (*Continued*)

He suggests that beginners try to develop the ability to sense change in the freedom or restriction of tissues, some distance from the point which is being contacted. Thus, if the ankles are being grasped and traction introduced, an attempt should be made to feel 'through the extremities' to the knee, hip, sacroiliac joint up into the spine itself. Concentration and practice can allow this skill to develop.

In his text Dr Greenman describes exercises which will allow the practitioner to develop the skills necessary to perform myofascial release techniques. These involve palpation of a body area, starting from above the skin, moving to a light contact which attempts 'to sense the inherent movement of the patient's tissues under your hand' (an 'inherent oscillation') – a concept which we have seen described in other ways, many times in this chapter.

A first step in being able to do this involves the ability to apply pressure or make contact, without movement, followed by being able to palpate the motions which are constantly at work within the tissue, without influencing them. These skills are precisely what the various exercises given in this chapter should allow you to do.

Greenman gives a concluding exercise, palpation of the motion of the sacrum, with the patient first supine and then prone. This you should by now also be able to perform, based on previous exercises.

As Greenman says:

> When you have been able to identify inherent soft tissue and bony movement you are well on your way to being able to use myofascial release technique.

It is hoped that the methods described above, based on the work of these marvellous researchers into human physiology, will allow greater skill in your diagnostic and therapeutic endeavours.

REFERENCES

Bassett C 1978 Pulsing electromagnetic fields. In: Buchwald H, Varco R (eds) Metabolic surgery. Grune and Stratton, New York

Baule G, McFee R 1963 Detection of the magnetic field of the heart. American Heart Journal 66:95–96

Becker A 1973 Parameters of resistance. Academy of Applied Osteopathy, Newark, OH

Becker R 1963 Diagnostic touch (part 1). Yearbook of the Academy of Applied Osteopathy Newark, OH, vol 63, pp 32–40

Becker R 1964a Diagnostic touch (part 2). Yearbook of the Academy of Applied Osteopathy, Newark, OH, vol 64, pp 153–160

Becker R 1964b Diagnostic touch (part 3). Yearbook of the Academy of Applied Osteopathy, Newark, OH, vol 64, pp 161–165

Becker R 1965 Diagnostic touch (part 4). Yearbook of the Academy of Applied Osteopathy, Newark, OH, vol 65 (2), pp 165–177

Burr H 1957 'Harold Saxton Burr'. Yale Journal of Biology and Medicine 30(3): 161–167

Burr H 1972 Blueprint for immortality. CS Daniel, Saffron Walden

Chaitow L 1999 Cranial manipulation: theory and practice. Churchill Livingstone, Edinburgh

Cohen D 1967 Magnetic fields around the torso. Science 156:652–654

Cohen D 1972 Magnetoencephalography. Science 175:664–666

Erlinghauser R 1959 The circulation of CSF through the connective tissue system. Yearbook of the Academy of Applied Osteopathy, Newark, OH

Ford C 1989 Where healing waters meet. Station Hill Press, New York

Frymann V 1963 Palpation. Yearbook of Selected Osteopathic Papers. Academy of Applied Osteopathy, Newark, OH

Greenman P 1989 Principles of manual medicine. Williams and Wilkins, Baltimore

Josephson B 1965 Supercurrents through barriers. Advances in Physics 14:419–451

Kennedy J 1955 Tubular structure of collagen fibrils. Science 121: 673–674

Korr I 1986 Somatic dysfunction, osteopathic manipulative treatment and the nervous system. Journal of the American Osteopathic Association 76:9

MacGinitie L 1995 Streaming and piezoelectric potentials in connective tissue. In: Blank M (ed) Electromagnetic fields. Advances in Chemistry Series 250. American Chemical Society, Washington, DC

Milne H 1995 The heart of listening. North Atlantic Books, Berkeley, CA

Nordenstrom B 1983 Biologically closed electric circuits: clinical, experimental and theoretical evidence for an additional circulatory system. Nordic Medical Publications, Stockholm

Oschman J 2001 Energy medicine. Churchill Livingstone, Edinburgh

Pick M 2001 Presentation 'Beyond the neuron'. Integrative Bodywork Conference, JBMT/University of Westminster, London

Richardson M 1988 Book review. The DO September

Selye H 1976 The stress of life. McGraw-Hill, New York

Seto A, Kusaka C, Nakazato S 1992 Detection of extraordinary large biomagnetic field strength from the human hand. Acupuncture and Electro-Therapeutics Research International Journal 17:75–94

Smith F 1986 Inner bridges – a guide to energy movement and body structure. Humanics New Age, New York

Speransky AD 1944 A basis for the theory of medicine. International Publishers, New York

Sutherland WG 1948 The cranial bowl. Sutherland, Mankato, MN

Upledger J 1987 Craniosacral therapy II: beyond the dura. Eastland Press, Seattle

Upledger J, Vredevoogd W 1983 Craniosacral therapy. Eastland Press, Seattle

Varma D 1935 The human machine and its forces. Health for All Publications, London

Wyckoff R 1952 Fine structure of connective tissues. Foundation Conferences on Connective Tissues 3:38–91

Zimmerman J 1990 Laying-on-of-hands and therapeutic touch: a testable theory. BEMI Currents (Journal of Bio-electro-magnetics Institute) 2:8–17

SPECIAL TOPIC 7
Assessing dural restriction

Dr John Upledger (Upledger & Vredevoogd 1987) explains how difficult it is to prescribe techniques used to localise restrictions imposed upon the spinal dural tube. It is not that the techniques themselves are difficult, it is describing them that is hard. The dura is firmly attached along the entire circumference of the foramen magnum as well as to the posterior bodies of the second and third cervical vertebrae. From there it is free until it reaches the second sacral segment (anterior portion). After this it attaches, via the filum terminale, to the periosteum of the coccyx.

Adhesions and restriction can occur, not only at the points of attachment but anywhere along its length, notably at intervertebral foramina. Simultaneous testing of motion at the occiput and sacrum allows mobility of the dura to be assessed, movements of which will be synchronous if normal mobility exists. Any 'lag' of one bone or the other indicates restriction. (See Exercise 6.2 and Figure 6.3 for a side-lying version of this palpation.)

Upledger suggests palpating the motion in these bones simultaneously as the patient lies supine. If a normal synchronous motion is palpated, he advocates experimentally slightly inhibiting the motion of either the occiput or the sacrum with one hand and noting the effect on the motion being perceived by the other hand.

If, in this assessment, dural drag is presumed, due to a 'lag' between the occipital and sacral motions, he asks you to see whether you can tell if this drag is coming from one end or the other or from somewhere in between (within the dural tube or on one of its spinal nerve sleeves).

A further assessment is possible by simply introducing gentle occipital traction (patient supine) in order to cause the mobile dural tube to move gently towards you. If there is any restriction in this 'glide', ask yourself how far down the tube the restriction is taking place (see Special Topic Fig. 7A).

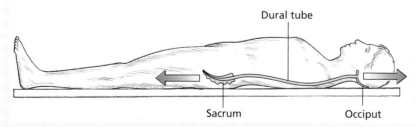

Special Topic Fig. 7A   Traction on the sacrum (or legs) will ensure a direct pull, via the dura, on the occiput, while traction from the occiput will ensure direct pull on the sacrum via the dura.

SPECIAL TOPIC EXERCISE 7.1

Time suggested: 4–6 minutes

Upledger describes an effective training exercise which sharpens perception of such restrictions as may be present.

Take a good length of clingfilm and flatten this along the length of a smooth, clean table. The polyethylene will cling to the surface to a degree, offering resistance to any movement along the length of the table as you pull on one end (see Special Topic Fig. 7B).

Initially he suggests you apply traction and see how much effort is required to cause some movement of the film. After establishing this he suggests placing an object (e.g. a glass of water) on the film before repeating the exercise to see how the degree of traction needs to be increased, to take account of the weight of the object.

Repetitive exercising in this way, with the weight in different positions, will increase perception of how motion is restricted in different localities.

After becoming familiar with variations in position of any restriction, he suggests you perform a series of exercises of this sort blindfolded (someone else places the object on the film) to see whether you can assess how far down the table the object has been placed, purely by assessing the resistance in the film as you pull on it. 'You will be surprised how quickly you can develop accuracy at touching the object which offers the restriction to your traction while you are blindfolded.' After this, retest the 'feel' of dural resistance with a patient or model supine, as you apply light traction to the occiput or sacrum.

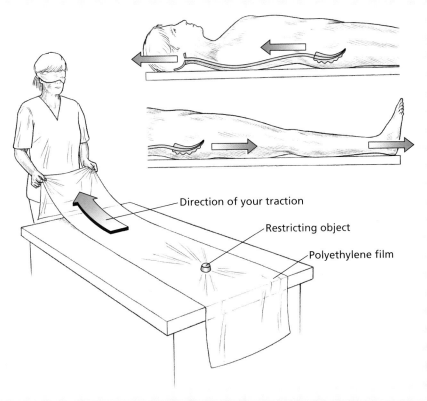

Direction of your traction

Restricting object

Polyethylene film

Special Topic Fig. 7B Upledger's skill training exercise for assessment of dural restrictions. This utilises polyethylene clingfilm (to represent the dura) and a 'restricting' object (to represent adhesion or restriction in the dural sheath). By standing at the feet (or by using the sacrum) or the head, restrictions can be assessed via gentle and highly focused traction.

Light traction pulls on the tube closer to your hands (upper cervical) and as force builds up, this influences the dura further down its course. With practice, one segment at a time can be palpated by gently stretching the dura. Of course, traction from the sacral end is also possible in the same manner.

REFERENCE

Upledger J, Vredevoogd W 1987 Craniosacral therapy. Eastland Press, Seattle

7

Assessment of 'abnormal mechanical tension' in the nervous system

In this chapter we will be examining some extremely important assessment techniques relating to what has been described as 'abnormal tension in the neural structures'. Before doing so it is necessary to look at some of the potential implications, other than pain, which such 'abnormal tensions' hold. We need therefore to briefly examine one physiological component which may be involved: the trophic function of nerves.

Irvin Korr, the primary researcher into the neurological and pathophysiological processes involved in osteopathic medicine over the past half century, has studied the phenomenon of the transport and exchange of macromolecular materials along neural pathways. Among his pertinent (to our study) findings are that the influence of nerves on target organs and muscles depends largely upon the delivery to them of specific neuronal proteins. There is also evidence of a return pathway by means of which messenger substances are transferred back from target organs to the central nervous system and brain along neural structures.

In one of Korr's examples (Korr 1981) it is shown that red and white muscles, which differ morphologically, functionally and chemically (and as we have seen in Chapter 5, differently in response to stress), can have all these differences reversed if their innervation is 'crossed', so that red muscles receive white muscle innervation and vice versa. 'This means, in effect that the nerve instructs the muscle what kind of muscle to be, and is an expression of a neurally mediated genetic influence,' says Korr.

In other words, it is the nerve which determines which genes in a muscle will be suppressed and which expressed and this information is carried in the material being transported along the axons. When a muscle loses contact with its nerve (as in anterior poliomyelitis, for example) atrophy occurs, not as a result of disuse but because of the loss of the integrity of the connection between nerve cells and muscle cells at the myoneural junction, where nutrient exchange occurs irrespective of whether or not impulses are being transmitted.

These and other functions depend upon the flow of axonally transported proteins, phospholipids, glycoproteins, neurotransmitters and their precursors, enzymes, mitochondria and other organelles.

Korr's words can help us to appreciate this phenomenon further.

- The rate of transport of such substances varies from 1 mm/day to several hundred mm/day, with 'different cargoes being carried at different rates'.
- 'The motor powers (for the waves of transportation) are provided by the axon itself.'
- Retrograde transportation seems to be 'a fundamental means of communication between neurons and between neurons and non-neuronal cells'.

Korr believes this process to have an important role in maintenance of 'the plasticity of the nervous system, serving to keep motor-neurons and muscle cells, or two synapsing neurons, mutually adapted to each other and responsive to each other's changing circumstances'.

Implications

What are the clinical implications of this knowledge and, more specifically, how is this related to our study of palpation? For a start, we certainly ought to understand what influences are operating on the tissues we palpate. For example, as discussed in previous chapters, knowledge of the craniosacral rhythmic fluid fluctuations, and of the tubular structure of collagen fibrils which many researchers believe are transport channels for CSF, gives us an awareness of what we might be feeling as we palpate for these rhythms.

Similarly, awareness of the trophic influence of neural structures on the structural and functional characteristics of the soft tissues they supply carries at least as much importance, especially when we realise just how vulnerable these nutrient highways are to disruption. Korr explains:

> Any factor which causes derangement of transport mechanisms in the axon, or that chronically alters the quality or quantity of the axonally transported substances, could cause the trophic influences to become detrimental. This alteration in turn would produce aberrations of structure, function, and metabolism, thereby contributing to dysfunction and disease.

Among the negative influences frequently operating on these transport mechanisms, Korr informs us, are: 'deformations of nerves and roots, such as compression, stretching, angulation and torsion'. These stresses occur all too often in humans, says Korr, and are particularly likely where neural structures are most vulnerable:

> In their passage over highly mobile joints, through bony canals, intervertebral foramina, fascial layers, and tonically contracted muscles (for example, posterior rami of spinal nerves and spinal extensor muscles).

Korr further amplifies his concern over negative influences on neural trophic function when he discusses 'sustained hyperactive peripheral neurons (sensory, motor and autonomic)'. For when there is a high rate of discharge from neural structures (facilitated segments and trigger points, for example) the metabolism of neurons is affected 'and almost certainly their synthesis and turnover of proteins and other macromolecules'.

These thoughts (and others of Korr's given below) relating to the vital trophic role of the nervous system, over and above its conduction of impulses, should be borne in mind as we examine methods of assessing adverse mechanical tension in the nervous system.

Assessment of adverse mechanical tension (AMT) in the nervous system

Testing for, and treating, 'tensions' in neural structures offers us an alternative method for dealing with some forms of pain and dysfunction, since such adverse mechanical tension is often a major component cause of musculoskeletal dysfunction as well as more widespread pathology (bear Korr's research in mind).

Maitland (1986) suggests that we consider this form of assessment and treatment to involve 'mobilisation' of the neural structures, rather than simply stretching them. He and others recommended that these methods be reserved for conditions which fail to respond adequately to normal mobilisation of soft and osseous structures (muscles, joints and so on). Maitland and Butler (Butler & Gifford 1989) have over the years discussed those mechanical restrictions which impinge on neural structures in the vertebral canals and elsewhere.

There is no general agreement as to the terminology which should be used in describing such biomechanical changes in the neural environment. Maitland et al (2001), for example, suggest that 'abnormal neural movement' is a more accurate description than 'neural tension'. Whatever we term the dysfunctional pattern, Butler & Gifford's focus on those 'adverse mechanical' changes which negatively influence neural function, and which cause a multitude of symptoms, including pain, has been a singular contribution to our understanding of some aspects of pain and dysfunction.

Base tests

Butler & Gifford (1989) have outlined a series of 'base tests' which can be used to discover precise mechanical restrictions relating to the nervous system. Five of the 'base (tension) tests' which will be described are useful not only for diagnosis but for passive mobilisation of the structures involved. The tissues involved in 'mechanical tension' often include the nerve itself, as well as its surrounding muscle, connective tissue, circulatory structures, dura and so on.

The five tension test methods which will be described are:

- straight leg raising (SLR)
- prone knee bending (PNB)
- passive neck flexion (PNF)
- a combination of these called 'slump' position
- the upper limb tension test (ULTT).

These tests are often performed in conjunction with each other (for example, 'slump' together with PNB). Despite some of these tests being familiar in other settings, if reliable results are wanted it is vital that the methodology for their use, as described in this particular context, is followed closely.

Simple examples

Butler & Gifford report that studies have shown that changes in tension in lumbar nerve roots have been demonstrated during PNF stretching manoeuvres and that there is often an instant alteration in neck and arm (and sometimes head) pain via the addition of ankle dorsiflexion during SLR. Additional stretches, such as ankle dorsiflexion performed during SLR, are described in this work as 'sensitising' manoeuvres.

Correct positioning vital

The Butler & Gifford approach calls for careful positioning of the region being tested, as changes in pain are assessed, as well as the use of passive stretches as a means of inducing release of restrictions when they are discovered. The developers of tension tests for adverse mechanical tension in the nervous system point out that body movements (and therefore these tests) not only produce an increase in tension within the nerve but also move the nerve in relation to surrounding tissues.

Meet the mechanical interface (MI)

The tissues which surround neural structures have been called the mechanical interface (MI). These adjacent tissues are those which can move independently of the nervous system (e.g. supinator muscle is the MI to the radial nerve, as it passes through the radial tunnel).

Any pathology in the MI can produce abnormalities in nerve movement, resulting in tension on neural structures with unpredictable ramifications. Good examples of MI pathology are nerve impingement by disc protrusion or osteophyte contact and carpel tunnel constriction. These problems would be regarded as mechanical in origin as far as the nerve restriction is concerned. Any symptoms resulting from mechanical impingement on neural structures will be more readily provoked in tests which involve movement rather than pure (passive) tension.

Chemical or inflammatory causes of neural tension also occur, resulting in 'interneural fibrosis' which leads to reduced elasticity and increased 'tension', which would become obvious with tension testing of these structures. (See Chapter 5, discussion of progression from acute to chronic in soft tissue dysfunction under the heading 'Local adaptation syndrome', p 110.)

Pathophysiological changes resulting from inflammation or from chemical damage (i.e. toxic) are noted as commonly leading on to internal mechanical restrictions of neural structures in a different manner to mechanical causes such as those imposed by a disc lesion, for example.

Adverse mechanical tension changes (or 'abnormal neural movement') do not necessarily and automatically affect nerve conduction, according to Butler & Gifford. However, Korr's research shows it to be likely that axonal transport would be affected by such changes.

AMT and pain sites not necessarily the same

When a tension test is positive (i.e. pain is produced by one or another element of the test – initial position alone or with 'sensitising' additions) it indicates only that there exists AMT somewhere in the nervous system and not that this is necessarily at the site of reported pain.

Butler & Gifford report on research indicating that 70% of 115 patients with either carpal tunnel syndrome or lesions of the ulnar nerve at the elbow showed clear electrophysiological and clinical evidence of neural lesions in the neck. This is, they maintain, because of a 'double crush' phenomenon in which a primary and often long-standing disorder, perhaps in the spine, results in secondary or 'remote' dysfunction at the periphery.

This phenomenon can also work in reverse, for example where wrist entrapment of the ulnar nerve leads ultimately to nerve entrapment at the elbow (they term this 'reversed double crush').

Neural vulnerability

Let us again refer to Korr's evidence of retrograde transportation of axonal flow, as this is one possible factor influencing such changes. In one of his texts (Korr 1970) he says:

> To appreciate the vulnerability of the segmental nervous system to somatic insults it must be understood that much of the pathway taken by nerves, as they emerge from the cord, is actually through skeletal muscle. The great contractile forces of skeletal muscles, with the accompanying chemical changes, exert profound influences on the metabolism and excitability of neurons. In this environment the neurons are subject to quite considerable mechanical and chemical influences of various kinds, compression and torsion and many others . . . slight mechanical stresses may, over a period of time, produce adhesions, constrictions and angulations imposed by protective layers. [Perhaps involving friction protectors such as meningeal extensions including nerve sheaths or nerve sleeves.]

Such mechanical stresses also, of course, interfere with axoplasmic flow:

> Flowing down every single nerve fibre is a stream of nerve cell cytoplasm in a volume so great that the nerve is said to 'turn over' its material completely three or four times a day, and this flow is essential to the continual nourishment of the fibres themselves along their entire length.

Since this axoplasmic flow also nourishes target tissues, in addition to which the nerves are known to carry back chemical messages from the tissues towards the cord in the same way, interference with the flow of chemical messages due to increased 'tensions' has major health implications. Korr further elaborated on four types of disturbance of nerve function which can result from local tissue impingement.

1. Increased neural excitability at the point of disturbance.
2. Triggering of supernumerary impulses (frequency of discharge from and into the spinal cord, as well as to the periphery increases, the patterns becoming 'garbled').
3. 'Cross-talk' which occurs when nerve fibres pick up electrical stimuli from neighbouring nerves.
4. Local stresses continually report to the spinal cord, thus 'jamming' normal transmission of patterned feedback.

Tension points and test descriptions

Butler & Gifford (1991) note that certain anatomical areas where the nervous system moves only a small amount relative to the surrounding interface during motion or where the system is relatively fixed are the most likely regions for AMT to develop. This is often noted where nerves branch or enter a muscle. Such areas are called 'tension points' and these are referred to in the test descriptions.

1. A positive tension test is one in which the patient's symptoms are reproduced by the test procedure and where these symptoms can be altered by variations in what are termed 'sensitising manoeuvres', which are used to 'add weight to', and confirm, the initial diagnosis of AMT. Adding dorsiflexion during SLR is an example of a sensitising manoeuvre.

2. Precise symptom reproduction may not be possible, but the test is still possibly relevant if other abnormal symptoms are produced during the test and its accompanying sensitising procedures. Comparison with the test findings on an opposite limb, for example, may indicate an abnormality, worth exploring.

3. Altered range of movement is another indicator of abnormality, whether this is noted during the initial test position or during sensitising additions.

Variations of passive motion of the nervous system during examination and treatment

1. An increase in tension can be produced in the *interneural component*, where tension is being applied from both ends, so to speak, as in the 'slump' test.

2. Increased tension can be produced in the *extraneural component*, which then produces the maximum movement of the nerve in relation to its mechanical interface (such as in SLR) with the likelihood of restrictions showing up at 'tension points'.

3. Movement of *extraneural tissues* in another plane can be engineered.

Before beginning the exercises below, look at Box 7.1, which gives some general precautions and contraindications for their use.

Box 7.1   General precautions and contraindications for Exercises 7.1–7.5

1. Take care of the spine during the 'slump test' if disc problems are involved or if the neck is sensitive (or the patient is prone to dizziness).
2. Take care not to be excessive in side-bending of the neck during ULTT.
3. If any area is sensitive, take care not to aggravate existing conditions during performance of tests (arm is more likely than leg to be 'stirred up').
4. If obvious neurological problems exist, take special care not to exacerbate by vigorous or strong stretching.
5. Similar precautions apply to diabetic, MS or recent surgical patients or where the area being tested is much affected by circulatory deficit.
6. Do not use the tests if there has been recent onset or worsening of neurological signs or if there is any cauda equina or cord lesion.

EXERCISE 7.1: STRAIGHT LEG RAISING (SLR) TEST

Time suggested: 3–4 minutes for each 'sensitising' addition

It is suggested that this test should be used in all vertebral disorders, all lower limb disorders and some upper limb disorders to establish the possibility of AMT in the nervous system in the lower back or lower limb.

See the text relating to hamstring test (for shortness) in Chapter 5 (Exercise 5.17A) and its accompanying figure (5.25).

The leg is raised in the sagittal plane, with the knee extended, until a barrier or resistance is noted or symptoms are reported.

Sensitising additions might include:

● ankle dorsiflexion (this stresses the tibial component of the sciatic nerve)
● ankle plantarflexion plus inversion (this stresses the common peroneal nerve, which may be useful with anterior shin and dorsal foot symptoms)
● passive neck flexion
● increased medial hip rotation
● increased hip adduction
● altered spinal position (the example is given of left SLR being 'sensitised' by lateral flexion to the right of the spine).

Perform the SLR test and incorporate each sensitising addition, in order to assess changes in symptoms, new symptoms, restrictions, etc.

Can the leg be raised as far as it should normally go (approximately 80°), and as easily, without force and without symptoms (new or old) appearing when the sensitising additions are incorporated?

Notes on SLR test

On SLR there is caudad movement of the lumbosacral nerve roots in relation to interfacing tissue (which is why there is a 'positive' indication – pain and limitation of leg-raising potential – from SLR if a prolapsed intervertebral disc exists).

Less well known is the fact that the tibial nerve, proximal to the knee, moves cuadad (in relation to the mechanical interface) during SLR, whereas distal to the knee it moves cranially. There is no movement of the tibial nerve behind the knee itself, which is therefore known as a 'tension point'.

The common peroneal nerve is attached firmly to the head of the fibula (another 'tension point').

EXERCISE 7.2: PRONE KNEE BEND (PKB) TEST

Time suggested: 3–4 minutes for each 'sensitising' addition in each position (1 and 2)

Method 1

Your palpation partner should be prone. You flex the knee, taking the heel towards the buttock, in order to assess reproduction of existing symptoms or other abnormal symptoms or altered range of movement (heel should approximate buttock easily).

During the test the knee is flexed while the hip and thigh are stabilised and this moves the nerves and roots from L2, 3, 4 and, particularly, the femoral nerve and its branches.

Method 2

If, however, the test is conducted with the person side-lying, the hip should be maintained in extension during the test (this alternative position is thought more appropriate for identifying entrapped lateral femoral cutaneous nerve problems).

The PKB test stretches rectus femoris and rotates the pelvis anteriorly, thus extending the lumbar spine, which can confuse interpretation of nerve impingement symptoms.

Reliance on sensitising manoeuvres helps with such interpretation. These include (in either prone or side-lying use of the test) the addition of:

- cervical flexion
- adopting the 'slump' position (Exercise 7.3) – but only in the side-lying variation of the test
- variations of hip abduction, adduction, rotation.

Can the knee easily be fully flexed, without force and without symptoms (new or old) appearing, when the sensitising additions are incorporated?

EXERCISE 7.3: THE 'SLUMP TEST'

Time suggested: 3–4 minutes for each 'sensitising' addition

This is regarded by Butler as the most important test in this series. It links neural and connective tissue components from the pons to the feet and requires care in performance and interpretation (see Fig. 7.1).

This test is suggested for use in all spinal disorders, most lower limb disorders and some upper limb disorders (especially those which seem to involve the nervous system).

The test involves your palpation partner introducing the following sequence of movements.

- Thoracic and then lumbar flexion, followed by
- Cervical flexion
- Knee extension
- Ankle dorsiflexion
- Sometimes also with hip flexion (produced by either bringing the trunk forwards on the hips or by increasing SLR)

continues

Sensitising manoeuvres during 'slump testing' are achieved as a rule by changes in the terminal positions of joints. Butler gives examples:

- Should the 'slump position' reproduce (for example) lumbar and radiating thigh pain, a change in head position – say away from full neck flexion – could result in total relief of these symptoms.
- A change in ankle and knee positions could significantly change cervical, thoracic or head pain.

In both instances this would confirm that AMT was operating, although the site would remain obscure.

Additional sensitising movements, with the person in the slump position, might involve the addition of trunk side-bending and rotation or even extension, hip adduction, abduction or rotation and varying neck positions.

The 'slump test' involves *tension* on the nervous system rather than *motion*.

Notes on 'slump' position

Cadaver studies demonstrate that neuromeningeal movement occurs in various directions, with C6, T6 and L4 intervertebral levels being regions of constant state (i.e. no movement, therefore 'tension points').

Butler reports that many restrictions, identified during the 'slump' test, may only be corrected by appropriate spinal manipulation and that SLR is more likely to pick up neural tension in the lumbosacral region.

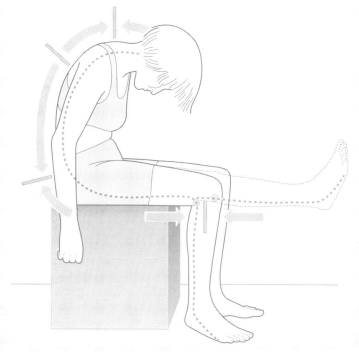

Fig. 7.1   The slump test position stretches the entire neural network from pons to feet. Note the direction of stretch of the dura mater and nerve roots. As the leg straightens, the movement of the tibial nerve in relation to the tibia and femur is indicated by arrows. No neural movement occurs behind the knee or at levels C6, T6 or L4 (these are the 'tension' points).

continues

EXERCISE 7.3: (Continued)

It is possible for SLR to be positive (e.g. symptoms are reproduced) and 'slump' negative (no symptom reproduction) and vice versa, so both tests should always be performed.

The following findings have been reported in research using the 'slump test'.

1. Mid-thoracic to T9 are painful on trunk and neck flexion in 50% of 'normal' individuals.
2. The following are considered normal if they are symmetrical:
   ● hamstring and posterior knee pain, occurring with trunk and neck flexion, when the knees are extended and increasing with ankle dorsiflexion
   ● restrictions in ankle dorsiflexion during trunk/neck flexion, while the knee is in extension
   ● there is a common decrease in pain and an increase in range of knee extension or ankle dorsiflexion on release of neck flexion.

If the patient's symptoms are reproduced by the slump position and can be relieved by sensitising manoeuvres, you have a positive test.

This is further emphasised if, as well as symptom reproduction, there is a symmetrical decrease in the range of motion which does not happen when tension is absent. For example, bilateral ankle dorsiflexion is restricted during slump, but disappears when the neck is not flexed.

In some instances, anomalous reactions are observed in which, for example, pain increases when the neck is taken out of flexion or when trunk on hip flexion decreases symptoms. Mechanical interface (MI) pathology may account for this.

EXERCISE 7.4: PASSIVE NECK FLEXION (PNF) TEST

Time suggested: 1–2 minutes for each variation

As with SLR, this test takes up slack from one end only. It allows movement of neuromeningeal tissues in relation to the spinal canal, which is its mechanical interface (MI).

Twenty two percent of patients with back pain were shown to have a positive PNF test in an industrial survey.

The head and neck are supported by your hands as you take the chin toward the chest. In a normal neck the chin should approximate the sternum without force or symptoms.

Variations such as neck extension, lateral flexion and PNF, in combination with other tests, should be used for screening purposes for AMT.

ULTT 1

Your palpation partner should be supine. Place the tested arm into abduction, extension and lateral rotation of the glenohumeral joint. Once these positions are established supination of the forearm is introduced together with elbow extension. This is followed by addition of passive wrist and finger extension.

If pain is experienced at any stage during placement of the person into the test position or during addition of sensitisation manoeuvres (below), particularly reproduction of neck, shoulder or arm symptoms previously reported, the test is positive and confirms a degree of mechanical interference affecting neural structures.

Additional sensitisation is performed by:

- adding cervical lateral flexion away from the side being tested
- introduction of ULTT 1 on the other arm simultaneously
- the simultaneous use of straight leg raising, bi- or unilaterally
- introduction of pronation rather than supination of the wrist.

Notes on ULTT 1

A great deal of nerve movement occurs during this test. In cadavers, up to 2 cm movement of the median nerve in relation to its mechanical interface has been observed during neck and wrist movement.

'Tension points' in the upper limb are found at the shoulder and elbow.

ULTT 2

Butler developed this test and finds it more sensitive than ULTT 1.

He maintains that it replicates the working posture involved in many instances of upper limb repetition disorders ('overuse syndrome').

In using ULTT 2, comparison is always made with the other arm.

Example of right-side ULTT 2:
For a right side test the person lies close to the right side of the table, so that the scapula is free of the surface. The trunk and legs are angled towards the left foot of the bed so that the patient feels secure.

The practitioner stands to the side of the person's head, facing the feet with the practitioner's left thigh depressing the shoulder girdle (see Fig. 7.2).

The person's fully flexed right arm is supported at both elbow and wrist, by the practitioner's hands.

Slight variations in the degree and angle of shoulder depression ('lifted' towards ceiling, held towards floor) may be used, by alteration of thigh contact.

Holding the shoulder depressed, the practitioner's right hand grasps the patient's right wrist while the upper arm is held by the practitioner's left hand.

continues

With these contacts sensitisation manoeuvres can be introduced to the tested arm – see below:

- shoulder internal or external rotation
- elbow flexion or extension
- forearm supination or pronation.

The practitioner then slides his right hand down onto the open hand and introduces supination or pronation or stretching of fingers/thumb or radial and ulnar deviations.

Further sensitisation may involve:

- neck movement (side-bend away from tested side, for example), or
- altered shoulder position, such as increased abduction or extension.

A combination of shoulder internal rotation, elbow extension and forearm pronation (with shoulder constantly depressed) is considered to offer the most sensitive test position.

Notes

Cervical lateral flexion away from the tested side causes increased arm symptoms in 93% of people and cervical lateral flexion towards the tested side increases symptoms in 70% of cases (Butler & Gifford 1991).

Butler & Gifford report that ULTT mobilises the cervical dural theca in a transverse direction, whereas the 'slump' mobilises the dural theca in an anteroposterior direction as well as longitudinally.

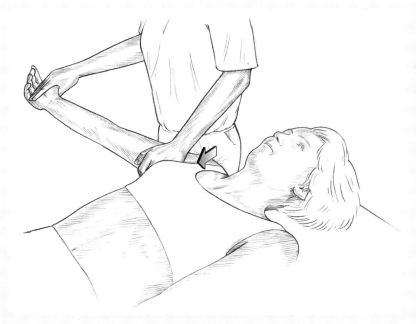

Fig. 7.2   Upper limb tension test (2). Note the practitioner's thigh depresses the shoulder as sensitising manoeuvres are carried out.

Implications of AMT

Bearing in mind Korr's evidence as to the many ways in which soft tissue (and osseous) dysfunction can impinge on neural structures, it is logical that maximum relaxation of any muscle involved in interface tissue should be achieved, by normal methods, before such tests (or subsequent treatment based on such tests) are considered.

It is not within the scope of this text to describe methods for releasing abnormal tensions except to suggest that, as in (most of) the examples of tests for shortened postural muscles given in Chapter 5, the treatment positions are a replication of the test positions.

Butler suggests that, in treating adverse mechanical tensions in the nervous system in this way, initial stretching should commence well away from the site of pain in sensitive individuals and conditions.

Re-testing regularly during treatment is also wise, in order to see whether gains in range of motion or lessening of pain provocation during testing are being achieved.

CAUTION: It is critical that any sensitivity provoked by treatment should subside immediately. If it does not the technique/test should be stopped or irritation could be caused to the neural tissues involved.

DISCUSSION REGARDING EXERCISES 7.1–7.5

The inclusion of these tests, in a text primarily aimed at enhanced palpatory literacy, may be questioned. What have they to do with palpation?

I consider that the tests previously described (Chapter 5), evaluating muscle length, as well as those for joint play (Chapter 9 and Special topic 9 on joint play) and those in this chapter, which evaluate possible AMT in neural structures, are all logical extension of palpation of the skin (and indeed of the region just above the skin) as well as of muscles and fascia.

The concepts of 'end-feel', range of motion and restrictive barriers are discussed elsewhere and assessment of such barriers and restrictions, as well as normal 'end-feel', requires a delicacy of touch which is a major element of palpatory literacy. These skills are likely to be enhanced if the tests described in this chapter are performed with delicacy and care.

Awareness of what Butler calls 'tension' points can be added to the knowledge we hold in mind as we palpate and test in other ways than those described above. As we use the methods developed by Lief, Nimmo, Lewit, Beal, Smith or Becker (or any other method of palpation) such knowledge is potentially very useful indeed.

If, for example, on NMT palpation or application of Becker's palpation methods, soft tissue changes were palpated in 'tension' point areas, as described by Butler, the possibility of neurological entrapment would be clear only if the concepts of AMT were understood. Use of one or all of the tests described above might then either confirm or deny this possibility.

Use of additional tests to assess for shortened muscle structures (Chapter 5) and joint restrictions (Chapter 9) would also be appropriate, as such changes could easily be the cause of adverse tension in the nervous system.

The inclusion of these tests is intended to encourage a different way of evaluating somatic dysfunction, using some familiar procedures (such as straight leg raising) as well as the enhancement of the palpation skills required in the performance of some quite complex manual procedures (ULTT 2, for example).

continues

DISCUSSION REGARDING EXERCISES 7.1–7.5 (*Continued*)

Clinical use of the tests involved in, as well as the underlying concepts of, AMT in neural structures, requires adequate professional training in these methods.

If you have succeeded in performing these tests, and their sensitising additions, and have acquired useful feedback and information which points towards AMT in the nervous systems of the model(s) you have worked with, then you may feel inspired towards further training in this subject, which has emerged out of physiotherapy methodology in recent years.

REFERENCES

Butler D, Gifford L 1989 Adverse mechanical tensions in the nervous system. Physiotherapy 75: 622–629

Butler D, Gifford L 1991 Mobilisation of the nervous system. Churchill Livingstone, Edinburgh

Korr I 1970 Physiological basis of osteopathic medicine. Postgraduate Institute of Osteopathic Medicine and Surgery, New York

Korr I 1981 Axonal transport and neurotrophic function in relation to somatic dysfunction. In: Korr I (ed) Spinal cord as organizer of disease processes, Part 4. Academy of Applied Osteopathy, Newark, Ohio, pp 451–458

Maitland G 1986 Vertebral manipulation. Butterworths, London

Maitland G, Hengeveld E, Banks K, English K 2001 Maitland's vertebral manipulation, 6th edn. Butterworth Heinemann, London

SPECIAL TOPIC 8
Source of pain – is it reflex or local?

Palpation of an area which the patient reports to be painful will usually produce increased sensitivity or tenderness if the pain is originating from that area. If, however, palpation produces no such increase in sensitivity, then the chances are strong that the pain is being referred from elsewhere.

But where is it coming from? knowledge of the patterns of probable distribution of trigger point symptoms can allow for a swift focusing on suitable sites in which to search for an offending trigger (if the pain is indeed coming from a myofascial trigger). The discomfort could, however, be a radicular symptom coming from the spine. Grieve (1984) reports:

> When pain is being referred into a limb due to a spinal problem, the greater the pain distally from the source, the greater the index of difficulty (the further distal, the more difficult) in applying quickly successful treatment.

Dvorak & Dvorak (1984) state:

> For patients with acute radicular syndrome there is little diagnostic difficulty, which is not the case for patients with chronic back pain, some differentiation for further therapy is especially important, although not always simple.

Noting that a mixed clinical picture is common, Dvorak & Dvorak then say:

> When testing for the radicular syndrome, particular attention is to be paid to the motor disturbances and the deep tendon reflexes. When examining sensory radicular disorders, the attention should be towards the algesias.

However, the referred pain may not be from either a trigger or the spine. Kellgren (1938, 1939) showed that:

> The superficial fascia of the back, the spinous processes and the supraspinous ligaments induce local pain upon stimulation, while stimulation of the superficial portions of the interspinous ligaments and the superficial muscles results in a diffused (more widespread) type of pain.

Mense & Simons (2001) give clear guidelines as to what the practitioner needs to be aware of when seeking the source of muscular pain:

> Because muscle pain and tenderness can be referred from trigger points, articular dysfunctions, and enthesitis [inflammation associated with musculotendinous junctions], the examiner must examine these sites for evidence of a condition that would cause referred muscle pain and tenderness.

Mense & Simons maintain that 'Local pain and tenderness in muscle is commonly caused by trigger points', but suggest that it is necessary to separate such local pain from other possible sources including projected, referred and central sources:

- projected pain (deriving from 'peripheral nerve irritation that initiates sensory action potentials at the site of irritation' – for example, the lightning pain felt when the ulnar nerve at the elbow is bumped

● referred pain, which commonly has a 'diffuse aching quality'. However, at times there may be a sharper 'projected pain', deriving from a nerve lesion, as in Tinel's sign.

Additionally visceral lesions may refer pain into muscle, such as in the pain noted in the lower left abdomen with appendicitis, which is very much the same type of pain noted when trigger points are present in that region. Central pain derives from sources such as a spinal cord injury, surgery involving the CNS or a peripheral injury which interrupts the connection to the CNS, such as occurs in amputation and subsequent phantom limb pain. Mense & Simons report that 'apparently, a peripheral pain experience can produce a central imprint that can serve as a central source of pain and also modifies peripheral referral patterns'.

Pain can also be referred to a muscle from:

● unknown sensitive locations which are not trigger points. For example, pressure on areas several inches from active and latent trigger points can produce referred pain. Mense & Simons (2001) state 'The reason for this spot sensitivity in normal muscle is unexplored'

● joints, particularly the capsules, zygapophyseal (facet) joints. This can lead to confusion when local trigger points produce similar patterns of pain. Mense & Simons report that 'The muscles crossing involved [blocked] joints are . . . likely to develop trigger points producing secondary muscle-induced pain because of the joint problem'.

Thus, ligaments and fascia must be considered as sources of referred pain and this is made clearer by Brugger (1960), who describes a number of syndromes in which altered arthromuscular components produce reflexogenic pain. These are attributed to painfully stimulated tissues (origins of tendons, joint capsules and so on) producing pain in muscles, tendons and overlying skin.

As an example, irritation and increased sensitivity in the region of the sternum, clavicles and rib attachments to the sternum, through occupational or postural patterns, will influence or cause painful intercostal muscles, scalenes, sternomastoid, pectoralis major and cervical muscles. The increased tone in these muscles and the resultant stresses which they produce may lead to spondylogenic problems in the cervical region, with further spread of symptoms. Overall, this syndrome can produce chronic pain in the neck, head, chest wall, arm and hand (even mimicking heart disease).

Dvorak & Dvorak have charted a multitude of what they term 'spondylogenic reflexes' which derive from (in the main) intervertebral joints. The palpated changes are characterised as:

> Painful swellings, tender upon pressure and detachable with palpation, located in the musculofascial tissue in topographically well defined sites. The average size varies from 0.5 cm to 1 cm and the main characteristic is the absolutely timed and qualitative linkage to the extent of the functionally abnormal position (segmental dysfunction). As long as a disturbance exists, the zones of irritation can be identified, yet disappear immediately after the removal of the disturbance.

The Dvoraks also see altered mechanics in a vertebral unit as causing 'reflexogenic pathological change of the soft tissue, the most important being the "myotendinoses", which can be identified by palpation'.

Some would argue that the soft tissue changes precede the altered vertebral states, at least in some instances (poor posture, overuse, misuse, abuse). Wherever you stand in this debate, this brief survey of some opinions as to 'where the pain is coming from' shows clearly that we need to keep many possibilities in mind.

As we palpate and evaluate, the question that we need to be asking ourselves almost constantly is 'which of this patient's symptoms, whether of pain or other forms of dysfunction, are the result of reflexogenic activity such as trigger points?'. In other words, what palpable, measurable, identifiable evidence is there which connects what we can observe, test and palpate to the symptoms (pain, restriction, fatigue, etc.) of this patient?

And what, if anything, can be done to remedy or modify the situation, safely and effectively, and what can the person do (or be taught to do) to prevent recurrence?

REFERENCES

Brugger A 1960 Pseudoradikulara syndrome. Acta Rheumatologica 18: 1
Dvorak J, Dvorak V 1984 Manual medicine: diagnostics. George Thieme Verlag, New York
Grieve G 1984 Mobilisation of the spine. Churchill Livingstone, Edinburgh
Kellgren J 1938 Observation of referred pain arising from muscles. Clinical Science 3: 175
Kellgren J 1939 On the distribution of pain arising from deep somatic strictures. Clinical Science 4:35
Mense S, Simons D 2001 Muscle pain. Williams and Wilkins, Philadelphia

8

Introduction to functional palpation

The learning experience in acquiring palpation skills depends upon the development of an awareness of what 'normal' feels like. Without that baseline for comparison it is hard to know what 'abnormal' feels like. Remembering what normal feels like offers an instant sense of 'this is not right'.

In this chapter we will look at functional palpation which, at its most basic, asks you to feel tissues as normal physiological demands are made of them, as you assess the response.

Healthy, well-adjusted and soundly functioning tissues will respond in a certain way and unhealthy, dysfunctional tissues in another. It is up to you to start to recognise, and imprint on your proprioceptive memory, what these responses – normal and abnormal – feel like.

The following series of exercises includes reference to, and thoughts derived from, the research work of: Edward Stiles (Johnston et al 1969), CA Bowles (1955), William Johnston (1966, 1988a, b, 1997), John Glover and Herbert Yates (1997), Philip Greenman (1989, 1996), as well as descriptive observations from British osteopath Laurie Hartman (1985). Also included later in this section (Exercises 8.3, 8.8) is a functional exercise based on the work of the developer of functional technique, HV Hoover (1969).

Hartman analyses this 'indirect palpation technique' saying that the practitioner's objective is to palpate the affected tissues, seeking 'a state of ease and release, rather than looking for the point of bind and barrier', which characterises so many other manipulative approaches (high-velocity thrust, articulation, muscle energy methods and so on). We have already experimented with an indirect form of assessment/palpation in Chapter 4, Box 4.4, where skin was moved on its underlying fascia in various directions, seeking a combined position of comfort/ease. That was a 'functional' exercise.

Finding dynamic neutral

The term 'functional technique' grew out of a series of study sessions held in the New England Academy of Applied Osteopathy in the 1950s under the general heading of 'a functional approach to specific osteopathic manipulative problems'.

In the 1950s and 1960s, research, most notably by Irvin Korr (1947), coincided with a resurgence of interest in this approach, largely as a result of the clinical and teaching work of Hoover. In functional work, palpation attempts to find a 'position of ease' and this involves a subjective appreciation of tissue as it is brought, by means of positioning, towards a state of 'comfort', 'ease', 'dynamic neutral'. This position is sensed by palpation, rather than relying on a report by the patient as to reduction in pain as positioning is pursued, as is the case in Laurence Jones's strain/counterstain (SCS) methods, as discussed in Chapter 5

(Jones 1981). An exercise will be described in this chapter (Exercise 8.9) in which a functional palpation for ease of a particular area will be compared with using SCS methodology in the same area. Theoretically (and commonly in practice) the palpated position of maximum ease (reduced tone) in the distressed tissues, located using functional technique, should correspond with the position which would have been found were pain being used as a guide (SCS).

Bowles (1955) gives an example of functional palpation.

> A patient has an acute low back and walks with a list. A structural diagnosis is made and the fingertips palpate the most distressed tissues, within the area of most distress. The practitioner begins tentative positioning of the patient, preferably sitting. The fingertips pick up a slight change toward a dynamic neutral response, a little is gained, a little, not much, but a little. A little, but enough so the original segment is no longer the most distressed area within the area of general distress. The fingers then move to what is now the most acute segment. As much feeling of 'dynamic neutral' (ease) is obtained here as possible. Being temporarily satisfied with slight improvements here and there, this procedure continues until no more improvement is detectable. That is the time to stop. Using [palpated] tissue response to guide the treatment, the practitioner has step by step eased the lesioning, and corrected the structural imbalance, to the extent that the patient is on the way to recovery.

Functional objectives

Hoover (1957) summarises the key elements of functional technique.

- Diagnosis of function involves passive evaluation, as the part being palpated responds to physiological demands for activity, made by the practitioner or the patient.
- Functional diagnosis determines the presence, or absence, of normal activity of a part, which is required to respond to normal body activities (say, respiration or the introduction of passive or active flexion or extension). If the participating part has free and 'easy' motion, it is normal; however, if it responds to activity by demonstrating palpated restricted or 'binding' motion, it is dysfunctional.
- The degree of ease and/or bind present in a dysfunctional site when motion is demanded is a fair guide to the severity of the dysfunction.
- The most severe areas of dysfunction are the ones to treat first.
- The directions of motion which induce ease in the dysfunctional tissues indicate precisely the most desirable pathways of movement.
- Use of these guidelines automatically prevents undesirable manipulative methods, since bind would result from any movement towards directions of stress for the tissues.
- Treatment using these methods is seldom, if ever, painful and is well received by patients.
- The application requires focused concentration on the part of the practitioner and may be mentally fatiguing. Functional methods are suitable for application to the very ill, the extremely acute and the most chronic situations.

Bowles (1955) is definite in his instructions to those attempting to use their palpating contacts in ways which will allow the application of functional methods.

- The palpating contact ('the listening hand') must not move.
- It must not initiate any movement.
- Its presence, in contact with the area under assessment/treatment, is simply to derive information from the tissue beneath the skin.
- It needs to be 'tuned into' whatever action is taking place beneath the contact and must temporarily ignore all other sensations such as 'superficial

tissue texture, skin temperature, skin tension, thickening or doughiness of deep tissues, muscle and fascial tensions, relative positions of bones and range of motion'.

● All these signs should be assessed and evaluated and recorded separately from the functional evaluation, which should be focused single-mindedly on tissue response to motion. 'It is the deep segmental tissues, the ones that support and position the bones of a segment, and their reaction to normal motion demands, that are at the heart of functional technique specificity.'

Terminology

Bowles explains the shorthand use of these common descriptive words.

> Normal somatic function is a well-organised complexity, and is accompanied by an easy action under the functionally-orientated fingers. The message from within the palpated skin is dubbed a sense of 'ease', for convenience of description. Somatic dysfunction could then be viewed as an organised dysfunction, and recognised under the quietly palpating fingers as an action under stress, an action with complaints, an action dubbed as having a sense of 'bind'.

In addition to the 'listening hand' and the sensations it is seeking, of ease and bind, Bowles suggests we develop a 'linguistic armament' which will allow us to pursue the subject of functional technique without 'linguistic embarrassment' and without the need to impose quotation marks around the terms each time they are used.

He therefore asks us to become familiar with the additional terms 'motive hand', which indicates the contact hand, which directs motion (or fingers, or thumb or even verbal commands for motion-active or assisted); and also 'normal motion demand' which indicates what it is that the motive hand is asking of the body part. The motion could be any normal movement such as flexion, extension, side bending, rotation or combination of movements – the response to which will be somewhere in the spectrum of ease and bind, which will be picked up by the 'listening hand' for evaluation.

At its simplest, functional technique sets up a 'demand-response' situation, which allows for the identification of dysfunction – as bind is noted – and for therapeutic intervention, as the tissues are guided into ease. Functional technique, palpation or treatment (there is really no difference) seeks the loose, free, easy, comfortable directions of movement and avoids anything which produces feelings, in the palpated tissues, of increased tone, tension, restriction, bind or pain.

Bowles's summary of functional methods

In summary, whatever region, joint or muscle is being evaluated by the listening hand, the following results might occur.

1. The motive hand makes a series (any order) of motion demands (within normal range), which includes all possible physiological variations. If the response noted in the tissues by the listening hand is ease in all directions symmetrically, then the tissues are functioning normally.

2. The motive hand makes a series of motion demands, which includes all possible variations; however, some of the directions of movement produce bind, although the demand is within normal physiological ranges. The tissues are responding dysfunctionally.

3. For therapy to be introduced, in response to an assessment of bind relating to particular motion demands, the listening hand's feedback is required so that,

as the motions which produced bind are reintroduced, movement is modified so that the maximum degree of ease possible is achieved. 'Therapy is monitored by the listening hand, and fine-tuned information, as to what to do next, is then fed back to the motive hand. Motion demands are selected which give an increasing response of ease and compliance, under the quietly palpating fingers.'

The results can be startling, as Bowles explains:

> Once the ease response is elicited, it tends to be self-maintaining in response to all normal motion demands. In short, somatic dysfunctions are no longer dysfunctions. There has been a spontaneous release of the holding pattern.

The palpating contact

Some practitioners mould the hand, part of the hand or palmar surface of the fingers to the tissues which are being evaluated for ease and bind as the area is moved actively or passively. Others use a method (termed a 'compression test') described by Johnston (1997) as follows.

> The compression test is the application of pressure, through the finger(s), to sense any increased tissue tension, at one segment, compared with adjacent segments. Even at rest, a compression test of a dysfunctional segment will register the local increased resistance of that segment's deep musculature . . . The segment's tissues change during motion testing. This provides a palpable measure of the degree of disturbed motor function . . . During motion testing, palpatory cues of increasing resistance in one direction are sensed *immediately*, along with an immediate sense of decreasing resistance (increasing ease) in the opposite direction. (Johnston's italics)

EXERCISE 8.1: BOWLES' SELF-PALPATION METHOD

Time suggested: 3–4 minutes

Stand up and place your fingers on your own neck muscles, paraspinally, so that the fingers lie, very lightly, without pressing but constantly 'in touch' with the tissues, approximately over the transverse processes.

Start to walk for a few steps and try to ignore the skin and the bones under your fingers. Concentrate all your attention on the deep supporting and active tissues as you walk.

After a few steps, stand still and then take a few steps backwards, all the while evaluating the subtle yet definite changes under your fingertips. Repeat the process several times, once while breathing normally and once while holding the breath in, and again, holding it out.

Standing still, take one leg at a time backwards, extending the hip and then returning it to neutral, before doing the same with the other leg.

What do you feel with your listening hands in all these different situations?

Comment

This exercise should help to emphasise the 'listening' role of the palpating fingers and of their selectivity about what they wish to listen to. The listening hand contact should be 'quiet, non-intrusive, non-perturbing', in order to register the compliance of the tissues and evaluate whether there is a greater or lesser degree of ease or bind on alternating steps and under different circumstances, as you walk, stand still, move your leg.

8.2A

Stand behind your seated palpation partner, resting your palms and fingers over their upper trapezius muscle, between the base of the neck and shoulder. The object is to evaluate what happens under your hands as your partner takes a deep breath.

Note: This is not a comparison between inhalation and exhalation, but is meant to help you assess how the areas being palpated respond to inhalation.

Do the tissues under your hands stay easy or do they bind?

You should specifically not try to define the underlying structures, or their status, in terms of tone or fibrosity. Simply assess the impact, if any, of inhalation on the tissues.

Do the tissues resist, restrict, bind or do they stay relaxed on inhalation?

Compare what is happening under one hand with what is happening under the other, during inhalation only – specifically avoiding comparison of the feel of the tissues during inhalation and exhalation.

8.2B

Your palpation partner should be seated with you standing behind.

The objective this time is to 'map' the various areas of 'restriction' or bind in the thorax, anterior and/or posterior, during the time your partner is inhaling.

In this exercise, try not only to identify areas of bind but map the territory, by assigning what you find into large (several segments of near the spine) and small (single segment) categories.

To commence, place a single hand, mainly fingers, on (say) the upper left thoracic area, over the scapula, and have your partner breathe deeply several times, first while seated comfortably hands on lap and then with the arms folded on the chest (exposing more the costovertebral articulation).

After several breaths, with your hand in one position, resite it a little lower or more medially or laterally, as appropriate, until the entire back has been 'mapped' in this way.

Most importantly for this exercise, remember that you are not comparing how the tissues 'feel' on inhalation as compared with exhalation, but how different regions compare (in terms of ease and bind) with each other, in response to inhalation.

Map the entire back and/or front of the thorax, in this way, for location of areas of bind and for the size of these areas.

Return and repalpate any large areas of bind and, within them, see whether you can identify any small areas, using the same simple contact, with inhalation as the motion component.

Individual spinal segments can also be mapped by sequentially assessing them, one at a time, as you evaluate their response to inhalations.

How would you normally handle the information you have uncovered if this were a 'patient'?

Would you try in some way to mobilise what appears to be restricted? If so, how?

continues

EXERCISE 8.2 *(Continued)*

Would your therapeutic focus be on the large areas of restriction or the small ones?

Would you work on areas distant from or adjacent to the restricted areas?

Would you attempt release of the perceived restriction by trying to move it mechanically towards and through its resistance barrier or would you rather be inclined to use some indirect approach, moving away from the restriction barrier?

Or, would you try a variety of approaches, mixing and matching, until the region under attention was free or improved?

There are no correct or incorrect answers to these questions. However, the various exercises in this section should open up possibilities for a variety of treatment options to be considered, ways which do not impose a solution but allow one to emerge.

8.2C
Your palpation partner should be seated, arms folded on the chest, with you standing behind, with your listening hand/fingertips placed on the upper left thorax, on or around the scapula area.

Your motive hand should be placed at the cervicodorsal junction, so that it can indicate to your partner your request that he move forward of the midline (dividing the body longitudinally in the coronal plane), not into flexion but in a manner which carries the head and upper torso anteriorly.

The movement will be more easily accomplished if your partner has arms folded, as suggested above.

The repetitive movement forward into the position described, and back to neutral, is initiated by the motive hand, while the listening hand evaluates the palpated tissues' response to the movements.

The comparison which is being evaluated is of one palpated area with another, in response to this normal motion demand.

As Johnston and his colleagues (1969) state, in relation to this exercise:

> It is not anterior direction of motion, compared with posterior direction, but rather a testing of motion into the anterior compartment only, comparing one area with the ones below, and the ones above, and so on.

Your listening hand is asking the tissues whether they respond easily or with resistance to the motion demanded of the trunk. In this way, try to identify those areas, large and small, which bind as the movement forward is carried out.

Compare these areas with those identified when the breathing assessment was used.

Comment

The patterns elicited in Exercise 8.2C involve movement initiated by you as the practitioner, whereas the information derived from 8.2A and 8.2B involved intrinsic motion, initiated by exaggerated respiration.

Johnston and his colleagues (1969) have, in these simple exercises, taken us through the initial stages of palpatory literacy, in relation to how tissues respond to motion, self-initiated or externally induced. You should, by these means, have become able to localise (map) areas of dysfunction (bind), large and small, and, within large areas, become able to identify small dysfunctional tissue localities. These localities can then be used as monitors in subsequent treatment, as the area is moved into positions which minimise the restrictions you are able to palpate in them.

Hoover's 'experiments'

Hoover (1969) poses a number of questions in the following exercises ('experiments' he calls them), the answers to which should always be 'yes'. If your answers are indeed positive at the completion of the exercise, then you are probably sensitive enough in palpatory skills to be able to effectively utilise functional technique.

EXERCISE 8.3: HOOVER'S THORACIC EXPERIMENT

Time suggested: 7–10 minutes (8.3A), 3–4 minutes each (8.3B and 8.3C)

8.3A
You should be standing behind your seated partner, whose arms are folded on their chest.

Having previously assessed by palpation, observation and examination the thoracic or lumbar spine of your partner, lightly place your listening hand, or finger pad contact, on those segments which you judge to be the most restricted or in which the tissues are most hypertonic.

Wait and do nothing as your hand 'tunes in' to the tissues. Make no assessments as to structural status. Wait for at least 15 seconds.

Hoover says:

> The longer you wait, the less structure you feel. The longer you keep the receiving fingers still, the more ready you are to pick up the first signals of segment response, when you proceed to induce a movement demand.

With your other hand, and by voice, guide your partner into flexion and then extension. The motive hand should apply very light touch, just a suggestion, to indicate to your partner in which direction you want movement to take place.

The listening hand does nothing but wait to feel the functional response of ease and bind, as the spinal segments move into flexion and then extension.

A wave-like movement should be noted as the segment being palpated is involved in the gross motion demanded of the spine.

A change in the tissue tension under palpation should be noted as the various phases of the movement are carried out.

Can you feel this?

Practise the same assessment of tissue response, at various segmental levels.

Try to feel the different responses of the palpated tissues during the phases of the process, as bind starts and then becomes more intense as the first barrier approaches, then eases somewhat as the direction of movement reverses, becoming ever easier, before a hint of bind reappears and then becomes intense again, as the opposite barrier is approached.

continues

EXERCISE 8.3 *(Continued)*

Decide where the maximum bind is felt and where maximum ease occurs. These are the key pieces of information required for functional technique, as you assiduously avoid bind and home in on ease.

Can you feel this?

Can you locate the point where the distressed tissues are at their most comfortable in response to whatever movement you are using as the challenge?

Try also to distinguish between that bind response which is a normal physiological result of an area coming towards the end of its normal range of movement and the bind which is a response to dysfunctional restriction.

Can you feel this?

8.3B
Return to the starting position as in 8.3A and while palpating an area of restriction or hypertonicity, induce straight side-flexion to one side and then the other, while assessing for ease and bind in exactly the same way as in 8.3A.

Can you locate the position of maximum ease during these movements?

8.3C

Return to the starting position and, while palpating an area of restriction or hypertonicity, induce rotation to one side and then the other, while assessing for ease and bind, in exactly the same way as in 8.3A and 8.3B.

Can you locate the position of maximum ease during these movements?

Comment

Hoover (1969) describes variations in what might be felt as the response of the tissues palpated during these various positional demands.

1. *Dynamic neutral.* This response to motion is an indication of normal physiological activity. There is minimal signalling during a wide range of motions in all directions. Hoover states it in the following way: 'This is the pure and unadulterated unlesioned (i.e. not dysfunctional) segment, exhibiting a wide range of easy motion demand-response transaction'.

2. *Borderline response.* This is an area or segment which gives some signals of some bind fairly early in a few of the normal motion demands. The degree of bind will be minimal and much of the time ease, or dynamic neutral, will be noted. Hoover states that 'most segments act a bit like this'; they are neither fully 'well' nor 'sick'.

3. *The lesion response.* Note that the use of the word 'lesion' predates the introduction of the term 'somatic dysfunction', to describe abnormally restricted segments or joints. To update this term we should call this a 'dysfunctional response'. This is where bind is noted almost at the outset of almost all motion demands, with little indication of dynamic neutral.

Hoover suggests that you:

> Try all directions of motion carefully. Try as hard as you can to find a motion demand that doesn't increase bind, but on the contrary, actually decreases bind, and introduces a little ease. This is possible. This is an important characteristic of the lesion [dysfunction].

Indeed, he states that the more severe the restriction, the easier it will be to find one or more slight motion demands which produce a sense of ease, dynamic neutral, because the contrast between ease and bind will be so marked.

Hoover's summary

Practice is suggested with dysfunctional joints and segments, in order to become proficient. Three major ingredients are required for doing this successfully, according to Hoover.

1. A focused attention to the process of motion demand and motion response, while whatever is being noted is categorised, as 'normal', 'slightly dysfunctional', 'frankly or severely dysfunctional' and so on.

2. A constant evaluation of the changes in the palpated response to motion, in terms of ease and bind, with awareness that this represents increased and decreased levels of signalling and tissue response.

3. An awareness that, in order to thoroughly evaluate tissue responses, all possible variations in motion demand are required, which calls for a structured sequence of movement demands. Hoover suggests that these be verbalised (silently):

> Mentally set up a goal of finding ease, induce tentative motion demands until the response of ease and increasing ease is felt, verbalise the motion-demand which gives the response of ease in terms of flexion, extension, side-bending and rotation. Practise this experiment until real skills are developed. You are learning to find the particular ease-response to which the dysfunction is limited.

In addition, depending upon the region being evaluated, the directions of abduction, adduction, translation forwards, translation backwards, translation laterally and medially, translation superiorly and inferiorly, etc., *all* need to be factored into this approach.

Bowles describes the goal

Bowles's (1955) words summarise succinctly what is being sought:

> The activity used to test the segment (or joint) is largely endogenous, the observing instrument is highly non-perturbational, and the information gathered is about how well or how poorly our segment (being palpated) of structure is solving its problems.
>
> Should we find a sense of ease and non-distorted following of the structures we diagnose the segment as normal. If we find a sense of binding, tenseness, tissue distortion, a feeling of lagging and complaining in any direction of the action, then we know the segment is having difficulty properly solving its problems.

The diagnosis would be of dysfunction.

The treatment would be functional; by holding a segment, an area, in its position of ease, resolution of dysfunction begins.

The whole key to successful normalisation of dysfunction lies in the finding of the position of dynamic neutral, of ease, and the degree of your palpatory sensitivity is what decides whether this will be achieved or not.

Spinal application of functional technique palpation

In order to practise functional evaluation and treatment of the spine or a joint, an area (of the spine, for example) needs to be identified as being dysfunctional, different or abnormal, as compared with the rest of the spine, using one of the many forms of assessment already described.

The identification of areas of muscle fullness during the seated and standing spinal flexion tests (see Chapter 9) or the neuromuscular assessment methods, or of 'flat' spinal areas as described in the assessment sequence for tight muscles in Chapter 5 or the previous exercises in this chapter, could all direct you to such a 'different' area, requiring further investigation or normalisation.

Hartman (1985) suggests another possibility, after initial suspicion has been alerted:

> Diagnosis of textural abnormality in the tissues is made in the normal way with palpation. A gradient of abnormality can be felt in a particular area and the centre of this area is made a focus.

Hartman suggests light tapping be introduced over the spinous processes and paravertebral musculature, to emphasise and localise the area of difference. There will be a variation in the resonance noted which, he suggests, will be subjectively picked up by the patient and which can guide you to the most central portion of the dysfunctional tissues. (See Special topic 10, Percussion palpation.)

Johnston's views on the barrier

Johnston (1966) explains the terms 'direct' and 'indirect' as follows.

> When the incremental aspects of these cues [directions of motion restriction] are appreciated as an immediately increasing resistance towards a sense of barrier in one direction, and an immediate increasing ease towards a sense of potential release, in the opposite direction, then the terms direct [towards the sense of resistance] and indirect [away from the sense of resistance] offer a classification of osteopathic manipulative procedures, based on diagnosed asymmetry, to be addressed.

It is easy to move from such a diagnostic assessment into active treatment.

Johnston's protocol

Johnston's summary of the planning and criteria involved in a functional approach to assessment and treatment can be expressed as follows.

- It is necessary to introduce motion in any one direction at a time which involves minimal force.
- Motion direction is towards a sense of increasing ease, which is manifested by a lessening in the sense of resistance to pressure from the palpating fingers.
- Different direction elements are combined, such as rotation and translation, producing variations in torsion.
- Active respiration is also monitored for its influence on ease.
- The examiner follows the continuous flow of information, signalling increasing ease/decreasing resistance during all procedures.

EXERCISE 8.4: FUNCTIONAL SPINAL PALPATION

Time suggested: 10–15 minutes

Evaluate the spine of your seated palpation partner, assessing areas of flatness or fullness, as you observe the flexed spine from the side or from in front.

Palpate the area and seek out the central site of tissue dysfunction, greatest hypertonia or sensitivity, using one of the previous exercises such as 8.3A. Using the flexed fingertips of one hand, tap lightly and steadily on the tissues identified, as well as on those surrounding the area. (See Special topic Figure 10A).

Can you identify a different sound in the most affected tissues?

Once a suitably 'different' (from adjacent segments) sound has been identified, one hand (the listening hand) should be placed on these tissues. The other hand is used to introduce motion into the region, passively or with some active cooperation, but only if directed to do so by you.

A sequence of normal physiological motions should be introduced to the region and in each instance (in each direction) the palpating hand, on the tense dysfunctional tissues, should be feeling for greater ease or greater bind, trying to find a point where a combination of the greatest directions of ease (see below) are summated, in order to achieve maximal relaxation of the tissues.

This, says Hartman, is a form of inhibition for the tense tissues, 'in that areas of irritability are quieted, the practitioner constantly looking for the state of ease and release'.

The movements introduced (sequence is irrelevant) for assessment of ease and bind should include:

- flexion and extension
- side-flexion, left and right
- rotation, left and right
- translation, anterior and posterior
- translation (shift), left and right
- translation, cephalad and caudad (involving traction and compression) followed by:
- respiration, involving both inhalation and exhalation.

Greenman describes the process of achieving the point of ease, involving the first six motions, as 'stacking' (the order in which these are applied is not significant; simply it is useful to apply them sequentially so that none is forgotten). This should be followed by the final respiratory screening, seeking the phase of the cycle which produces maximum ease.

Johnston (1997) has described this:

> The final component step of the functional procedure involves a request for a specific direction of active respiration, whichever direction (inhalation or exhalation) contributes further to the increasing ease. For example, if inhalation, the request is for the subject to take a deep breath slowly, and to hold briefly.

After a position of greatest ease has been established using one of the planes of movement (say, flexion and extension), that position of ease is used as the starting point for the next direction (say, rotation left and right) or plane (say, side-flexion left and right) to be assessed for its position of greatest ease.

continues

When this is discovered you will have found a combined position of ease for the first two directions of movement tested, say extension and side-flexion or rotation.

You will have 'stacked' the second onto the first and from that combined position of ease you would then introduce the next direction for assessment, say translation right and left . . . and so on, until all directions have been evaluated and their positions of ease 'stacked', one onto the other (see Fig. 8.1).

Then the respiratory assessment is introduced and the final position of ease held for 60–90 seconds or so, before complete reevaluation of previously identified restrictions.

A sense of a wider range of normal (greater ease) should be felt by the practitioner as these releases occur.

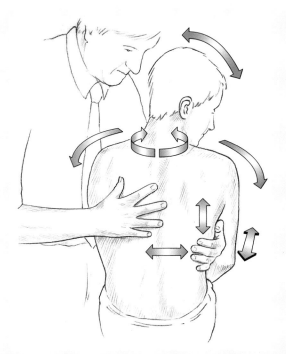

Fig. 8.1   Arrows show directions of movement, as ease and bind are assessed by the 'listening' hand on the spinal tissues during functional evaluation of spinal segments. Movements are: Flexion-extension, Rotation left and right, Side-bending left and right, Translation to each side, Translation forward and back, Translation up and down (traction and compression).

EXERCISE 8.5: GREENMAN'S FUNCTIONAL LITERACY PALPATION

Time suggested: 15–20 minutes for the three phases of the exercise

Greenman describes a sequence of exercises for achievement of 'functional literacy'. The following is a modified summary of his sequence.

8.5A

Stand behind and to the side of your seated palpation partner, whose arms should be folded, so that the hands are holding the opposite shoulders. Place a 'listening' hand, or finger pads, onto the upper thoracic spine, where tissue tightness or fullness has been identified.

Allow the hand to be very still. Wait until it feels 'nothing' (no movement).

Your other hand ('motor' hand) should be placed on your partner's head, in order to lead it through specific motions, such as flexion or extension (very slowly performed, without jerking).

The palpating hand tries to identify tissue changes, in terms of increased ease or increased bind.

Keep repeating a single movement of the head into slow flexion, back to neutral, into flexion, back to neutral . . . noting where the point of maximum ease is located in this plane of movement.

Then introduce slow repetitive backward bending of the head as you palpate for ease. Extend slowly, return to neutral, extend, back to neutral.

Is the ease greater with the head in a flexed or extended direction?

8.5B

Return to neutral and introduce side bending right and rotation to the left of the head and neck on the trunk, several times (back to neutral after each excursion).

Then introduce side bending left and rotation to the right of the neck and head on the trunk, all the while palpating the area being assessed for alterations in their ease and bind characteristics.

In which parts of this compound series of movements do the tissues relax most or become most tense?

Is there a symmetrical range of ease and bind in both directions?

Find the point – somewhere between extreme side bending left, rotation right, and side bending right, rotation left – in which the palpated tissues feel at their most relaxed.

8.5C

Return the neck and head to neutral and introduce, and try to combine, the following movements, as you palpate for ease and bind:

- small amount of forward bending, accompanied by right side bending and right rotation of the head and neck on the trunk
- follow this with slight flexion, left side bending and left rotation of the head and neck on the trunk.

Palpate constantly for ease in the thoracic segment under your listening hand. Evaluate the symmetry of the findings.

Was ease/bind found at the same place moving the head and neck to the left and to the right?

Comment

Greeman (1996) suggests that similar palpation exercises be performed in various regions of the spine. In each case what you are looking for in normal tissue, or where there is only minimal dysfunction, is a wide range of motion accompanied by minimal signalling (i.e. most of the tissue being palpated is in relative ease).

Where a significant degree of dysfunction exists, there will be narrow ranges which produce signals of ease or decreased bind.

Experience is the only teacher as to what is and what is not significant clinically in this information.

EXERCISE 8.6: GREENMAN'S FUNCTIONAL SPINAL PALPATION

Time suggested: 20 minutes

Note that this is more or less the same exercise as 8.5, with the difference that you should first practise it on a dysfunctional segment and then a normal one.

8.6A

Your palpation partner should be seated. You stand behind and to one side, palpating a previously identified area of dysfunction in the thoracic spine.

Adopt a contact where the patient has their arms folded and you embrace the shoulder furthest from you with one hand, drawing the opposite shoulder into your axilla, so that you can control the various directions of motion.

Sequentially introduce the elements of:

- forward bending, followed by backward bending
- left side bending, right side bending
- rotation left, rotation right
- a combination of side bending in one direction, with rotation to the same side, during flexion and then extension.

Then introduce side bending in the other direction, with rotation to the opposite side during flexion and then extension.

Add to a combination of positions of ease discovered during these assessments elements such as translation anterior and posterior, translation from side to side and translation cephalad and caudad, in order to discover where the maximum point of ease occurs.

Can you sense ease positions in any of these motions?

Can you find a 'most easy' position, by combining elements of these motions?

Maintain the final position of ease and after a minute return the area to neutral.

Reevaluate the positions of ease. Have they changed?

8.6B

Perform exactly the same sequence on a segment lower down the spine which does not display evidence of dysfunction.

Compare your findings of range, and positions of ease and bind, with those discovered during the previous exercise.

8.7A
Repeat all the components of Exercise 8.6A but now introduce a long-held (as long as is comfortable to the person) breath, in both inhalation and exhalation, in each of those positions in which maximum ease was previously palpated.

Is there any additional release (or increase) of resistance during or after either phases of held breath?

The secret of this approach is learning to apply all suitable directions of motion which enhance ease, together with the respiratory component which produces maximal ease.

8.7B
Repeat the sequence of Exercise 8.6A but this time identify the most extreme positions of bind, so that you can eventually engage the restriction barrier.

In this position (whatever combination of movements has led to maximal bind), have the patient gently try to return to the starting position (normal) against your resistance for a 10-second hold.

Repalpate the area of dysfunction after this isometric contraction and see whether you have increased the range, pushed back the barrier, increased ease? This is a muscle energy procedure, in which an isometric contraction of the tense soft tissues has encouraged a reduction in tone and an increase in elasticity, after the contraction.

Which approach appeals to you most, seeking ease or obliging the barrier to retreat after engaging it?

Hoover's clavicle 'experiment'

The developer of functional technique, HV Hoover, explained the essence of this approach in the words of the founder of osteopathy, Andrew Taylor Still: 'I am doing what the body tells me to do'.

Hoover (1969) asks the beginner to perform the following three 'experiments', grouped together in Exercise 8.8. In each case a question is posed, the answer to each being 'yes'.

Your answers will tell you whether you are ready to use this method – whether you have achieved palpatory literacy.

8.8A
Question 1: Does the clavicle move in a definite and predictable manner, when demands are made upon it by definite movements of an adjacent part?

Stand facing your seated palpation partner and place the pads of the (relaxed) fingers of your right hand lightly over the right clavicle, just feeling the skin overlaying it (see Fig. 8.2). This hand is the listening hand. It is there to evaluate what happens.

continues

With your left hand, hold the right arm close to the elbow (this is your motor or moving hand).

Your partner must be relaxed, passive and cooperative, not helping or hindering the introduction of movements by your motive hand.

The listening hand should barely touch the skin, no pressure at all being applied to the clavicle.

Raise and lower the arm slowly, several times, until you are certain that it is relaxed, that you have the weight of the arm without assistance. The exercise can now begin.

Slowly take the arm backwards from the midline, introducing shoulder extension, just far enough to sense a change in the tissues under the palpating hand. Then return the arm to its starting position.

Do not move quickly or jerk the arm, so ensuring that the sensations being picked up by both the motive and the listening hand are accurate.

Repeat this several times, slowly, so that you become aware of the effect of a single, simple, movement (remember the question you are asking your partner's body).

Now take the arm forward of the midline (shoulder flexion) and again assess the effect on the palpated tissues (clavicle and surrounding tissue).

Subsequently, in no particular sequence, abduct and then adduct the arm; rotate the arm externally and subsequently internally, each time slowly and if necessary repeatedly, each time noting the tissue response to a single direction of movement.

What response was noted to each of these single physiological movements?

Remember this was not an exercise in which you were meant to compare the effect of one movement with another (that comes next), but a time to evaluate what effect single movements produced, as perceived by your palpating hand and also by the motive hand.

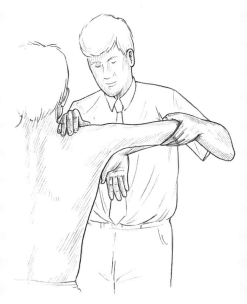

Fig. 8.2 Assessing positions of the arm which induce ease or bind at the acromioclavicular joint (after Hoover 1969).

continues

EXERCISE 8.8 *(Continued)*

Revisit Exercises 5.16A and B, where you evaluated the feeling of resistance as you moved the leg into abduction, as well as the palpated feeling of 'bind' in the medial hamstrings and other adductors.

8.8B

Question 2: Are there differences in ease of motion, and feeling of ease and bind in the tissues associated with this clavicle, when it is caused to move in different physiological motions?

Follow the same starting procedure until the exercise proper begins (i.e. ensure a relaxed, supported arm, with your palpating contact in place).

Move the arm backwards into extension very slowly, as you palpate the changes in the tissues around the clavicle.

Compare the feeling of the tissues when this is done with what happens as you take the arm into flexion, bringing it forwards.

Now compare the feelings in the listening hand as you abduct and then adduct the arm, slowly, deliberately, gently.

Compare the tissue changes (ease/bind) as you first internally and then externally rotate the arm.

Did there appear to be directions of motion which produced enhanced feelings of ease in the tissues? What were they?

8.8C

Question 3: Can the differences of ease of motion, and tissue texture, be altered by moving the clavicle in certain ways?

Repeat the introductory steps up until the exercise proper begins.

Flex the patient's arm, bringing it forward of the midline, slowly and gently until you note the clavicle moving or the tissue texture under your palpating hand changing. Stop at that point.

Now extend the arm backwards from the midline, slowly and gently until you note the clavicle moving or the tissue texture under the palpating hand changing. Stop at that point.

Find a point of balance between these two states, a point of balance from which movement, in any direction, causes the clavicle to move, along with a change in tissue texture.

Hold this point of physiological balance, which Hoover called 'dynamic neutral'. Starting from this first position of ease, you should next find the point of balance between adduction and abduction.

Once this has been established you will have found a combined position of ease between flexion and extension, as well as adduction and abduction.

Starting from this combined ease position you should then move on to find the point of balance between internal and external rotation.

You will then have achieved a state of reciprocal balance between the arm and the clavicle.

From here Hoover leads you to another important finding.

continues

8.8D

Holding the arm and clavicle in reciprocal balance, dynamic neutral, as at the end of 8.8C above, test to see whether any of the six physiological motions (flexion/extension/adduction/abduction/internal and external rotation, as in 8.8B), on its own, gives a sensation of improved tissue texture, compared with the other physiological motions.

One of the directions may be found which does not increase bind or which increases ease more than the others.

Having found this motion, slowly and gently continue to repeat it for as long as the sensory hand continues to report that tissue conditions, motion of the clavicle, are gaining in ease.

Should bind begin to be noted as this is done, Hoover suggests that the various directions of motion should all be rechecked, to find that which introduces the most ease. If none do, then stop at this point, noting what it is that you have been feeling.

If a further direction of motion producing ease is found, this is repeated until bind seems to occur again.

Repeat the retesting procedure of all the directions of motion.

Hoover says:

> This process of finding the easy physiological motion, and following it until bind starts, and then rechecking, may go on through two or more processes, until a state of equilibrium is found from which tissue texture indicates ease in all [directions of] physiological motion.

8.8E

In order to perform this final part of Hoover's experiment, the untreated, opposite clavicle should be taken through stages 8.8A, B and C.

When you have reached a reciprocal balance between arm and clavicle, reliance is placed on the tissues to 'tell' you what movements are required by it to achieve maximum ease.

You need to relax and become entirely passive as the sensory (or listening) hand detects any change in the clavicle and its surrounding tissues. Such a change if felt by the listening hand, sends the information to the reflex centres, which relay an order to the motor hand to move the arm so as to maintain the reciprocal balance or neutral. If this is the appropriate move, there will be a feeling of increasing ease of motion and improved tissue texture.

This process continues through one or more motions until the state of maximum ease or quiet is attained.

This is a process known as fascial unwinding, which is the natural culmination of functional technique when patiently applied.

This functional palpation/treatment approach can be employed, with the addition of translation motions, for any extremity or spinal joint, as a means of identifying directions of ease and bind.

EXERCISE 8.9: COMBINED FUNCTIONAL AND SCS PALPATION OF ATLANTOOCCIPITAL JOINT

Time suggested: 10–15 minutes

8.9A

Your palpation partner is supine. You sit at the head of the table, slightly to one side, so that you are facing the corner. One hand (your caudal hand) cradles the occiput, with opposed index finger and thumb palpating the soft tissues adjacent to the atlas. The other hand is placed on the forehead or the crown of the head.

The caudal hand assesses for feelings of 'ease', 'comfort' or 'release' in the tissues surrounding the atlas, as the hand on the head directs it into a compound series of motions, one at a time.

As each motion is 'tested', a position is identified where the tissues feel at their most relaxed or easy. This position of the head is used as the starting point for the next element in the sequence of assessment.

In no particular order (apart from the first movements into flexion and extension) the following directions of motion are tested, seeking always the position of the head and neck which elicits the greatest degree of ease in the tissues around the atlas, to 'stack' onto the previously identified positions of ease:

- flexion/extension (suggested as the first directions of the sequence)
- side bending left and right
- rotation left and right
- anteroposterior translation (shunt, shift)
- side-to-side translation
- compression/traction.

Once three-dimensional equilibrium has been ascertained (known as dynamic neutral) in which a compound series of ease positions have been 'stacked', the person is asked to inhale and exhale fully, to identify which stage of the breathing cycle enhances the sense of palpated 'ease', and then to hold the breath in that phase of the cycle for 10 seconds or so.

The final combined position of ease is held for 90 seconds before *slowly* returning to neutral.

Note that the sequence in which directions of movements are assessed is not relevant, providing as many variables as possible are employed in seeking the combined position of ease.

This held position of ease is thought to allow neural resetting to occur, reducing muscular tension, and also to encourage improved circulation and drainage through previously tense and possibly ischaemic or congested tissues.

8.9B

With your palpation partner lying supine and with you seated at the head of the table, palpate the tissues around the atlantooccipital joint, using drag palpation, and locate what you consider to be the area of greatest sensitivity/tenderness.

Apply a single-digit pressure to this sensitive area, sufficient to evoke a reported score of '10' on the pain scale (where 10 = marked discomfort and 0 = no pain).

Maintain this pressure as you carefully reposition (fine-tune) the head and neck, in order to reduce the pain score to 3 or less.

continues

EXERCISE 8.9 *(Continued)*

The most likely position to ease reported pain of this sort is slight extension, followed by slight side bending toward, and slight rotation away from, the painful point.

If such a combination is not effective, fine-tune until you identify the head/neck position which reduces the score most.

Once you have established this position of ease, hold it for 90 seconds and then, on release, repalpate to see whether the tissues are less sensitive.

Pay particular attention to the final position of ease and decide whether it is in any way similar to the final position achieved when you sequentially stacked positions of ease, in Exercise 8.9A.

This exercise offers you the chance to explore the two major methods of positional release technique and also gives you a very useful method for easing distressed tissues in this sensitive and vulnerable area.

Conclusion

The exercise in this chapter are extremely important. They are elegant in their objectives (to locate comfort/ease/balance), apparently simple and yet demanding of intense focus.

They also represent, as clearly as it is possible, the objective of a seamless transition from assessment to treatment. This is so because once the point of optimal ease has been identified, for as long as this is held, self-generated, homeostatic, normalisation processes are operating. The tissues take advantage of being held in a state of ease to commence normalisation, of circulation, neural status, tone. Everything negative that is taking place when tissues are tense and contracted (increased pain perception, ischaemia, drainage impairment, mechanical and chemical irritation, etc.) is put into reverse. So finding the point of 'ease' by palpation is the task of the practitioner, while using that position advantageously is the prerogative of the body itself.

If these concepts excite you then you are urged to investigate further by studying the practice of positional release (Chaitow 2002, D'Ambrogio & Roth 1997, Deig 2001).

REFERENCES

Bowles C 1955 Functional orientation for technic. American Academy of Applied Osteopathy Yearbook, Newark, OH
Chaitow L 2002 Positional release techniques, 2nd edn. Churchill Livingstone, Edinburgh
Clover J, Yates H 1997 Strain and counterstrain techniques. In: Ward R (ed) Foundations for osteopathic medicine. Williams and Wilkins, Baltimore
D'Ambrogio K, Roth G 1997 Positional release therapy. Mosby, St Louis, MI
Deig D 2001 Positional release technique. Butterworth Heinemann, Boston
Greenman P 1989 Principles of manual medicine. Williams and Wilkins, Baltimore
Greenman P 1996 Principles of manual medicine, 2nd edn. Williams and Wilkins, Baltimore
Hartman L 1985 Handbook of osteopathic technique. Hutchinson, London
Hoover H 1957 Functional technique. Yearbook of the Academy of Applied Osteopathy, Newark, OH
Hoover H 1969 A method for teaching functional technique. Yearbook of the Academy of Applied Osteopathy, Newark, OH
Johnston W 1966 Manipulative skills. Journal of the American Osteopathic Association 67:
Johnston W 1988a Segmental definition, Part I. Journal of the American Osteopathic Association 88:
Johnston W 1988b Segmental definition, Part II. Journal of the American Osteopathic Association 88:
Johnston W 1997 Functional technique. In: Ward R (ed) Foundations for osteopathic medicine. Williams and Wilkins, Baltimore
Johnston W, Robertson A, Stiles E 1969 Finding a common denominator. Yearbook of the American Academy of Applied Osteopathy, Newark, OH
Jones L 1981 Strain and counterstrain. Academy of Applied Osteopathy, Colorado Springs
Korr I 1947 The neural basis for the osteopathic lesion. Journal of the American Osteopathic Association 47:191

SPECIAL TOPIC 9
Joint play/'end-feel'/ range of motion: what are they?

Joint play refers to the particular movements between bones associated with either separation of the surfaces (as in traction) or parallel movement of joint surfaces (also known as translation or translatoric gliding).

Some degree of such movement is possible between most joints, restricted only by the degree of soft tissue elasticity. Any change in length of such soft tissues, therefore, automatically alters the range of joint mobility – also known as the degree of 'slack' – which is available.

Joint separation or 'degrees of traction'

Grades can be ascribed to the range of separation possible between joint surfaces.

- When traction is applied to a joint (at right angles to the joint surface) a slight separation, merely removing the intrinsic compressive force of surrounding tissues, is known as a Grade I degree of traction.
- When the 'slack' is removed by further separation, tightening the surrounding tissues, this is a Grade II degree of traction.
- This increases to a Grade III when actual stretch of the tissues is introduced.

Glide or translation

When a gliding translation between joint surfaces occurs, this takes place with the surfaces parallel to each other (also called 'rollgliding') (see Special Topic Fig. 9A).

Only a portion of the joint will be able to move parallel with its opposing surface in this way, at any given time. Since the surfaces of joints are never completely flat, only one part is parallel with the other at any moment (technically this is described as due to the surfaces being incongruent). Once again grading is possible.

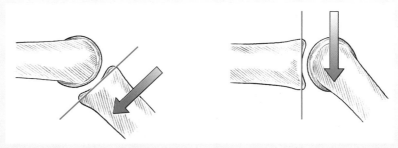

Special Topic Fig. 9A   Parallel displacement of a bone involving translatoric gliding (after Kaltenborn). One bone is moved parallel to the treatment plane until the tissues surrounding the joint are tightened (grade II) or the tissues crossing the joint are stretched (grade III).

- A Grade I glide involves slack being taken up and a degree of tightening of the soft tissues.
- Grade II involves actual stretching of these tissues as translation continues.

Convex and concave rule

An important rule, relating to whether the joint surface is concave or convex, is described by Kaltenborn (1985). This states that if a concave surface moves in relation to another surface, then the direction of gliding and the direction of the movement of the bone are the same. This means that the moving bone and the concave surface of the joint are on the same side as the axis of motion (see Special Topic Fig. 9B).

However, when a convex joint surface is in a gliding motion the bone movement will be in the opposite direction to the glide. This means that the moving surface and the bone lie on opposite sides of the axis of rotation. Thus, when there is a joint restriction, ascertained by careful assessment of joint play (i.e. gliding), it is essential to know the relative shape of the articulation. In the case of a convex joint surface (for example, the head of the humerus) the bone will need to be moved by the therapist in a direction opposite to the direction of restricted bone motion in order to increase or improve the range of motion in the joint.

In the case of a concave joint surface (for example, the proximal head of the ulna) the bone will need to be moved in the same direction as the direction of

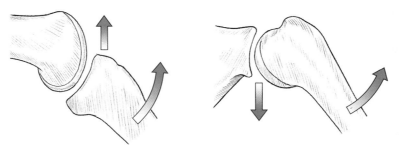

Special Topic Fig. 9B   The direction of gliding in a joint depends upon whether the surface on which movement is occurring is concave or convex. If concave gliding occurs it is in the same direction as the bone movement (left) while convex gliding occurs in the opposite direction to the movement of the bone (right) (after Kaltenborn).

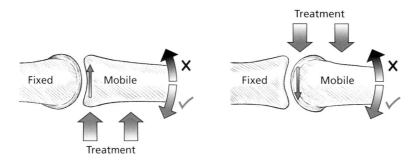

Special Topic Fig. 9C   This figure illustrates the 'convex-concave rule' in which a mobile bone moves on a fixed structure. *Left*: the joint surface is concave (as would be the case in the tibia, ulna or a phalangeal joint). If the mobile bone was restricted in an upward direction (striped arrow), a gliding mobilisation made during treatment would also be in an upward direction (as indicated by the two large arrows). *Right*: there is a mobile bone associated with a convex surface (as in the head of the humerus, the femur or talus). If this was restricted in an upward direction (striped arrow), a gliding mobilisation made in treatment would be in a downward direction (large arrows) (after Kaltenborn).

restriction of bone movement, in order to improve the range of motion in the joint (see Special Topic Fig. 9C).

Importance of joint play

Just how vital joint play is to the body is made clear in the example given by Kuchera & Kuchera (1994), discussing the subtalar joint. This is a 'shock-absorber', a designation earned, they say, because 'in coordination with the intertarsal joints, it determines the distribution of forces upon the skeleton and soft tissues of the foot'.

Mennell (1964) graphically describes this shock-absorbing potential,

> Its most important movement is a rocking movement of the talus upon the calcaneus, which is entirely independent of voluntary muscle action. It is this movement which takes up all the stresses and strains of stubbing the toes, and that spares the ankle from gross trauma, both on toe-off and at heel-strike, in the normal function of walking, and when abnormal stresses . . . are inflicted on the ankle joint. If it were not for the involuntary rocking motion at the subtalar joint, fracture dislocations would be more commonplace.

Similar shock-absorbing potential exists at the sacroiliac joint which, when this is lost as in cases where the joint has fused, can result in fractures of the sacrum (Greenman 1996).

Barriers

All joints have 'normal' ranges of motion and some guidelines as to these are found in Chapter 9. Palpation should involve a screening of these for abnormal restriction or for hypermobility.

The end of a joint's range of motion may be described as having a certain feel and this is called 'end-feel'.

If a joint is taken actively or passively to its maximum range of normal motion it reaches its physiological barrier. This has a firm but not harsh end-feel. If this is taken to its absolute limit, the anatomical barrier is engaged and this has a hard end-feel, beyond which any movement would produce damage.

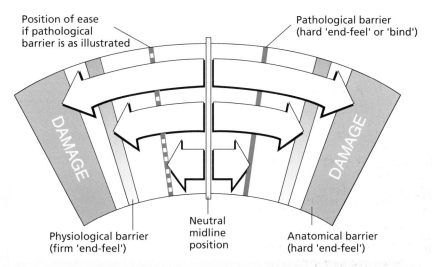

Special Topic Fig. 9D Schematic representation of a range of motion indicating normal restriction barriers (anatomical and physiological) as well as a pathological barrier and a position of maximal ease. The quality of the 'end-feel' of each of these will vary markedly.

If there is, for any reason, a restriction in the range of motion then a pathological barrier would be apparent on active or passive movement in that direction.

If the reason for the restriction involved interosseous changes (arthritis, for example) the end-feel would be sudden or hard. However, if the restriction involved soft tissue dysfunction the end-feel would have a softer nature (see Special Topic Fig. 9D).

Kaltenborn summarises normal end-feel variations thus.

- Normal soft end-feel is due to soft tissue approximation (such as in knee flexion) or soft tissue stretching (as in ankle dorsiflexion).
- Normal firm end-feel results from capsular or ligamentous stretching (internal rotation of the femur, for example).
- Normal hard end-feel occurs when bone meets bone, as in elbow extension.

However, pathological end-feel can involve a number of variations such as:

- a firmer, less elastic feel when scar tissue restricts movement or when shortened connective tissue exists
- an elastic, less soft end-feel when increased muscle tonus restricts movement
- an empty end-feel is one in which the patient stops the movement (or asks for it to be stopped) before a true end-feel is reached, as a result of extreme pain (fracture or active inflammation) or psychogenic factors.

Hypermobile joints

Ligaments and muscles which are hypermobile do not adequately protect joints and therefore fail to prevent excessive ranges of motion from being explored. Without this stability, overuse and injury stresses evolve and muscular overuse is inevitable.

Janda (1984) observes that in his experience:

In races in which hypermobility is common there is a prevalence of muscular and tendon pain, whereas typical back pain or sciatica are rare.

Logically, the excessive work rate of muscles which are adopting the role of 'pseudoligaments' leads to tendon stress and muscle dysfunction, increasing tone in the antagonists of whatever is already weakened and complicating an already complex set of imbalances, including altered patterns of movement (Beighton et al 1983).

What to do with abnormal barriers when you find them

One objective of palpation of restrictions is to define the degree of limitation by establishing the range of motion in various directions.

Another is assessment of the nature of those restrictions through, among other factors, determination of the softness or hardness of the end-feel. Some manipulative techniques involve engaging the pathological barrier before any of a variety of methods are employed to increase the range of motion; pushing the barrier back, so to speak.

This might involve the use of isometric contractions of the agonist (shortened muscle or group of muscles) or of their antagonists, as in muscle energy technique (MET), or it might involve active high-velocity thrust (HVT) adjustment/manipulation as in chiropractic and some osteopathic treatment. Or it might involve mobilisation, using long leverage or use of joint play techniques. A different approach would be to move towards the direction opposite the direction of restriction, easing away from the barrier(s) of restriction, as in functional osteopathic techniques such as strain/counterstrain.

Whichever approach is used, there remains the importance of knowing how to 'feel' the end of range of motion in any direction, without provoking sensitive tissues further. Practising on normal tissues and joints makes recognition of restricted ones simpler.

Kaltenborn states:

> The ability to see and feel the quality of movement is of special significance in manual therapy, as slight alterations from the normal may often be the only clue to a correct diagnosis.

Active and passive movements

If pain occurs anywhere in a range of movement (active or passive) which is both preceded and followed by pain-free motion, the range in which the pain is noted is called a painful arc.

Deviations of normal pathways during such a painful arc indicate avoidance strategies and are important diagnostically.

As a rule, active movements test all anatomical structures as well as the psychological willingness of the patient to move the area. Passive movements test only non-contractile tissues with such movements being compared with

SPECIAL TOPIC EXERCISE 9.1: ASSESSING JOINT PLAY AT THE PROXIMAL TIBIOFIBULAR JOINT

Time suggested: 3–4 minutes

Your palpation partner should be supine with hip and knee flexed so that the sole of the foot is flat on the table. You sit so that your buttock rests on the patient's toes, stabilising the foot to the table. The head of the fibula is grasped between thumb and index finger of one hand, as the other hand holds the tibia firmly, inferior to the patella.

Care should be taken to avoid excessive pressure on the posterior aspect of the fibula head, as the peroneal nerve lies close by (Kuchera & Goodridge 1997). The thumb resting on the anterior surface of the fibula should be reinforced by placing the thumb of the other hand over it.

A movement which takes the fibular head firmly posteriorly and anteriorly, in a slightly curved manner (i.e. not quite a straight backward and forward movement, but more back and slightly curving inferiorly, followed by forward and slightly curving superiorly, at an angle of approximately 30°), determines whether there is freedom of joint glide in each direction.

If restriction is noted in either direction, repetitive rhythmical but gentle springing of the fibula, at the end of its range, should restore normal joint play.

It is worth noting that when the fibular head glides anteriorly there is automatic reciprocal movement posteriorly at the distal fibula (lateral malleolus), while posterior glide of the fibula head results in anterior movement of the distal fibula. Restrictions at the distal fibula are, therefore, likely to influence behaviour proximally and vice versa.

Are you able to feel the glide?

accepted norms as well as the corresponding opposite joint. End-feel, painful arcs, shortened muscles, restricted or exaggerated joint function are all assessed in this way. As a general rule, a greater degree of motion is achieved passively rather than actively.

Many of the exercises in Chapter 9 will provide the opportunity for you to refine your skills in 'reading' end-feel.

REFERENCES

Beighton P et al 1983 Hypermobility of joints. Springer Verlag, Berlin
Greenman P 1996 Principles of manual medicine, 2nd edn. Williams and Wilkins, Baltimore
Janda V 1984 Low back pain – trends, controversies. Presentation, Turku, Finland, 3–4 September
Kaltenborn F 1985 Mobilization of the extremity joints. Olaf Norlis Bokhandel, Oslo
Kuchera M, Goodridge J 1997 Lower extremity. In: Ward R (ed) Foundations for osteopathic medicine. Williams & Wilkins, Baltimore, MD
Kuchera W, Kuchera M 1994 Osteopathic principles in practice. Greyden Press, Columbus, OH
Mennell J 1964 Joint pain. T and A Churchill, Boston

9

Palpation and assessment of joints (including spine and pelvis)

The assessment of the functional integrity, or otherwise, of joints has been exhaustively covered in many osteopathic, orthopaedic and chiropractic textbooks over the past half century or more. The intent in this chapter is not to duplicate such information, but rather to summarise some of the most important elements of joint palpation, together with the provision of guides as to what some 'normal' ranges of motion might be expected to be.

In addition, some novel, sequential approaches will be covered, as will an assessment/palpation approach which was developed in the context of osteopathic medicine, which claims to evaluate the current degree of adaptive potential of the individual (Zink & Lawson 1979).

Serious students of joint palpation should seek elsewhere for more comprehensive descriptions of clinical joint assessment.

Observe, palpate, actively and passively test

Dysfunction of joints can be demonstrated in three different ways, all of which form part of a comprehensive assessment of the musculoskeletal system: observation, palpation and testing of function (which is itself separated into active and passive movements).

We have already seen (Chapters 4 and 5) that there exist useful sequential screening patterns for uncovering evidence of shortened muscles (postural muscle screening) or changes within those muscles (NMT assessment, Nimmo's method, etc.).

Mitchell et al (1979) provide further useful guidance on succinct methods for eliciting information as to where to focus attention or where more detailed examination is required. Such an approach is necessary, since it is patently impossible during any normal consultation examination to cover each and every muscle, joint and test. As Mitchell puts it: 'The purpose . . . is to identify a body region, or body regions, which deserve(s) more detailed evaluation'.

The following process of evaluation contains elements of the methods suggested by Mitchell et al, with many other researchers' ideas also being incorporated.

Notes

Each of the segments numbered below can be seen as an individual exercise for developing and practising the palpation and observational skills necessary for enhancing the ability to evaluate the mechanical and functional integrity of the musculoskeletal system.

As expertise and confidence are gained in the application of the skills described in each individual exercise below, the sequence should be combined with others, so that a comprehensive evaluation process emerges.

Note that not all joints, or functions of joints, are covered, since this book is not meant to provide detailed instruction in structural and functional analysis, but rather to enhance the skills needed to do so.

Symptoms

When palpating and assessing dysfunction it is very important to identify what eases symptoms, as well as what worsens them, as this may reveal patterns which 'load' and 'unload' the biomechanical features out of which the symptoms emerge. The patient's own viewpoint as to what helps, and what worsens, symptoms, as well as the practitioner's evaluation as to where restrictions and abnormal tissue states exist, and how dysfunction manifests during standard testing and palpation, should together form the basis, with the history, for making a tentative initial assessment.

Repetitions are important

In performing assessments (testing a shoulder for internal rotation, for example), if performing a particular action produces no symptom, it may be useful to have the movement performed a number of times. As Jacob & McKenzie (1996) explain:

> Standard range of motion examinations and orthopedic tests do not adequately explore how the particular patient's spinal [or other area of the body] mechanics and symptoms are affected by specific movements and/or positioning.

Perhaps the greatest limitation of these examinations and tests is the supposition that each test movement needs to be performed only once to fathom how the patient's complaint responds. The effects of repetitive movements or positions maintained for prolonged periods of time are not explored, even though such loading strategies might better approximate what occurs in the 'real world'.

Assessments should evaluate symptoms in relation to posture and position, as well as to function or movement. Function needs to be evaluated in relation to quality, as well as symmetry and range of movement involved.

Any assessment needs to take account of the gender, age, body type and health status of the individual being assessed, as these factors can all influence a comparison with the 'norm'.

Attention should be paid to the effect of movement on symptoms (does it hurt more or less when a particular movement is performed?), as well as to the degree of functional normality revealed by the movement.

EXERCISE 9.1: OBSERVATION OF THE CLIENT

Time suggested: 10–12 minutes (reducing to 3–5 with practice)

Observe your palpation partner walking, both slowly and briskly. Look for:

- normal and equal length of stride
- good weight transfer from heel to lateral foot, to metatarsal joints, with a push-off from the big toe
- evidence of external or internal rotation of the legs
- normal flexion and extension of hips, knees and ankles.

Pay particular attention to the presence, or otherwise, of a well-developed arch during mid-stride on the weight-bearing foot.

Normal gait should involve the following.

- Weight placed evenly on each foot.
- Pelvis virtually horizontal, with a slight sway being normal (more so in women).
- The spinal column curves, when observed from behind, should move from side to side, in a wave-like manner, with the greatest range in the mid-lumbar area.
- The thoracolumbar junction should remain above the sacrum at all times (see notes on long leg/short leg later in this chapter).
- A swing of the arms should come from the shoulder with little head motion.
- Asymmetry of arm position.
- The upper shoulder fixators should appear relaxed.

Look for:

- asymmetrical patterns, stiffness and any tendency to rock or limp
- symmetrical levels of knees and malleoli
- morphological asymmetries – scars, bruises, etc.

Lewit (1992) suggests listening to the sounds made as the patient walks. He also points out that 'certain faults become more marked if the patient closes her eyes, walks on tiptoe or on the heels, and these should be examined as required'.

Always ask patients to adopt their typical work posture as part of the evaluation.

Try to read any body language which hints at unresolved or somatised emotional issues – inhibited/withdrawn, extrovert, 'military', depressed or other stereotypical postures.

Record all findings.

EXERCISE 9.2: POSTURAL OBSERVATION – POSTERIOR AND LATERAL ASPECTS

Time suggested: 10–12 minutes (reducing to 3–5 with practice)

Posture should then be viewed from behind, attention being given to:

● head balance (are ear lobes at the same height?)
● neck and shoulder symmetry
● levels of scapulae
● any lateral spine curves
● the distance the arms hang from the side of the body
● the levels of the folds at waist level (are they symmetrical?)
● gluteal folds (are they the same height from the floor?)
● morphological changes.

The side view is examined for:

● normality of anteroposterior spinal curves
● head position relative to the body
● abdominal ptosis
● winging of the scapulae
● the angle of the feet
● morphological changes.

Record and chart all findings.

EXERCISE 9.3: POSTURAL OBSERVATIONS AND RANGE OF SPINAL MOTION

Time suggested: 10–12 minutes (reducing to 3–5 with practice)

Posture and symmetry are then observed from the front and the following are observed and recorded, evaluating symmetry or otherwise of:

● stance (foot placement)
● patella height
● intercostal angle
● clavicles.

The side view is then evaluated again.

Is the head/centre of gravity over the body or forward or backwards of it?

The person is asked to bend backwards – range should be around 35°, with a sharp bend at the lumbosacral junction or at the thoracolumbar junction (in cases of increased mobility).

Anteflexion has a normal range of around 60°, when the knees are extended. Hamstring shortness affects this test so seated anteflexion is a more accurate assessment of lumbar flexibility.

Side bending, with strict care that no ante- or retroflexion accompanies this, should achieve a range of 20° to each side.

Note that hypermobility of the lumbar spine is, according to Lewit (1992), indicated most strongly by hyperlordosis when standing relaxed, together with exaggerated lumbar kyphosis when sitting relaxed.

Record all findings.

EXERCISE 9.4: CREST HEIGHT PALPATION

Time suggested: 2–4 minutes

The barefoot person stands erect, with back to you (your eyes at the level of the iliac crests). Feet should be a little apart, ankles directly below the hip sockets (heels 10–15 cm apart), toes pointing straight ahead.

Place the radial border of your index finger (hands palm down) just inferior to the iliac crests and push firmly in a superomedial direction, until the index fingers rest on the pelvic crest.

If your hands are level, there is no anatomical leg length difference. If there is a difference (and there is no iliac rotation or spinal scoliosis), then an anatomical leg length difference is possible (see also later in this chapter for discussion of leg length discrepancy).

A slim book should be placed under the heel of the short side, to equalise leg length, until symmetry of pelvic crest heights is achieved, so that the following tests (below) can be performed.

Could there be an anatomical leg length difference?

Can you balance the iliac crest heights by 'building up' the short leg?

EXERCISE 9.5: PALPATION FOR PSIS POSITION

Time suggested: 2–3 minutes

Assessment of the posterior superior iliac spine (PSIS) position is achieved by palpating just below the sacral dimples, for osseous prominences. These are palpated for symmetry. Is one anterior or posterior, in relation to the other?

If one PSIS is anterior to the other, then there is shortness of either

- the ipsilateral external rotators, possibly including iliopsoas, quadratus femoris, gemellus (superior and/or inferior) and obturator (internal and/or external) if the hip is not flexed, and piriformis, if the hip is flexed, or
- the contralateral internal rotators, possibly including gluteus medius and minimus and hamstrings (if the hip is not flexed) or adductor magnus and hamstrings (if the hip is flexed).

Posterior displacement indicates the possibility of precisely the opposite pattern of shortening.

Is one PSIS superior or inferior to the other, as you palpate? Inferior displacement may involve short hamstrings, iliac or pubic dysfunction.

Record whether one PSIS is anterior or posterior, in relation to the other, and whether either PSIS appears superior or inferior, compared with the other.

Your palpation partner should be standing as in Exercise 9.4 above (iliac crests having been levelled by placing a slim book under the short leg if asymmetry was discovered). Your thumbs should be placed firmly on the inferior slopes of the PSIS. Your partner keeps his knees extended as he bends forwards towards the toes, while your contact thumbs retain their positions on the same tissues overlying the PSIS (see Fig. 9.1).

Is there movement of your thumbs? The practitioner observes, especially near the end of the excursion of the bend, whether one or other PSIS 'travels' more anterosuperiorly than the other. If one thumb moves a greater distance anterosuperiorly during flexion, it indicates that the ilium is 'fixed' to the sacrum on that side (or that the contralateral hamstrings are short or that the ipsilateral quadratus lumborum is short: therefore, all these muscles should have been assessed prior to the standing flexion test).

If both hamstrings are excessively short this may produce a false-negative test result, with the flexion potential limited by the muscular shortness, preventing an accurate assessment of iliac movement.

At the end of the flexion excursion, Lee (1999) has the patient come back to upright and bend backward, in order to extend the lumbar spine. 'The PSISs should move equally in an inferior [caudad] direction.'

The standing flexion test indicates iliosacral status, because the muscular influences from the lower extremity determine iliac relationships with the sacrum, when standing. This influence

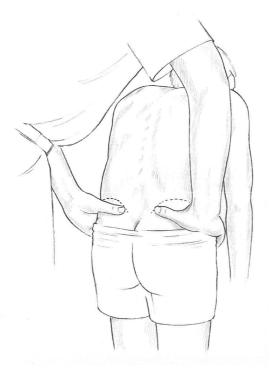

Fig. 9.1　Standing flexion test for iliosacral dysfunction. The restricted side is the one on which the thumb moves during flexion.

continues

EXERCISE 9.6: (Continued)

disappears when the patient is seated (see Exercise 9.8 below) at which time a positive test would indicate sacroiliac dysfunction (i.e. if asymmetry of PSIS movement occurs during flexion as evidenced by thumb movement).

Did your thumbs move symmetrically during flexion or not at all? Which iliosacral joint, if any, is dysfunctional?

Note

Both the standing flexion test (above) and the 'stork' test (see Exercise 9.10 below) are only capable of demonstrating which side of the pelvis is most dysfunctional, restricted or hypomobile. They do not, however, offer evidence as to what type of dysfunction has occurred (i.e. whether it is an anterior or posterior innominate rotation, internal or external innominate flare dysfunction, or something else).

The nature of the dysfunction needs to be evaluated by other means, some of which will form exercises in this chapter.

EXERCISE 9.7: OBSERVATION OF ROTOSCOLIOSIS DURING STANDING FLEXION

Time suggested: 3–5 minutes

With the person standing fully flexed, you should move to a position so that the spine may be viewed from directly in front (looking down the spine), for paravertebral (erector spinae) symmetry and evidence of greater 'fullness' on one side.

Note what is found for comparison with subsequent evidence noted when the patient is seated (Exercise 9.9).

Mitchell suggests that:

- If there is greater paravertebral fullness on one side of the spine, this is probably evidence of a degree of rotoscoliosis, caused by the transverse processes being more posterior on the side of greater fullness.
- If this is more evident in standing flexion than in seated flexion, muscular tightness/shortness (postural muscles of the leg/pelvis, for example) is probably a primary factor, with the rotoscoliosis a compensatory feature.
- If, however, greater paraspinal fullness is displayed during seated flexion, then rotoscoliosis is probably primary, with pelvic imbalance and postural muscle shortness being compensatory.
- If the evidence of fullness on one side during flexion is the same when both seated and standing, then rotoscoliosis is primary, with no leg muscle compensation.

Is there increased 'fullness' in the paraspinal muscles during flexion?

If so, what does it relate to, according to Mitchell's guidelines described above?

EXERCISE 9.8: SEATED FLEXION TEST

Time suggested: 2–3 minutes

The seated flexion test evaluates sacroiliac dysfunction and adds to evidence relating to erector spinae tightness.

Your palpation partner should be seated on a low, firm surface, legs apart, hands behind neck. You should be behind, eyes at the level of the PSISs, while your thumbs palpate the inferior aspect of each PSIS (see Fig. 9.2). The person goes into a slow forward bend, as far as possible, as you observe the behaviour of your thumbs.

When sitting, the ischia are locked, making any motion between the sacrum and the ilia dependent on sacral freedom. This therefore helps to isolate sacroiliac dysfunction.

The thumbs should be stable or they might be 'dragged' upwards to an equal slight degree, if there is no restriction.

If one thumb (on the PSIS) travels superiorly more than the other, it indicates that there is a restriction of the sacroiliac articulation on that side.

Further tests (not described here) are needed to determine whether torsion or flexion of the sacrum is involved.

Did the PSIS (and your thumb) move more on one side than the other?

Is there a sacroiliac lesion and if so, on which side?

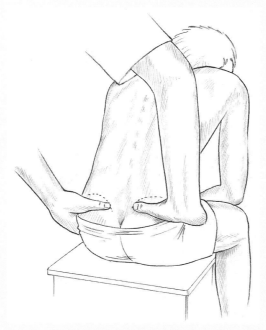

Fig. 9.2   Seated flexion test for sacroiliac dysfunction. The restricted side is the one on which the thumb moves during flexion.

EXERCISE 9.9: OBSERVATION OF ROTOSCOLIOSIS DURING SEATED FLEXION

Time suggested: 2–3 minutes on each side

In this same position (seated flexion) the fullness of the paravertebral muscles is again observed as you move to the front of the patient, with findings being interpreted as described in Exercise 9.7, above.

If paraspinal fullness is more apparent on one side during seated flexion and there is no appreciable degree of rotoscoliosis, suspect quadratus lumborum shortening on that side. This can produce a pelvic tilt, as well as interfering with respiration (through its influence on both 12th rib or diaphragm with which it merges).

The side-lying, hip abduction test described in Chapter 5 and/or direct palpation of the lateral border of quadratus can give evidence of overactivity and therefore shortness of QL, as well as possible spasm or trigger point activity above the iliac crest (see Exercise 5.14, Figs 5.21 and 5.22).

Is there asymmetry in the paraspinal muscles during this test?

If so, how do you interpret it?

Confirmation of standing flexion test findings

It is seldom wise to rely on a single test result as evidence of dysfunction (see Chapter 2 for discussion of this). Therefore, if there is an indication of iliosacral or sacroiliac dysfunction, based, for example, on the standing or seated flexion tests, it is wise to confirm dysfunction using other means.

The tests described in Exercises 9.10A&B, as well as 9.11A&B, offer opportunities to support or challenge the accuracy of previously gathered information.

Lee (2002) has noted that while individually, in isolation, some tests may fail evaluation as to their reliability and validity, when such tests are combined into a sequence, involving a number of evaluation strategies, and especially when 'a clinical reasoning process is applied to their findings', they offer a logical biomechanical diagnosis and 'without apology, they continue to be defended'.

As you perform the exercises in this (and other) chapters, you are urged to reread Chapter 2 with its in-depth discussion of the value and validity of palpation tests and the importance of ensuring that more than one piece of evidence is used, when deciding on the significance of tests. Clinical reasoning should be used as you weigh the relative importance of test and assessment results, in relation to each other, in relation to symptoms and in relation to the person's personal and medical history.

EXERCISE 9.10A: STANDING ILIOSACRAL 'STORK' OR GILLET TEST

Time suggested: 3–4 minutes (see Fig 2.2 p18)

You are behind your standing partner. Place one thumb on the PSIS and the other thumb on the ipsilateral sacral crest, at the same level. Your partner flexes the knee and hip and lifts the tested side knee, so that he is standing only on the contralateral leg.

The normal response would be for the ilium on the tested side to rotate posteriorly as the sacrum rotates toward the side of movement. This would bring the thumb on the PSIS caudad and medial.

continues

EXERCISE 9.10A: (Continued)

Lee (1999) states that this test (if performed on the right), 'examines the ability of the right innominate to posteriorly rotate, the sacrum to right rotate and the L5 vertebrae to right rotate/sideflex'.

If, however, upon flexion of the knee and hip, the ipsilateral PSIS moves cephalad in relation to the sacrum, this is an indication of ipsilateral pubic symphysis and iliosacral dysfunction. This finding can be used to confirm the findings of the standing flexion test (above). Petty & Moore (1998) also suggest that a positive Gillet test indicates ipsilateral sacroiliac dysfunction.

Lee (1999) reminds us that this test also allows assessment of 'the patient's ability to transfer weight through the contralateral limb and to maintain balance'.

EXERCISE 9.10B: STANDING HIP EXTENSION TEST

Time suggested: 3–4 minutes

The person stands with weight on both feet equally. You palpate the PSIS and sacral base, as in the Stork/Gillet test (9.10A) above.

The person extends the leg at the hip, on the side to be tested.

The innominate should rotate anteriorly and the thumb on the PSIS should displace superolaterally, relative to the sacrum. Failure to do so suggests a restriction of the innominate's ability to rotate anteriorly and to glide inferoposteriorly on the sacrum.

Did your thumb on the PSIS move appropriately, superolaterally?

If not, what does it mean?

Notes on form and force closure of the SI joint

Two mechanisms lock the SI joint physiologically and these are known as 'form closure' and 'force closure' mechanisms.

Form closure is the state of stability which occurs when the very close-fitting joint surfaces of the SI joint approximate, in order to reduce movement opportunities. The efficiency and degree of form closure will vary with the particular characteristics of the structure (size, shape, age) as well as the level of loading involved. Lee (1999) states:

In the skeletally mature, S1, S2 and S3 contribute to the formation of the sacral surface [of the SI joint] and each part can be oriented in a different vertical plane. In addition the sacrum is wedged anteroposteriorly. These factors provide resistance to both vertical and horizontal translation. In the young, the wedging is incomplete, such that the SI joint is planar at all three levels and is vulnerable to shear forces until ossification is complete (third decade).

Force closure refers to the support offered to the SI joint by the ligaments of the area directly, as well as the various sling systems which involve both muscular and ligamentous structures (see discussions within this chapter) (Vleeming et al 1997).

Examples of force closure are:

● during anterior rotation of the innominate or during sacral counternutation, the SI joint is stabilised by a tightening of the long dorsal sacroiliac ligament
● during sacral nutation or posterior rotation of the innominate, the SI joint is stabilised by the sacrotuberous and interosseous ligaments.

EXERCISE 9.11: FORCE AND FORM TESTS

Time suggested: 3 minutes

9.11A: prone active straight leg raising test

This functional assessment enhances information deriving from the seated flexion test (Exercise 9.8).

The prone person is asked to extend the leg at the hip by approximately 10°. Hinging should occur at the hip joint and the pelvis should remain in contact with the table throughout.

Excessive degrees of pelvic rotation in the transverse plane (i.e. anterior pelvic rotation) indicate possible dysfunction.

If form features (i.e. structural components) of the SI joint are at fault, the prone straight leg raise will be more normal when medial compression of the joint is applied. This is achieved by you bilaterally applying firm medial pressure toward the SI joints, with hands on the innominates, during the procedure.

Force closure may be enhanced during the exercise if latissimus dorsi can be recruited to increase tension on the thoracolumbar fascia. Lee (1999) states: 'This is done by [the practitioner] resisting extension of the medially rotated [contralateral] arm prior to lifting the leg'.

If force closure enhances more normal SI joint function, the prognosis for improvement is good, to be achieved by means of exercise and reformed use patterns.

9.11B: supine leg raising test for pelvic stability

This functional assessment enhances information deriving from the seated flexion test (Exercise 9.8).

The person is supine and is asked to raise one leg.

If there is evidence of compensating rotation of the pelvis toward the side of the raised leg during performance of the leg raising, dysfunction is confirmed. The same leg should then be raised as you impart compressive force, directed medially across the pelvis, with a hand on the lateral aspect of each innominate, at the level of the ASIS (this augments form closure of the SI joint).

If this form closure enhances the person's ability to easily raise the leg, this suggests that structural factors within the joint (form) may require externally enhanced support, such as a supporting belt.

To enhance force closure, the same leg is raised with the person slightly flexing and rotating the trunk toward the side being tested, against your resistance, which is applied to the contralateral shoulder. This activates oblique muscular forces and force-closes the ipsilateral SI joint (which is being assessed).

If the initial leg raising effort suggests SI dysfunction and this is reduced by means of force closure, the prognosis is good, if the patient engages in appropriate rehabilitation exercise.

Did either the prone or supine leg raising test suggest sacroiliac dysfunction?

Were any such indications reduced when form closure was applied by you?

Were any such indications reduced when force closure was created by resisted muscular efforts, as described?

Do any of these findings support suggested SI joint dysfunction findings, based on the seated flexion test, the stork or standing hip extension tests?

EXERCISE 9.12: THE F-AB-ER-E TEST

Time suggested: 3–4 minutes (see Fig 2.1 p17)

You should now perform the F-AB-ER-E test, so called because it simultaneously assesses flexion-abduction-external rotation-extension of the hip, in that sequence.

This test pinpoints hip pathology but also adds information which might be useful in other aspects of pelvic dysfunction.

Your palpation partner lies supine and you stand on the side of the table closest to the leg being tested. The person flexes the hip, allowing external rotation, so that the foot of that leg rests just above the opposite knee.

The knee on the tested leg is allowed to drop towards the table. It should reach a position where the lower leg is horizontal with the table. If this is not possible, carefully try to take it to that position by depressing the knee towards the floor.

Compare the range with the other side.

If there is pain in the hip as the knee drops (or is taken) towards the floor, there is probably hip pathology.

Is there any hip dysfunction evidenced by this test in your patient (model)?

EXERCISE 9.13: PUBIC TUBERCLE PALPATION

Time suggested: 3–4 minutes

Mitchell and his colleagues (1979) also suggest other assessments be made of this region, specifically for pubic tubercle height.

Ask the supine person to find the pubic crest on himself and to maintain a finger-pad contact on the superior surface of the bone, close to the symphysis. You should stand to one side, at upper thigh level, facing cephalad.

Once the person has located the bony surface of the pubic bones, the palm of your table-side hand is placed on the lower abdomen, finger tips close to the umbilicus. The heel of your hand is slid caudally, until it comes into contact with the superior aspect of the pubic bone.

Having located this landmark, you should place both index fingers on the anterior aspect of the symphysis pubis and slide each of these laterally (to opposite sides) approximately 1–2 finger-tip widths, in order to evaluate the positions of the pubic tubercles.

Is one tubercle more cephalad or caudad than the other?

Is there evidence of increased tension one side or the other at the attachment of the inguinal ligament?

Is one side more tender than the other?

If one side is more cephalad it is only possible to discover which side is dysfunctional (i.e. is one side too cephalad or is the other too caudad?) by referring to the standing flexion test (Exercise 9.6 above). The side of dysfunction is shown by relative motion of the palpating PSIS (thumb) in that test.

Does one side of the pubis palpate as being nearer the head than the other?

If so, is that side superior or is the other side inferior?

EXERCISE 9.14: PALPATION FOR ISCHIAL TUBEROSITY HEIGHT

Time suggested: 3–4 minutes

Place the heels of your hands over the ischial tuberosities, fingers directed towards the head of your prone palpation partner. The most inferior aspect of the tuberosities is located with your thumbs and the relative height is assessed with your eyes directly above them. (See notes in Special topic 3, on use of the dominant eye.)

If the tuberosities are level there is no dysfunction. If one side is more cephalad than the other, it is presumed to involve a superior subluxation/dysfunction on that side.

This can be confirmed by assessment of the status of the sacrotuberous ligaments. To test these, the thumbs now slide in a medial and superior direction (towards the coccyx) bilaterally, until they meet the resistance of the sacrotuberous ligament.

If there is a superior ischial subluxation/dysfunction, the ligament on that side will palpate as being slack compared with its pair.

Are the ischial tuberosities level?

If not, which is superior?

EXERCISE 9.15: PALPATION OF INTERNAL MALLEOLI

Time suggested: 3–4 minutes

Apparent ('functional') short leg assessment is based initially on assessment of the levels of the internal malleoli.

Stand at the foot of the table and compare the levels of the internal malleoli, with your palpation partner supine. If there is a discrepancy in the levels of the malleoli this may signify a short leg due to iliosacral and pubic dysfunction.

Ask the person to lie prone and reexamine the internal malleoli. If there is a discrepancy when prone, the short leg is likely to be due to sacroiliac or lumbar dysfunction.

Note: These concepts and others will be expanded on later in this chapter when the short leg/long leg question will be examined in more detail.

Is there an apparent short leg? If so, is this due to iliosacral or sacroiliac problems?

Do these findings tally with the standing/seated flexion tests? Or the stork/standing leg extension tests? Or the form/force closure tests?

Tests of ASIS positions indicate iliac rotation dysfunction and iliac flare patterns. The side of dysfunction, when comparing the levels of the ASISs, relates to the side on which the thumb moved cephalad during the standing flexion test.

9.16A

Your palpation partner lies supine and straight. You should locate and palpate the inferior slopes of the ASISs, with your thumbs and view from directly above the pelvis with your dominant eye (see Special topic 3 on eye dominance) in order to compare the levels for superior/inferior symmetry/asymmetry.

If the ASISs are level, there is no imbalance. Conversely, if there was a right-side dysfunction indicated by the standing flexion test and the left-side ASIS is superior in this assessment, it indicates a right-sided anteriorly rotated ilium. Spend a little time (draw a sketch or examine the patient) working out why this is so, if it appears confusing.

If one ASIS is more superior than the other it could indicate a posterior iliac restriction on that side or an anterior iliac restriction on the other side (see Fig. 9.3). This is differentiated by comparison with the results of the standing flexion test (Exercise 9.6 above). For example, if the flexion test revealed a left-side iliosacral dysfunction and the ASIS test showed left-side superior, this would indicate that there was a left-side, posterior, iliac restriction.

Is one ASIS more superior than the other? If so, does it relate to a posterior iliac lesion on that side or to an anterior iliac lesion on the other side (see Fig. 9.4)?

9.16B

Now palpate, and place your thumbs on, the medial slopes of ASIS, with your eyes above and directly over the midline.

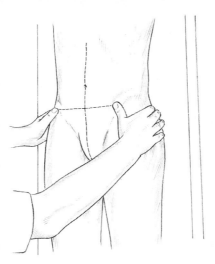

Fig. 9.3 Practitioner adopts a position offering a bird's-eye view of ASIS prominences on which rest the thumbs.

continues

EXERCISE 9.16 *(Continued)*

Compare the distances from the umbilicus (if scars make this unreliable use the xiphoid as a landmark instead) to ASIS contacts on both sides.

If the distances are equal there is no imbalance. If there is a difference it could mean that on the greater side (longer distance from umbilicus to ASIS) an outflare of the ilium has occurred or that an inflare has occurred on the shorter distance side.

Once again, reference to the standing flexion test (9.6) gives the answer.

If the flexion test showed an iliosacral restriction on the right and the ASIS umbilicus distance is greater on the right, there is indeed an iliac outflare on that side.

What would it indicate if the flexion test (9.6) had shown an iliosacral restriction on the right and the ASIS–umbilicus distance was greater on the left side?

What difference, if any, is there in the distances from ASIS to umbilicus (or other landmark) as you view them?

What does this indicate in relation to your palpation partner, if there was an indication of a iliac dysfunction when you performed Exercise 9.6?

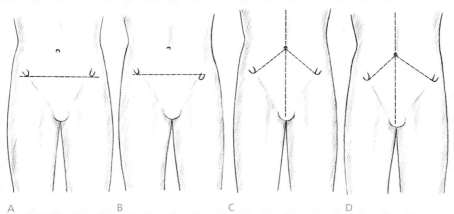

A   B   C   D

Fig. 9.4   (A) The ASISs are level and there is no rotational dysfunction involving the iliosacral joints. (B) The right ASIS is higher than the left. If a thumb 'travelled' on the right side during the standing flexion test this would represent a posterior right iliosacral rotation dysfunction. If a thumb 'travelled' on the left side during the test this would represent an anterior left iliosacral rotation dysfunction. (C) The ASIS are equidistant from the umbilicus and the midline, and there is no iliosacral flare dysfunction. (D) The ASIS on the right is closer to the umbilicus/midline which indicates that either there is a right side iliosacral inflare (if the right thumb moved during the standing flexion test) or there is a left side iliosacral outflare (if the left thumb moved during the standing flexion test).

DISCUSSION REGARDING EXERCISES 9.1–9.16

If you have comfortably and competently completed the exercises in this chapter, up to this point, then you should be able to observe your patient for signs of asymmetry and functional imbalance and decide whether or not an iliosacral or sacroiliac restriction exists and what type it is. Your confidence in the assessment results will be amplified by various tests confirming each other. If there are contradictions between the various test results, the possibility exists that either the tests are not being carried out well or that any dysfunctional pattern which is present does not relate to anything these tests might reveal. The variations in the presence or otherwise of increased paraspinal muscle fullness in seated and standing flexion tests may have alerted you to the presence of rotoscoliosis and the possible influence of postural muscle shortness on whatever patterns you have observed or palpated.

Spinal dysfunction

The next few test exercises focus on identification of spinal dysfunction. Individual spinal segments may be assessed for a variety of restrictions and motions: flexion, extension, side bending (left and right), rotation (left and right) as well as such translatory movements as separation (traction), compression and lateral and anteroposterior translations. These were all discussed in the context of 'functional analysis' in Chapter 8. General observation assessment is made by viewing the patient standing upright, standing flexed, seated and seated flexed, as well as in such other positions (extension and so on) as you may think useful.

The following exercises, which are not meant to provide a completely comprehensive spinal assessment, include methods derived from a number of texts, including: Sutton (1977), Lewit (1992) and Grieve (1984). Also much consulted in the devising of these exercises were the words of William Walton (1971).

EXERCISE 9.17: SPINAL PALPATION/ASSESSMENT SEQUENCE

Time suggested: 7 minutes 9.17A and 9.17B, 2–3 minutes 9.17C and 9.17D, 10–15 minutes 9.17E

9.17A: cervical spine palpation – supine

With your palpation partner supine, you should be seated at the head of the table. Palpate the posterior and anterior aspects of the transverse processes for local tenderness.

In this position, the pads of your middle fingers can be placed gently on the articular pillars of C2–7 successively, in order to palpate for any reduction in the symmetrical range of movement as the supporting palms of the hands guide the head into forward and backward bending.

Note any sense of bind on any movement as well as the quality of 'end-feel' as an indication of the presence of dysfunction/restriction.

9.17B: cervical spine palpation – seated

With your partner seated, assess gross ranges of motion of the cervical spine, in rotation right and left, side bending right and left, as well as flexion and extension.

Also attempt to evaluate individual segments during these same movements. Achieve this by placing the pads of your thumb and third finger of one hand over the articular pillars of each vertebrae in turn (C2–7) while the other hand introduces the sequence of normal motions, listed above, successively.

What do you feel – in terms of altered end-feel or increased bind – on any of these movements, at any segment or involving the entire cervical spine?

9.17C: atlantoccipital range of motion

With the head in full flexion (supine or seated) the atlantoaxial joint may be palpated for restrictions in rotation.

Full flexion locks all cervical joints below C2.

Can you sense any difference in rotation of the AO joint as you turn it left and then right?

9.17D: occipital deviation assessment

For occipitoatlantal joint assessment your partner should be supine, with you at the head of the table.

He is asked to first tilt the head backward and then to tip the chin towards the chest as you observe any deviation from the midline during these movements.

If the chin is seen to deviate to one side from the midline, that is the side towards which the occiput is deviated.

What restrictions in normal motion did you find in this region during application of these exercises in cervical function?

9.17E

Compare the results obtained from Exercises 9.17A–D with the following, more precise palpation approach (Walton 1971).

The supine person's head may be flat or on your flexed knee, which is placed appropriately on the table.

The occiput is cradled in the palms of both hands, leaving the pads of the fingers free to palpate the entire cervical spine, both lightly and deeply.

continues

First, the pads press lightly over the facets and transverse processes until palpable changes (tension, oedema, fibrosis, sensitivity, temperature changes, lessened skin elasticity and so on) have been noted.

Increased pressure is then introduced to investigate for deeper changes in these tissues, such as oedema, deep muscular tension, interosseous changes and restrictions in mobility.

Flexion and extension

Flexion or extension restrictions can be assessed by placing the pads of your fingers between the spinous processes of the vertebral segments being evaluated. The space is compared with that present in the segments above or below.

Where an increased degree of separation is palpated, check the segment by extending the head/neck at that level, to assess the relative range of movement.

If movement is less than in the segments above and/or below or a hard end-feel is noted, then that segment is 'locked in flexion' (unable to extend fully).

Similarly, if the space between segments (between their spinous processes, that is) palpates as narrower compared with those above and/or below, the implications can be simply checked by introducing flexion and monitoring the degree/range of movement.

If flexion range seems less than it should be as compared with its neighbours, or a hard end-feel is noted, it is 'locked in extension' (unable to flex fully).

Side bending

Side bending is assessed by placing the pads of the palpating fingers between the transverse processes, while laterally flexing the cervical spine down to the segment being checked.

If this suggests that transverse processes on one side (say, the left) are overapproximated, then side bend the head and neck to the right, until the segment being checked should move (i.e. the transverse processes on the left should separate). If they fail to do so, then that segment is 'lesioned', 'subluxated' or 'locked' in side bending to the left.

Rotation

Rotation is assessed through use of deeper palpation, over the articular facets. If one facet feels more posterior than the one above or below it, the cervical spine should be rotated towards the opposite side (away from the palpated posterior transverse process).

If this fails adequately to rotate (compared with its neighbours) or even if it does rotate but with signs of increased tissue resistance or bind, then it is said to be lesioned, or restricted, in rotation to the side of the posterior transverse process.

What findings did you make using this last assessment (9.17E) as compared with the previous ones (9.17A–D)?

Record your findings.

EXERCISE 9.18: THORACIC PALPATION

Time suggested: 7–12 minutes for each method

9.18A: upper thoracic spine, seated assessment
Your palpation partner should be seated.

You place both thumbs on the transverse processes of T1 to T3 successively, as the person first flexes, returns to neutral and then extends the head/neck repetitively, slowly, until evaluation is complete.

Was there any asymmetry or one-sided or bilateral sense of excessive bind during any of the movements?

9.18B: mid-thoracic spine, prone assessment
Your palpation partner should be prone, with his chin resting on the table, head in the midline.

Your thumbs should be placed sequentially on the transverse processes of T4 to T9. Firm ventral pressure is exerted, after soft tissue slack has been removed, in order to evaluate resistance of each segment to hyperextension.

Any sense of unilateral or bilateral resistance or bind should be noted.

A rotation restriction, towards the side of maximum resistance, may be suspected.

9.18C: sphinx position, mid-thoracic palpation
The prone person arches his back by supporting the upper body on the elbows, chin resting on the heels of hands.

You are at the head of the table, palpating the tips of the transverse processes from T7 to L5 with your thumbs, noting any increased posteriority, which indicates rotation towards that side of the involved segment.

Note also any sense of tissue tension/bind.

9.18D: seated thoracic assessment/palpation
An alternative or additional evaluation might involve having the seated person (straddling the table for stability or on a high, fixed stool) in a variety of positions as follows.

With the arms folded, you stand at the side, grasping the far shoulder and fixing the other shoulder with your axilla. This leaves a hand free to palpate the tips of the thoracic spinous processes for tenderness. Periosteal pain points on the spinous processes (see Chapter 5) indicate chronically increased tonus in the attaching muscles.

The patient then places the hands behind the neck, elbows together in front of the face. Both elbows are grasped in one of your hands, from below, allowing spinal extension to be easily introduced, as a finger of the other hand palpates between the spinous processes for the degree of movement and the quality of the end of the range of motion, at each segment sequentially. The person is taken from neutral into retroflexion (backwards bending) and back to neutral, repetitively, slowly, until evaluation is complete. If the spinous processes fail to 'close', then a flexion restriction is probable (i.e. it cannot extend) (see Fig. 9.5).

The elbows are then held from above and sequential flexion is introduced as the tension of the end of the range of movement, of each segment, is palpated with your other hand. The person is taken from neutral into anteflexion (forward bending) and back to neutral,

continues

repetitively, slowly, until evaluation is complete. Any failure to easily flex indicates an extension restriction (i.e. it cannot flex) (see Fig. 9.6).

For side-bending assessment you stand behind, with one thumb resting on the interspace to be tested, as the other hand introduces pressure towards the palpated side, through the contralateral shoulder, to produce side bending over your palpating digit. This palpating hand therefore acts as a fulcrum. The end range of motion of each segment is assessed in the thoracic spine. Any sense of increased bind or altered quality of 'end-feel' may indicate an inability to side bend and therefore a restricted segment (see Fig. 9.7).

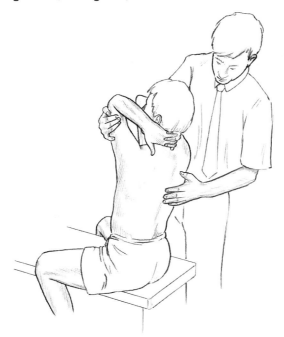

Fig. 9.5   Palpation of retroflexion (extension) of the thoracic spine.

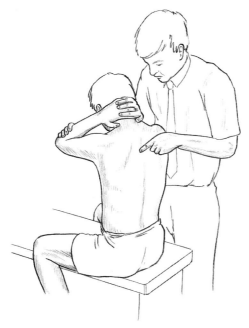

Fig. 9.6   Palpation of gapping of spinous processes during flexion.

continues

EXERCISE 9.18 *(Continued)*

Rotation is examined with the person seated astride the table, hands behind the neck. You stand to one side and pass a hand across the chest to grasp the opposite shoulder, forearm lying across the chest. Flexion is introduced and the trunk is sequentially rotated, as the individual segments are palpated. (Note that rotation must be around the body's axis, so that the palpating fingers – one each side of the spine – can palpate accurately the degree of rotation available in each direction.) Any sense of bind or altered end-feel might indicate a rotation restriction in the segment being evaluated.

What restrictions in normal motion or altered quality of end-feel did you find in this region using these methods?

Record your findings.

9.18E: Walton's thoracic palpation

Compare the findings from the previous evaluations in this exercise with those you achieve using Walton's approach as follows.

After use of a superficial stroking palpation of the seated person's thoracic spine and paraspinal tissues, any suspicious areas (evidenced by tension, tenderness, skin changes, oedema) are palpated more deeply, into the periaxial structures.

One side at a time is examined. You should be standing to the side of the seated individual, so that if the right side of the thoracic spine is being examined, you will stand slightly behind and to the right. Your right hand is placed on the left shoulder, with your forearm crossing behind the neck, allowing your elbow to rest on the right shoulder. This gives the contact arm the ability to introduce a great variety of possible directions of movement, controlling the person into flexion, extension, side bending and rotation with relative ease. The free (in this case, left) hand is able to palpate any segment (spinous process intervals and transverse processes, as well as facet prominences), while motions are

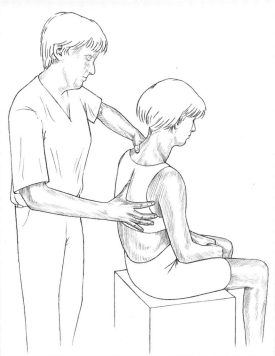

Fig. 9.7   The patient is side-bent (towards the right in this instance) over the palpating thumb which assesses the nature of the 'end-feel'. A sense of unusual 'bind' might indicate a restriction.

continues

introduced by the right hand/arm. Obviously, all hand positions (and your position) are reversed for checking the opposite side.

After assessing the relative space between spinous processes, any which appear more widely separated than their neighbours are checked by you moving the contact arm to the front of the patient, grasping the opposite axilla and introducing extension over the palpating thumb or finger(s). If the spinous processes fail to approximate when this is done, then the superior vertebral segment is probably locked in flexion.

With the control arm behind the patient's upper back once again, passive flexion is used to test the range of motion of any segments where overapproximated spinous processes have been palpated. Any which fail to flex adequately are probably restricted in extension.

Palpation with your finger or thumb between the transverse processes allows you to identify segments where approximation seems greater than in neighbouring segments. Side bending is easily introduced (via the control hand or elbow) away from the palpating digit. If the transverse processes fail to separate, then a side-bending restriction towards that side is probable.

Rotation can be assessed by fixing, with a thumb pad, the transverse process and articular facet of the vertebra below the one being checked. The control arm then introduces rotation up to the vertebra being tested. If it fails to move normally in rotation, say to the left, then it is said to probably be locked in rotation to the right. The articular facet of that vertebra will be posterior on the side in which rotation is locked.

Walton wisely warns that any restrictions in this area may be linked to viscerosomatic reflex activity producing paraspinal muscular tension (see Chapter 5).

9.18F: Denslow's thoracic palpation

Denslow (1960) suggests the following thoracic palpation exercise.

> The patient is sitting. Palpate the spinous processes of T1, T6 and T12 and note whether or not bony prominences appear to be hard and clean cut (as would be felt if a similarly shaped piece of metal with rounded edges were palpated through a velvet cloth) or if the tissues over, and investing the spinous processes appear to be thickened . . . Examination for motion under voluntary control is achieved by placing the tip of the middle finger of one hand between the spinous processes at the cervicothoracic area. With the other hand flex and extend the patient's neck. Move the finger from interspace to interspace until the spines of C7 and T1 are identified. Check for the ease and range of motion . . . Examination for motion not under voluntary control is achieved by repeating the procedure described above, and at the end of the range of motion, which is under voluntary control, spring the joint to produce further flexion or extension and check for 'give' in the restraining tissues.

This last element, the springing of the joint, allows you to evaluate the quality of the end of the range of motion. Is it elastic, hard, spongy, firm but not excessively so . . . or what?

Which of the diagnostic methods gave you the best results?

Which of the positions allowed you the most sensitive assessment contacts?

Record your findings.

Time suggested: 7–10 minutes for each method

9.19A: springing palpation of the lumbar segments
Your palpation partner should lie prone.

This palpation exercise involves sequential 'springing' of individual segments and is performed with two fingers of one hand resting on the transverse processes of a segment, while the hypothenar eminence of the other, extended, arm rests over them.

Slack is taken out and a springing movement to the floor is made as the intrinsic resistance of the segment is assessed. A yielding springiness should be felt.

If, however, resistance is sensed and if there is pain, a restriction exists. If only pain is felt, a disc lesion is possible.

With the person side-lying these segments are again palpated by gentle springing of each lumbar segment, first with the patient anteflexed and then retroflexed. (See methods 9.19B & C, below.)

This palpation method tells you whether a segment is not moving freely, i.e. that it is 'blocked', but does not tell you what form that restriction takes (locked in flexion, rotation, etc.).

What restrictions in normal motion did you find in this region so far?

9.19B: side-lying extension palpation of the lumbar spine
Your partner lies on one side, close to the edge of the table, facing you, with knees and hips flexed.

You lean across the person and your hands palpate individual segments, stabilising with your cephalad hand the lumbar spinous process above the segment to be assessed, while a finger of the caudad hand lies between the spinous processes, to palpate for movement.

The person's bent knees should be in contact with either your abdomen or thighs so that direct pressure can be made through the long axis of the femurs, so introducing retroflexion (backwards bending) to the lumbar spine.

After taking out the slack, the segment is sprung by pressure through the long axis of the femurs, towards the palpating hands.

On springing, a movement of the vertebrae below the one being fixed by the cephalad hand should be felt. If a 'blocked' segment exists, then little or no motion will be palpated. Once again, such palpated restrictions tell you that there is a problem, but not what the problem is.

9.19C: side-lying flexion palpation of the lumbar spine
The same position as 9.19B is adopted, so that the person lies on their side, knees and hips flexed, facing you as you lean across to fix (stabilise) the thoracic region with your cephalad forearm.

The knees and hips should be fully flexed so that the thighs press against the abdomen/chest, held there by the pressure against the lower legs, exerted by contact with your abdomen or thighs. This induces a great deal of anteflexion of the lumbar spine, rounding it maximally.

continues

Your caudad forearm should be used to contact the buttocks and with this contact you repetitively increase and decrease the degree of lumbar flexion, as both hands palpate individual segments for decreased, increased or normal ranges of flexion, as the region is gently sprung in this manner.

What restrictions in normal motion did you find in this region?

9.19D: Walton's lumbar palpation

Walton suggests having the person seated astride the end of the table with hands clasped behind the neck.

You stand to the side of and behind the patient, passing an arm through the 'loop' of the patient's arms on one side to rest the hand on the opposite upper arm.

This provides you with control over flexion, extension, rotation and side-bending motions while your other hand palpates for normal mobility in the same manner as in thoracic examination described in Exercise 9.18E.

Walton's palpation helps you to identify the form of any restriction/dysfunction you may have palpated when using Exercises 9.19A, B or C.

Which of the various methods of lumbar palpation have provided you with the most useful information?

Record your findings and repeat the exercises.

DISCUSSION REGARDING EXERCISES 9.17–9.19

Exercises 9.17, 9.18 and 9.19 provide a wide range of palpation possibilities for evaluating whether localised segmental dysfunction is present, as well as ways of identifying what the nature of such dysfunction is.

This text does not comprehensively describe all methods for such evaluation. It does, however, provide the tools which can enhance the skills necessary for using these, or other, methods of evaluation, in spinal assessment.

Semantics

In spinal palpation and evaluation, you should aim to be able to assess and describe the characteristics of a restricted spinal segment in a manner which other health-care professionals can understand.

The terminology used to describe restricted spinal joint may include the words 'blocked', 'dysfunctional', 'lesioned' or 'subluxated', depending upon whether the description emerges from physical medicine, osteopathy or chiropractic. The use of language extends to specifics as well. For example, when a flexion restriction exists in the thoracic spine (i.e. the segment is unable to extend fully or is 'locked in flexion'), you should be able to determine, and to describe, whether or not:

- the degree to which the spinous process of the vertebra in question is able to approximate to and/or to separate from the vertebrae above and below it

continues

DISCUSSION REGARDING EXERCISES 9.17–9.19 (Continued)

- there is a greater degree of protuberance of the spinous process of the vertebra in question, compared with those above and below it
- there is an overall increase in the degree of flexion in the area being evaluated
- there is an overall decrease in the degree of extension in the area in question
- there are any associated motion restrictions evident (side bending, rotation, etc.)
- there is any muscular hypertonicity, or spasm, or other palpable tissue changes (e.g. fibrotic, oedema, inflammation) in the area
- there is tenderness on palpation
- there is pain without palpation in the area
- the effect of the restriction, if any, on the associated ribs.

It should be possible to answer these questions during the sequence of assessment described above in all the joints of the spine, almost without thought, once your palpation skills are sufficiently sensitive.

Refer back to the previous chapter and those methods which focus on more 'functional' approaches and which ask the palpating hand to recognise both normal and abnormal responses in the region being assessed, when a normal function is being performed – whether this involves a movement or a function such as breathing.

Breathing

Our attention will now turn toward evaluation of aspects of breathing function and of individual rib restrictions.

EXERCISE 9.20: BREATHING WAVE ASSESSMENT

Time suggested: 2–3 minutes

Your palpation partner should be placed prone with a suitable pillow beneath the abdomen to prevent undue lumbar extension. In this position the breathing 'wave' should be observed. This is a wave-like motion, ideally starting at the sacrum or in the lumbar region, which spreads in a wave up to the upper thoracics when spinal mechanics are free.

If there is restriction in any of the spinal segments, the movement will seem to stop (see Fig. 9.8). If there are regions of the spine which are restricted, either intrinsically or by virtue of the paraspinal musculature, the segment may rise as a block on inhalation.

Observe the wave and if areas move in a block-like manner, palpate these to assess their tone and tissue status (fibrotic, etc.). Compare what you palpate with tissues in more functional areas, where the wave moves sequentially rather than as a block.

Does the wave start at the sacrum?

Does it start elsewhere?

Do some parts of the spine move in a block?

Chart this, as well as the directions in which the wave moves, after its commencement (cephalad, caudad, both directions?). Where does the wave cease – mid-thoracic area, base of neck?

continues

Compare what is observed with findings of restriction during palpation, as in the previous spinal assessment exercises or the observed paraspinal 'fullness' in earlier assessments or particularly in relation to areas of flatness as observed in Chapter 5, Exercise 5.19 A&B and Figure 5.23.

The breathing wave is not diagnostic but provides a 'snapshot' of the current response of the spine to inhalation and exhalation. It can be used to evaluate progress as restricted areas are treated, and the wave alters to a more normal pattern over time.

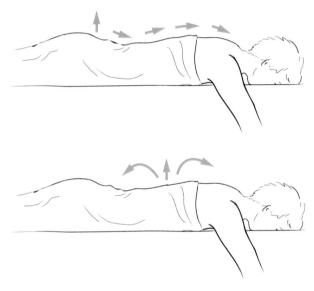

Fig. 9.8   Functional (top) and dysfunctional breathing wave patterns as the spine responds to inhalation.

EXERCISE 9.21: PALPATION FOR DEPRESSED RIBS

Time suggested: 5–7 minutes

Ribs restricted in exhalation are depressed (they cannot freely move into the inhalation phase).

Depressed ribs are identified by palpation, which should be performed from the side of the table which brings the dominant eye over the centre-line (see Special topic 3 on the dominant eye). The eyes should be focused between the palpating digits, so that peripheral vision picks up any variation in the movement of the ribs.

Motion of both bucket (up and down motion of upper ribs) and pump-handle (lateral and medial movement of lower ribs) movements should be assessed.

Examination is performed while the supine (knees flexed) patient breathes deeply and steadily. The rib positions (right and left, same level) at full inhalation and exhalation are compared for relative rise and fall (upper ribs), as well as lateral excursion (lower ribs).

Place your index fingers on the superior surface of a pair of ribs. If one of the pair fails to rise as far as the other (or to move laterally, if below the fifth rib), it is depressed.

continues

EXERCISE 9.21 (Continued)

There will usually be a series of such ribs forming a compensating group, rather than a single rib, unless it has been traumatically jarred out of place. It is necessary to identify the most cephalad of a group of ribs which fails to rise normally on exhalation. This is regarded as the key rib which is locked in its exhalation position (i.e. it is depressed).

Just as such a rib can affect those below it, so can one locked in inhalation (i.e. an elevated rib, see below) affect those above it, making the most cauded of a group of elevated ribs the key one.

First and second ribs are often depressed and may be associated with pain and numbness in the shoulder, suggesting thoracic outlet syndrome or scalene anticus syndrome (anterior and medial scalene insert into the first rib and posterior scalene inserts into the second rib).

Such depressed ribs are often found in patients with asthma or obstructive pulmonary problems or where there is a tendency to hyperventilation.

In Jones' SCS methodology (see Chapter 5) tender points for depressed ribs lie on the mid-axillary line, in the intercostal spaces above and/or below the rib in question.

What restrictions in normal rib motion did you find in this region?

Are there any depressed ribs?

Did you find a group of these and if so, did you identify the most cephalad of that group?

Do these findings correlate with tender points on the mid-axillary line at the same level?

Can you identify associated scalene and/or pectoral shortness relating to any depressed rib dysfunction, if you palpate these muscles?

EXERCISE 9.22: PALPATION FOR ELEVATED RIBS

Time suggested: 5–7 minutes

Ribs restricted in inhalation are described as 'elevated'. These are identified by palpation using one fingertip placed on the superior surface of the pair of ribs being assessed (as in the previous exercise). Slightly exaggerated breathing effort is called for, in both inhalation and exhalation, during testing.

Motion of both bucket (up and down motion of upper ribs) and pump-handle (lateral and medial movement of lower ribs) movements should be assessed. Your eyes should be focused between the palpating digits, so that peripheral vision picks up any variation in the movement of the ribs.

If a rib on one side fails to return to neutral to the same degree as its pair, it is an elevated rib, locked in an inhalation position.

When an elevated rib is identified, all pairs of ribs below should be checked until a normal pair are identified (i.e. both rise and fall equally). The abnormal rib cephalad to the normal pair is the key rib (this being the most caudad of the elevated group).

continues

It is essential to identify the most cauded of a group of elevated ribs. The intercostal muscles superior to an elevated rib will usually be sensitive and will palpate as tense.

The fifth rib is commonly noted to be locked in elevation. There may be an associated deep radiating chest pain on deep breathing and tightness in the pectoralis minor. Cardiac or pulmonary disease may need to be excluded. There may be swelling indicating costal chondritis.

Tender points for elevated ribs lie at the angles of the ribs posteriorly.

What restrictions in normal motion did you find in the ribs palpated?

Did you identify an elevated rib? If so, did you identify a group of these and, most importantly, the most caudad of this group?

Did these findings correlate with tender points in the intercostal spaces around the angles of the ribs, posteriorly?

Did you palpate any interspace sensitivity, especially in the space above an elevated rib and close to the sternum?

EXERCISE 9.23: GREENMAN'S RIB PALPATION

Time suggested: 3–5 minutes

Philip Greenman (1989) suggests additional palpation processes for assessment of rib dysfunction.

Sitting behind the seated or standing person, palpate the most posterior aspects of the rib cage, from above downwards, feeling for a 'smooth' convexity which gets wider from above downwards.

What is being felt for is any rib angle which seems to be more or less posterior than others. At the same time, any increase in tone in the muscles overlaying or between the ribs (as well as pain) is sought.

The muscles which attach to the angles of the ribs are the iliocostalis group and they become hypertonic when rib dysfunction occurs.

Can you identify any rib dysfunction using this form of palpation?

EXERCISE 9.24: RIB PALPATION SEATED

Time suggested: 5–7 minutes

Your palpation partner is seated or prone and you sit behind or stand to one side.

With fingertips, palpate along the shafts of the ribs, feeling for differences one from the other. The inferior margins of ribs are more easily palpated than the superior ones. Assess the intercostal width (space between the ribs), evaluate differences in symmetry and feel for changes in tone in the intercostal muscles. Trigger points and fibrous changes may be found.

Move towards the spine and locate the articulation between the ribs and the transverse processes. Palpate these, as the patient deeply inhales and exhales. Assess intercostal motion as well as rib mobility in relation to its spinal articulation.

Could you palpate all the elements described in this assessment?

Compare your findings with those established in your previous rib function assessments as outlined above.

Notes on acromioclavicular and sternoclavicular dysfunction

Whereas spinal/neck and most other joints are seen to be moved by and to be under the postural influence of muscles, and therefore to an extent to be capable of having their function modified by muscular influences, articulations such as those of the sternoclavicular, acromioclavicular and iliosacral joints seem far less amenable to such influences, although muscle energy techniques in particular are widely used in the osteopathic profession to help restore the functional integrity of these joints. Review the ideas of Fritz Smith in Chapter 6, regarding foundational joints, and also Special topic 9, on joint play.

Begin evaluation of AC dysfunction at the scapula, the mechanics of which closely relate to AC function.

Your palpation partner sits erect and the spines of both scapulae are palpated by you, standing behind.

Make finger contact with the medial borders of the scapulae and then identify the inferior angle. Using your palpating fingers on these landmarks, check the levels to see whether they are the same. Asymmetry suggests AC dysfunction, although the side of dysfunction remains to be determined.

To test the right-side AC joint, you stand behind the person, with your left hand palpating over the joint. Your right hand holds the patient's right elbow.

The arm should be lifted in a direction 45° from the sagittal and frontal planes and as the arm approaches 90° elevation, the AC joint should be carefully palpated for hinge movement between the acromion and the clavicle. When there is no restriction, the palpating hand/finger should move slightly caudad as the arm is abducted beyond 90°.

If the AC joint is restricted the palpating digit will move cephalad as the arm goes beyond 90° elevation.

The relative positions of the scapulae become important once dysfunction at the AC joint has been identified, as this determines the position the arm is held in when soft tissue manipulation is used – in either internal or external rotation of the shoulder (Chaitow 2001).

Were the scapulae symmetrically positioned or was one more cephalad than the other?

Do both your partner's AC joints respond normally to abduction of the arm, as described?

If not, is the scapula on the dysfunctional side superior or inferior to the normal side?

EXERCISE 9.26: ASSESSMENT OF RESTRICTED ABDUCTION IN THE STERNOCLAVICULAR JOINT ('SHRUG TEST')

Time suggested: 3–5 minutes

As the clavicle abducts, it rotates posteriorly.

To test for this motion the person lies supine or is seated, with arms at the side.

You place your index fingers on the superior surface of the medial end of the clavicle and ask the person to shrug the shoulders as you palpate for the expected caudal movement of the medial clavicle.

If either clavicle fails to fall caudad there is a restriction preventing normal abduction (see Fig. 9.9).

Do your patient's sternoclavicular joints respond normally to a shrug or does the joint remain static or even rise rather than falling as this action occurs?

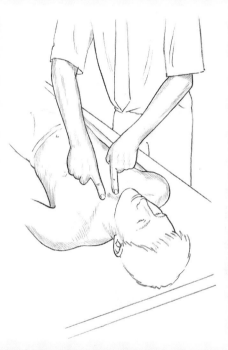

Fig. 9.9 Assessment ('shrug test') for restriction in clavicular mobility.

EXERCISE 9.27: ASSESSMENT OF RESTRICTED HORIZONTAL FLEXION OF THE UPPER ARM (STERNOCLAVICULAR RESTRICTION) – 'PRAYER' TEST

Time suggested: 1–2 minutes

Your palpation partner should lie supine and you stand to one side with your index fingers resting on the anteromedial aspect of each clavicle.

The person is asked to extend the arms forwards, palms together, pointing to the ceiling in a 'prayer' position.

On pushing the hands forwards towards the ceiling, the clavicular heads should drop towards the floor and not rise up to follow the hands (see Fig. 9.10).

If one or both fail to drop, there is a restriction (see Fig. 9.9).

Do your patient's sternoclavicular joints respond normally to the prayer test?

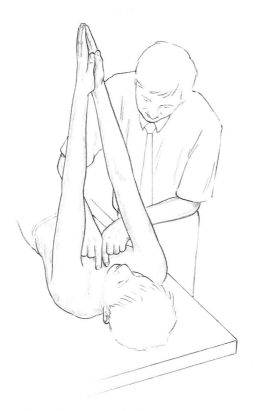

Fig. 9.10   Assessment ('prayer test') for restricted horizontal flexion of the sternoclavicular joint.

DISCUSSION REGARDING EXERCISES 9.20–9.27

This series of exercises started with breathing taking centre stage, first with an appreciation of the breathing wave, as a means of seeing how muscular and spinal restrictions might impinge on a normal function pattern, and then by introducing specific rib restriction characteristics, which can be both palpated and observed. The possibility of the presence of clavicular restrictions can be elicited by observation or palpation or both.

In this chapter, overall, it should have become clear that observation and palpation go together intimately and that general evaluation needs to provide a background to specific local restrictions and dysfunctions. You can also see that functional (such as the breathing wave observation) and structural (such as rib restriction) evaluations are inseparable.

Palpation of the skull

The next palpation exercise is a structural one, pure and simple, and focuses on the anatomy and landmarks of the skull.

In earlier chapters some of the exercises assessed elements of cranial and sacral rhythm function. The next palpation exercise is aimed specifically at learning more about cranial sutures and articulations.

Whether or not you intend to use cranial osteopathic (or craniosacral or sacrooccipital) methods, the exercise provides a useful way to enhance your palpatory skills and familiarise yourself with the amazing landscape of the skull.

This exercise should be performed on a living person but in order to derive maximum benefit it is suggested that a good reference manual and a disarticulated skull (human or plastic) be kept handy for reference and comparison of anatomical landmarks, suture patterns and general familiarisation with individual articulations.

Extensive osteopathic research has shown that the sutures of the skull permit a degree of plasticity, or motion, and that the sutures themselves, in life, contain connective tissue fibres arranged in specific patterns related to the functional motions of the area. There are also blood vessels and small neural structures (including free nerve endings and unmyelinated fibres).

The following palpation is not comprehensive as it leaves out most of the face and orbital structures. It is meant as a palpation exercise, not as a lesson in cranial work (Chaitow 1999).

Start by having your palpation partner lying supine, without a pillow. You are seated at the head of the table, forearms supported on the table, as you palpate, with pads of fingers, the vertex of the skull just over halfway posteriorly for the sagittal suture.

Before commencing the palpation observe the symmetry of the head and face from the perspective you now have. Does the nose seem centrally directed or does it slant one way or the other? Are the ears symmetrical? Are the eyebrows symmetrical? Is the slope of the forehead acute or fairly flat? Is the centre of the jaw in the midline or angled? Is the head as a whole symmetrical or distorted in any observable way?

Now begin to trace the path of the sagittal suture and note its pattern of serration which is wider posteriorly and narrows anteriorly.

A suture may be palpated by very lightly running the pad of a single digit from side to side, so as to sense the path of the meandering joint.

As you move from side to side along this suture, anteriorly, you will come to a depression or hollow, known as the bregma, where the coronal suture meets the sagittal suture.

Was one side of the suture more prominent than the other?

Were there any areas of unexpected rigidity?

Now, using one hand on each side (using the finger pads), palpate laterally from the bregma along the coronal suture (asking the same questions as to symmetry and rigidity or any unusual tissue changes) until you reach the articulation between the frontal and parietal bones.

Ask yourself also whether or not the sutures are symmetrical.

As your finger pads reach the end of the coronal sutures, they will palpate a slight prominence, after which the pterion is reached. This is the meeting point of the temporal, sphenoid, parietal and frontal bones.

Review these landmarks, sutures and bones on an atlas or model of the skull. Are the depressions and prominences symmetrical, on each side of the skull?

Moving slightly more inferiorly you will palpate, at the temple, the tip of the greater wing of the sphenoid, a most important contact in cranial work.

Is one great wing (temple) more prominent than the other?

Is one side higher or lower than the other?

Are there any areas of unusual rigidity?

Return to the pterion in order to follow the articulation between the parietal bone and the temporal squama (review your textbook or disarticulated model). This curves backwards over the ear (the temporal squama is bevelled on its interior surface to glide slightly over this articulation).

Follow this very subtle articulation on each side; these are best palpated by repetitively running a finger pad (very) lightly from the parietal bone down towards the ear (and so onto the temporal bone) and back again, noting the slight bump as you pass over the articulation.

continues

EXERCISE 9.28 *(Continued)*

As your finger pads progress posteriorly along the temporo-parietal articulations, they eventually reach the asterion on each side. The asterion is a star-shaped (hence its name) junction, where the occipital, temporal and parietal bones meet.

Ask yourself constantly the same questions regarding symmetry, prominences, depressions, rigidity. Make sure you identify each of the named landmarks and sutures.

Pass from the asterions superiorly (and medially) along the lambdoidal sutures, until you once again reach the midline. As you palpate the individual sutures, you should constantly compare side with side.

The lambdoidal sutures meet the sagittal suture at the L-shaped lambda. Now move each finger pad back again to the asterion and palpate your way towards the mastoid processes, along the occipito-mastoid sutures, which will vanish below soft tissues as you approach the neck.

Palpate this and become aware of the powerful muscular attachments inserting into the cranium from below (including upper trapezius and sternocleidomastoid) as well as the huge and powerful muscles which attach only to the cranium, such as temporalis. Have your partner activate some of these muscles as you palpate the sutures, in order to evaluate the slight movements they produce.

Now return up the lambdoidal sutures to the lambda, from where this palpation journey began, for it is from here that the sagittal suture runs anteriorly toward the bregma.

CAUTION: Never use more than a few grams of pressure on any sutures when palpating.

The time needed to perform this palpation exercise well is at least 15 minutes. Repeat the exercise many times, until these landmarks are familiar to you and you are instantly aware of the answers to the questions raised.

Knee palpation exercise

The following exercise is the only one in this chapter devoted to a joint which is not in some way associated with the spine or pelvis.

Denslow (1960) describes a series of useful functional tests for the knee.

Your palpation partner lies supine and you are standing at knee level.

Place the thumb and middle finger of your left hand in the groove between the femur and tibia of the person's right knee. Grasp the ankle with your right hand.

Have the person actively flex and extend the knee (with some assistance from you), while you check for the ease and range of motion and for changes in the width and depth of the grooves you are palpating.

Repeat this on the other leg and compare the ease of total motion on the two sides.

Now repeat the palpation exercise as described, but this time add slight springing force at the end of the extremes of flexion and extension of the knee.

Check the amount of elastic 'give' in the restraining (soft) tissues and compare your findings on both knees.

Finally, examine the knee by placing the heel of your left hand against the lateral aspect of the patient's straight (extended) right knee, with your middle finger in the groove between tibia and femur on the medial aspect.

Place your right hand on the ankle and spring the joint of the knee medially, by exerting force with your two hands in opposite directions (pushing medially with the right and laterally with the left).

Do the same on each leg.

Check and compare the degree of elastic 'give' in the restraining soft tissues and for changes in the configuration of the groove in each leg.

Could you sense symmetrical range of motion, freedom of movement and end-feel?

Could you sense joint play when you 'sprang' the joint?

Repeat this type of palpation on other extremity joints, looking for evidence of individual and symmetrical freedom of movement, full range of motion and freedom of joint play (see Special topic 9).

Palpation and evaluation of long leg/short leg problems

The following notes and exercises relate to an all-too-common musculoskeletal problem and are meant to help you to integrate your palpatory and assessment skills. These notes should not be considered to be definitive on this topic, although they do include the opinions and methods of many leading clinicians. They provide a starting point for using palpatory skills in a complex setting, for those who wish to explore body mechanics. The major usefulness of this section will be to encourage the use of palpatory skills to both joint and soft tissues, through the use of the various exercises.

Before coming to these, it is necessary to present the viewpoints of a number of experts (some of whom disagree on aspects of the problem) so that what is being palpated and evaluated makes some sense. Refer also to the pelvic and spinal assessments, discussed earlier in this chapter.

EXERCISE 9.30: SHORT LEG ASSESSMENT

Time suggested: 15 minutes

Mitchell et al (1979) offer the guidelines listed below regarding 'functional', or apparent, short leg assessment. They stress that the assessment is needed to give evidence of the success or otherwise of subsequent treatment, offering a 'baseline' from which to work.

For this exercise it is suggested that you carry out their suggested protocol.

- The height of the pelvic (iliac) crest should be assessed with the patient standing (see Exercise 9.4). This gives evidence suggesting an anatomical leg length difference.
- To assess for a functional (apparent) short leg the person is first placed supine, lying quite straight. The distances of the inferior slopes of the internal malleoli from the trunk are compared by placing the thumbs on them and the eyes directly over them. If one side appears shorter, i.e. the malleolus is closer to the trunk, there is probably an iliosacral lesion on that side producing this apparent shortness (presuming the iliac crests were level when the patient was standing).
- Retest for an iliosacral lesion with the patient performing the standing flexion test as PSIS excursion is noted (see Exercise 9.6).
- If no shortness is observed with the patient supine, place the patient in a prone position, lying straight. Again measure and compare by viewing the medial malleoli, with the thumbs on their inferior slopes.
  If the malleoli are level there is no functional shortness. If one side appears shorter, i.e. the malleolus is closer to the trunk, it is on the side of a possible sacroiliac lesion.
- Retest for a sacroiliac lesion by performing the seated flexion test with thumbs on the PSIS, looking for the one which has the greatest excursion on flexion of the seated patient (see Exercise 9.8).

A variety of iliosacral, sacroiliac, pubic and lumbar lesions may cause this apparent shortness, according to Mitchell et al.

Did either the supine or prone assessments of the relative levels of the malleoli confirm either iliosacral or sacroiliac restrictions, determined by standing or seated flexion tests?

Fryett's short leg observations (Fryett 1954)

1. Legs are usually of unequal length, in as many as 90% of people.
2. This is probably a major cause of sacroiliac dysfunction.
3. Other factors such as:
   - unilateral psoitis
   - unequal lumbar tension
   - shortened fascia in the hip region
   - shortened or relaxed ligaments
   - flat feet

may all make the legs appear to be of unequal length when actually they are not.

4. Measuring to identify short leg problems is best achieved by X-ray, according to Fryett. To avoid distortion, the tube must be absolutely in the centre

of the target, horizontal to the heads of the femur, patient standing still, knees extended. This gives accurate definition of the height of the trochanters (to within 0.5 cm) but distorts the sacrum and lumbar spine.

5. All individuals with leg length differences (no matter how slight) have a degree of functional disturbance of the SI joints, unless a heel-lift correction has been made.

6. Bone, young and old, is plastic and conforms with Wolff's Law which states: 'Every change in the use or static relations of a bone leads not only to a change in its internal structure and architecture but also to a change in its external form and function'.

7. In chronic cases [of short leg] the SI joint is not perfectly normal in form and cannot be treated as though it were. As a rule the problem has been present since the patient first began to walk.

8. Compensation always occurs, sometimes adequately, so that a severely lopsided, deformed pelvis, associated with leg length differences of up to 1 cm, may produce no pain whatever.

9. Fryett does not like the term 'short' leg, for often the problem is one of a long leg. He points out that the degree of load carried by a leg will influence its growth.

10. Some authorities believe that right-handed people brace themselves more on the left leg which develops more than does the right. Many right-handed people have a left foot which is larger than their right in consequence.

11. Janda has pointed out that we spend at least 80% of our time standing on one leg (when we are not sitting or lying down, that is).

12. The angle of the neck of the femur varies, normally being about $125°$. If it inclines towards the perpendicular (coxa valga), however, it would appear to make the leg longer than normal. The opposite situation, an inclination more to the horizontal (coxa vara), tends to make the leg shorter than normal.

Cailliet and the short leg

Cailliet (1962) says that measuring from the ASIS to the malleolus (as suggested by some experts) is, at best, inaccurate and offers little of significant value. He suggests three landmarks.

1. Standing barefoot, both legs close together, fully extended at the knees. Examiner places fingers on pelvic brim and determines the horizontal levels of his fingertips. This is quite accurate (see Exercise 9.4).

2. Note the dimples over the SI joints (where the gluteus maximus attaches to the periosteum over the sacrum) and estimate from these the pelvic level. This will only be difficult when the patient is very overweight or underweight (see Exercises 9.6 and 9.8 for more on pelvic palpation/assessment; Exercise 9.5 evaluates the position of the PSISs, which usually lie just inferior to these 'dimples').

3. Observe the lumbar spine at its 'take-off' from the sacrum. The postero-superior spines of the vertebrae are usually prominent and observable. If an oblique take-off is seen, this implies obliquity of the sacral base.

If these three clinical observations indicate a leg length discrepancy, the exact amount of this can be assessed by using a series of boards of varying thickness (0.25, 0.75, 1.25, 2 and 2.5 cm). These can be placed under the foot of the short leg until the pelvis reaches a balanced level.

Cailliet insists that it is, after all, a level pelvis (and therefore a straight spine) which we desire, rather than leg symmetry. He reminds us that a history of polio, genu valgum or varum or a previous fracture may all result in significant leg length discrepancies. It is only the effect on pelvic and spinal mechanics which matters.

Karel Lewit's views

Lewit (1985, 1992, 1999) has much to say on the subject of short legs. He reminds us that an artificial difference of more than 1 cm in leg length changes the balance in the coronal plane and is immediately felt and resented, whereas raising both heels is hardly noticed. Using a plumbline, Lewit observes for lateral shift of the pelvis from the midline.

Note: This can be used to test spinal mechanics in patients if we insert heelpads and watch the changes in deviation.

Physiological response to a short leg (Lewit)

Reaction (adaptation) to unequal leg length (as presented by the patient or initiated by the practitioner) is normal if:

1. there occurs a convex curve to the low side
2. there is rotation of the vertebral bodies to the low side (provided there is a lordosis and not a flat or kyphotic lumbar spine, in agreement with Fryett)
3. the lumbodorsal junction remains vertically above the sacrum
4. the pelvis as a whole shifts to the high side.

Note: If there is an obliquity of the sacral base on standing, this should always be observed again on sitting. If it remains when seated then the cause is not a short leg. (We should therefore compare sitting and standing sacral obliquity before using Cailliet's boards.)

Testing for equal weight distribution requires standing on two scales and ensuring that they display more or less equal weights. Only then can a plumbline assessment be valid. As heel lifts are placed for the assessment of deviation, the weight must be seen to be equally balanced. If weight is placed on one foot more than the other, the whole body deviates to that side, with the head deviating furthest.

The person should be assessed for weight distribution on two scales, with and without a heel pad on the lower side (of the pelvis). A subjective reaction should also be sought: do they feel happier with or without the pad? If there is a one-sided flat foot, an arch support is likely to be more effective than a heel lift.

Lewit agrees that leg length is of no concern unless it causes obliquity at the sacral base and the spine. How to measure differences, he says, is beside the point, for what is important is what we see on X-ray in relation to spinal mechanics.

Pathological findings related to short leg (Lewit)

1. A tilt (obliquity) without compensating scoliosis, or with insufficient scoliosis, so that the lumbodorsal junction does not find itself above the lumbosacral junction.
2. No pelvic shift to the high side.
3. No rotation of the vertebral bodies when there is a scoliosis and lordosis, or actual rotation to the opposite side from the scoliosis (away from the convexity), or scoliosis to the high instead of the low side.

Objectives of correction involving heel lifts

1. The achievement of a sufficient degree of compensation to bring the lumbodorsal junction over the lumbosacral junction (or close to this point).

2. A return of the pelvis from the high side to the centre.
3. A decrease in the degree of scoliosis.

In some instances of complex pelvic distortion a leg may appear shorter in the supine position, whereas on sitting this is reversed. There is usually a muscular 'blockage' involving spasm of the iliacus and/or there may be imbalance between the gluteals.

Lewit suggests that an assessment should also always be made of any difference in leg length below the knee, by having the supine patient bend both knees, feet on the table. The knee which is highest in relation to the table belongs to the long leg.

EXERCISE 9.31: SHORT LEG ASSESSMENT AND PALPATION

Time suggested: 15–20 minutes

Observe your standing partner's pelvic landmarks (level of pelvic brims, SI 'dimple' levels, spinal 'take-off' angle).

Is there a short leg and if so, which side is it on?

Do the spinal and pelvic changes reflect good or poor adaptation to a short leg (as per Lewit's criteria)?

- Is there a convex curve to the low side?
- Is there rotation of the vertebral bodies to the low side?
- Does the lumbodorsal junction remain vertically above the sacrum?
- Does the pelvis as a whole shift to the high side?

If you have a plumbline, assess lateral shift of the body.

Record your findings. Ask yourself what these findings mean in relation to short leg problems.

EXERCISE 9.32: CREATING AN ARTIFICIAL SHORT LEG TO ASSESS SPINAL AND PELVIC RESPONSE

Time suggested: 7–10 minutes

If your palpation partner has no leg length discrepancy when standing, use a pad, folded paper or other tool to raise first one heel (increasing the leg length) and then the other.

In each case observe for normal or abnormal changes, bearing in mind the differences which occur when there is a normal or exaggerated lumbar curve and when this is flat (see Fryett's notes above, p. 297).

When you 'create' a short/long leg situation artificially:

- is the lumbar spine convex towards the low side (short leg)?
- do the vertebral bodies rotate towards that side?
- is there a pelvic shift to the high side?
- is the lumbodorsal junction directly over the lumbosacral junction?

Decide whether the spinal mechanics are physiologically normal or not. Now go through De Jarnette's sequence below and compare results with the above (De Jarnette 1935).

De Jarnette and the short leg

Much of sacrooccipital technique (SOT) work depends upon assessment of a short leg and associated dysfunction.

Heel tension is usually assessed, since the Achilles with the greatest tension is thought to be the strong leg (in most cases). The complexities of defining category 1, 2 and 3 patients in SOT and the use of supporting blocks to normalise leg length, together with a host of odd 'signs' (dollar sign, crest sign, fossa signs, and so on) defy easy explanation, so this will not be attempted. If these concepts interest you, study SOT by attending professional seminars.

In a handbook of chiropractic first aid, De Jarnette provides the following insights into short leg problems.

Patient is supine, grasp ankles and pull these into extension and assess for the superior inner malleolus, thus identifying the short leg.

Correct the long leg first by placing the foot of that leg on the extended knee of the short leg, rotating the hip externally so that the knee of the flexed (long) leg falls towards the floor.

Hold this stretch until relaxation of the tense musculature is felt (30 seconds or more).

Go back to a normal supine position.

Next, hold the ankle of the short leg firmly with one hand, having flexed that leg at the knee, and adduct the knee so that it is forced across the extended knee of the long leg.

Pull the ankle laterally to increase stretch in the musculature around the pelvis/hip area, holding this position for 40 seconds (there may be some discomfort).

Patient lies with feet flat on table, knees flexed and well separated.

Hold the knees in this position as patient tries strongly to bring them together for 10 seconds or so.

Same position but this time knees are together, as patient tries strongly to separate these while you resist for 10 seconds or so.

The resisted approximation and separation are repeated alternately, 3 times each, in order to improve tone in the supporting soft tissues of the SI joints and pelvis.

This sequence is recommended by De Jarnette for **low back**, hip and leg problems of many types.

EXERCISE 9.33: DE JARNETTE'S SHORT LEG SEQUENCE

Time suggested: 25–30 minutes

Go through this entire De Jarnette sequence after you have performed Exercises 9.31 and 9.32. Then, see whether Exercises 9.31 and 9.32 give you any different information or indications.

Also, perform De Jarnette's sequence on someone in whom the standing and seated flexion tests (Exercises 9.6 and 9.8) were positive and then perform the tests again, to see whether the sequence changed the findings.

Note: Soft tissue dysfunction, for example involving hypertonic or shortened psoas or piriformis musculature, can create imbalances which produce apparent leg length discrepancies. The assessments relating to short leg imbalances in this chapter have ignored specific focus on muscle status (apart from De Jarnette's lengthy stretching suggestions). It should not, therefore, be assumed that what is included in this chapter is definitive, since the objective has been to enhance palpation and assessment skills and not to teach clinical methods of care for such dysfunctional states.

Assessing the body's compensation potential

In some of the tests associated with leg length imbalance, Lewit included evaluation of the manner in which the spine responds to the challenge of a short leg (see Exercises 9.31 and 9.32). In a very real way this provides a picture of the current degree of compensation potential of the spinal and pelvic structures, when faced with adaptive demands.

How well can the spine cope with being shoved off balance in this way? If it cannot cope very well (by virtue of not meeting Lewit's criteria), how well or badly might you expect it to cope with other demands, such as therapeutically designed modifications involving lengthening, strengthening, mobilisation, manipulation, etc.?

Zink & Lawson (1979) described methods for testing tissues' rotational preference at four crossover sites where fascial tensions can most usefully be noted:

- occipitoatlantal (OA)
- cervicothoracic (CT)
- thoracolumbar (TL)
- lumbosacral (LS).

They report that most people display alternating patterns of rotatory preference, with about 80% having a common pattern of L-R-L-R, which they termed the 'common compensatory pattern' (CCP), reading from the OA region downwards.

Zink & Lawson observed that the 20% of people whose CCP did not alternate had poor general health histories. Treatment of either CCP or uncompensated fascial patterns has the objective of trying, as far as is possible, to create a symmetrical degree of rotatory motion at these key crossover sites.

Fascial compensation is seen as a useful, beneficial and above all functional response (i.e. no obvious symptoms result) on the part of the musculoskeletal system, for example as a result of anomalies such as a short leg or to overuse. Decompensation describes the same phenomenon, where adaptive changes are seen to be dysfunctional, producing symptoms, evidencing a failure of homeostatic mechanisms (i.e. adaptation and self-repair).

Zink & Lawson (1979) have therefore described a model of postural patterning, resulting from the progression towards fascial decompensation. By testing the tissue 'preferences' (loose/tight) in these different transitional areas, Zink & Lawson maintain that it is possible to classify patterns in clinically useful ways:

- ideal, which are characterised by minimal adaptive load being transferred to other regions, as evidenced by, more or less, symmetrical degrees of rotation potential
- compensated patterns, which alternate in direction from area to area (e.g. atlantooccipital-cervicothoracic-thoracolumbar-lumbosacral) and which are commonly adaptive in nature (see Fig. 9.11A)
- uncompensated patterns which do not alternate and which are commonly the result of trauma (see Fig. 9.11B).

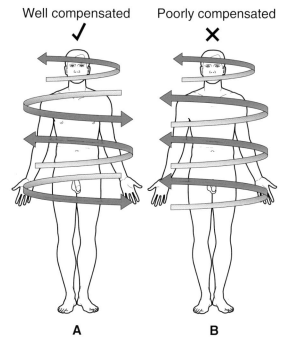

Well compensated ✓   Poorly compensated ✗

A   **B**

Fig. 9.11 Zink's postural (fascial) patterns. Tissue 'preferences' in different areas identify adaptation patterns in clinically useful ways: *ideal* = minimal adaptive load transferred to other regions; *compensated* (A) = patterns alternate in direction from area to area; atlantooccipital, cervicothoracic, thoracolumbar, lumbosacral; *uncompensated* (B) = patterns which do not alternate. Therapeutic objectives which encourage better compensation are optimal (adapted from Zink & Lawson 1979).

EXERCISE 9.34: ASSESSMENT OF TISSUE PREFERENCE (ZINK SEQUENCE)

Time suggested: 3–5 minutes

Occipitoatlantal area

Your palpation partner is supine and you stand at the head. Cradle the head as the neck is fully (but painlessly) flexed, so that any rotatory motion will be focused into the upper cervical area only.

Carefully introduce rotation left and right of the atlantooccipital structures. Is there a preference to turn easily to the left or the right or is rotation symmetrically free?

Cervicothoracic area

The person is supine and relaxed. You sit or kneel at the head of the table and slide your hands under the patient's scapulae. Each hand, independently, assesses the area being palpated for its 'tightness/looseness' preferences, by easing first one and then the other scapula area towards the ceiling.

Is there preference for the upper thoracic area to turn right or left?

Thoracolumbar area

The person is supine and you stand at waist level facing cephalad. Place your hands over the lower thoracic structures, fingers lying along the lower rib shafts, directed laterally.

Treating the structure being palpated as a cylinder, your hands test the preference of the cylinder to rotate around its central axis, one way and then the other.

In which direction does the thoracic 'cylinder' prefer to rotate?

continues

Lumbosacral area

The person is supine and you stand below waist level, facing cephalad, and place your hands on the anterior pelvic structures. This contact is used as a 'steering wheel' to evaluate tissue preference, as the pelvis is rotated around its central axis, seeking information as to its 'tight/loose' preferences.

In which direction does the pelvis prefer to rotate?

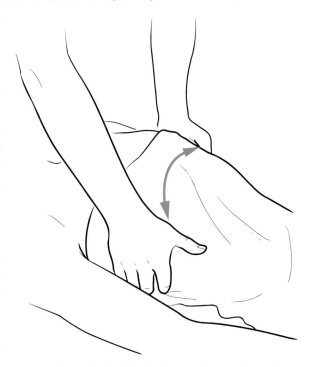

Fig. 9.12   Assessment of tissue rotation preference in thoracolumbar (diaphragm) region.

Reflections on possible learning outcomes from Exercise 9.34

Was there asymmetry in terms of the rotational preference of tissues in any of the four tested regions? If so, record these.

Based on Zink & Lawson's hypothesis, what are the implications of your findings regarding the rotational preferences of these four regions, in terms of the individual's adaptive capacity and overall health status?

Did you ensure that you were using the least possible effort to induce smooth and comfortable rotational movements?

Passive Gross motion testing

'Passive' clearly implies that the person being assessed is not (consciously) a party to the movement and that, as far as possible, this derives from the actions of the examiner. These tests (below) are in contrast to the often used, 'active' motion tests, in which the person is observed performing a particular movement, such as flexing and extending the spine or walking, sitting down and standing up again.

'Gross' suggests that large areas are involved in the assessment and not single joints. For example, the neck may be assessed as to its rotational range or spinal flexion. As Johnston (1982) points out:

> Whether any such test is completely passive may beg the point. The term 'induced gross motion' may be more accurate, since it correctly implies that the [practitioner] induces the movement and directs the specific motion desired.

Normal ranges of motion for any particular region, whether active or passive, vary considerably with body region, age, gender and somatotype.

Broad interpretations of specific tests

In this series of tests, palpation evaluates the tissues' willingness (or readiness) to move freely in different directions. The range of motions, whether these are symmetrical, and whether or not pain or discomfort is noted during the movement are all relevant.

The findings of the tests described below have been seen to have general postural, adaptational and even constitutional implications. As we have seen (Exercise 9.34), Zink & Lawson (1979) in particular described assessments which correlate uneven degree of rotation potential in specific regions to overall health status.

Other tests, such as those described by Johnston (1964, 1982), are seen as having implications related to postural adaptation status. Posture in this sense representing anything but a static series of parts, in relation to each other, with the centre of gravity as reference point. Instead, 'posture constantly functions to establish and maintain a "readiness to move" . . . the potential capacity of a complete cooperative participation of the body's various motive parts.'

It is when this cooperative participation and readiness to move freely are lost or diminished that dysfunction can be assumed. Johnston (1982) explains:

> The premise is that gross motion testing should play a significant role in the physical examination . . . palpation of a region's response to motion identifies the summation of [the] responses of individual parts, and when an individual part, or parts, are dysfunctional, that dysfunction is reflected in the overall response to the induced gross movements in which that part, or parts, should be participating, but cannot. A positive finding of asymmetry [during gross motion tests] will identify a region of the somatic system where segmental parts can then be individually examined, to define the locus of major dysfunction.

Cautions

1. A cautionary note needs to be introduced regarding standard methods when performing motion testing, for instance, of the effect of a particular movement on the patient's symptoms. Jacob & McKenzie (1996) in particular highlight the need in assessment for repetitive movement ('loading'), which simulates normal daily activities.

Standard range of motion examinations and orthopaedic tests may not adequately explore how the particular patient's spinal mechanics and symptoms are affected by specific movements and/or positioning. Perhaps the greatest limitation of these examinations and tests is the supposition that each test movement need be performed only once [in order] to fathom how the patient's complaint responds. The effect of repetitive movements, or positions maintained for prolonged periods of time, is not explored, even though such loading strategies might better approximate what occurs in the 'real world'.

During assessment movements should reproduce those actually performed in daily life, although it is, of course, appropriate to evaluate single directions of motion – abduction of the arm, for example – in order to gain information about specific muscles. In daily life, however, abduction of the arm is a movement seldom performed on its own; it is usually accompanied by flexion or extension and some degree of internal or external rotation, depending on the reason for the movement.

2. Your hand placement needs to be light when introducing passive movements. It is very important to avoid the individual receiving a sense from the contact hand(s) that the hands will move the part. Rather, there should be a sense that the hands initiate and guide but do not physically move the part. Johnston (1982) explains further: 'Light contact also complements the [practitioner's] need to sense response to motion throughout the test'.

3. You should be relaxed and be positioned so that proprioceptive sensory information received during the assessment is not distorted.

4. As noted in the early chapters, many palpation sensations are more readily noted when the eyes are closed.

Johnston's explanation of general ('gross') motion tests

Johnston (1964) explains that there is more to performing tests than simply looking for signs of 'something' specific (sacroiliac joint, hip joint, etc.) being dysfunctional, although this clearly has value when trying to make sense of a patient's symptoms.

A broader evaluation may be seen to be taking place, of 'general dynamic function', such as posture (see Hip shift test below).

In this particular assessment, and most similar passive motion tests, a simple 'yes–no' question is asked of the pelvis: whether it is able to move symmetrically when challenged to move toward the midline, by the practitioner. There is clearly more likelihood of symmetrical range of movement when there is no local or gross dysfunction, such as may be present if the individual is locked into a dysfunctional, distorted, pattern.

By evaluating the relative freedom of movement, or restriction, of the pelvis using the hip shift test (in this example), progress can be monitored after treatment has been applied. As Johnston (1964) explains:

> Either the postural midline is a point of freedom, from which gross movement is easily initiated in all directions, or it is a point from which only certain patterns of free motion are allowed; attempts in other directions encounter restrictive responses from within the body framework.

Concluding exercise

The final exercise in this chapter is once again based on the work of WL Johnston (1982). Johnston selected a number of areas, and methods, which he used to gain an 'initial impression' during physical examination, a screening for evidence of dysfunction in particular regions. Any evidence elicited by such gross testing called for further detailed investigation. Such tests do not say *what* is wrong, only that *something* is wrong.

Note: Johnston uses the term 'active' to mean practitioner induced, not patient induced (common terminology in Europe has this as passive, since that is the patient's role in the performance of the tests).

He selected his methods to, firstly, gain an initial impression of motion performance for each region of the body and, secondly, to sample the major movement patterns of the body. For example:

- rotational movement is introduced, with the patient seated, to the head/neck and shoulders, and with the patient standing, to the hips
- side bending is introduced to the neck with the shoulders stabilised on the side from which bending is occurring, and to the trunk by downward pressure on the shoulders
- translatory movements – side to side – are introduced at the femoral trochanters with the patient standing
- a lateral swing of the legs with the patient supine is followed by
- passive elevation of the arms (supine), which completes a sampling of motions for each spinal and extremity region.

Johnston points out that:

> Patient cooperation is gained by the practitioner briefly describing the procedure and asking the patient . . . to go along with it and not offer resistance.
>
> Placement of hands is light, and . . . the practitioner's active role is merely to initiate and guide the motion and complements the practitioner's need to sense response throughout the test.
>
> Position of the practitioner should be comfortable and flexible to minimise any additional proprioceptive sensory interference to reception of palpable cues. The movements introduced should not challenge the patient's sense of balance without the practitioner supplying an element of coordinated support. Postural challenge will evoke responses . . . that will reflect a false positive.

Criteria for a positive finding are palpatory. Once the practitioner has developed the palpable sense of a normal resistance barrier typically present at the end of a gross motion range, he or she applies this measure with respect to timing and quality; to go beyond this point will require additional practitioner force. For one example, with the patient supine, do the legs (supported together at the ankles by the practitioner's hands to just clear the table level) swing easily to right and left without encountering abnormal degrees of resistance? Is the endpoint encountered sooner in one direction than in the opposing direction? (Palpable cues are more sensitively measured by the hands with the eyes closed.)

Does the quality of the endpoint retain a normal sense of resilience or slight give or is it perceived as a hard, firm barrier?

EXERCISE 9.35: JOHNSTON'S 'GROSS MOTION' TESTS (see Exercises 9.35A–D)

Time suggested: 10–15 minutes

Seated
1. Rotation of the head left and right
2. Side bending of the neck with opposite shoulder stabilised (side bend left with the right shoulder stabilised)
3. Rotation introduced through the shoulders (arms folded)
4. Trunk side bending introduced through the shoulders (see Exercise 9.35A)

Standing
5. Rotation of the hips, left and right (see Exercise 9.35B)
6. Translation of the hips, left and right (see Exercise 9.35C)

Supine
7. Side-to-side motion (translation) applied from the trochanters
8. Lateral swing of the legs (see Exercise 9.35D)
9. Arms taken overhead

Perform these tests and record your results.

Your palpation partner is seated on a stool or chair, with arms folded. You stand behind and place your hands, one each side, over the region between the neck and shoulders (see Fig. 9.13).

Using minimal effort, you should introduce side-flexion to one side by means of downward pressure (to the floor) on one shoulder, until a sense of resistance is noted.

The person is eased back to the upright and the opposite direction of side-flexion is introduced.

If resistance is noted in one direction and not the other (or in both directions), the test is 'positive'.

The process is repeated several times, in order to assess any asymmetry in the range and quality of the movement, as well as the end-feel.

Reflections on possible learning outcomes

Were you able to sense any asymmetry when performing the test – either in range or in the quality of the end-feel when a barrier was reached on side-flexion? If so, record what the difference was and what you think the implications might be.

If there was asymmetry, where do you believe the restriction was located?

Did you ensure that you were using the least possible effort to induce smooth and comfortable movements during the test?

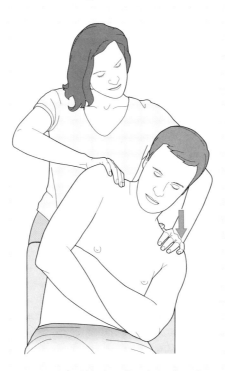

Fig. 9.13 Side-bending introduced through the shoulders.

EXERCISE 9.35B: HIP ROTATION TEST (JOHNSTON 1964)

Time suggested: 3–5 minutes

Your barefoot partner stands in front of you, with feet slightly apart, weight evenly distributed, arms hanging loosely.

You place your hands onto the lateral pelvis, over the hip joints 'so that the general area of prominence of the greater femoral trochanter is lightly contacted by the palmar surface of the digits at each side'.

The hips are used as contacts to guide the pelvis into rotation in one direction (to its easy end of range) and then the other (see Fig. 9.14).

You judge whether there is symmetry of rotational movement and also the quality of the end of range.

If resistance is noted in one direction and not the other (or in both directions), the test is 'positive'.

Reflections on possible learning outcomes

Were you able to sense any asymmetry when performing the test – either in range or in the quality of the end-feel when a barrier was reached?

If so, record what the difference was and what you think the implications might be.

If there was asymmetry, where do you believe the restriction was located? Did you ensure that you were using the least possible effort to induce smooth and comfortable movements involved in the test?

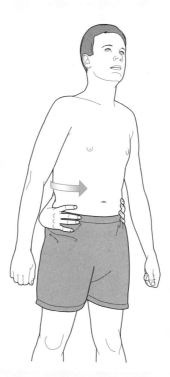

Fig. 9.14 Rotation of the hips for assessment of gross motion.

EXERCISE 9.35C: HIP SHIFT (TRANSLATION) TEST (JOHNSTON 1964)

Time suggested: 3–5 minutes

Your barefoot partner stands in front of you, with feet slightly apart, weight evenly distributed, arms hanging loosely.

You place your hands onto the lateral pelvis, over the hip joints, 'so that the general area of prominence of the greater femoral trochanter is lightly contacted by the palmar surface of the digits at each side'.

By means of a light but definite pressure of one hand and then the other, motion is initiated across the midline. This should involve a shunt/translation motion, not an attempt to induce side-flexion (see Fig. 9.15).

The degree of resistance of freedom of movement is evaluated one way and then the other, as well as the 'end-feel' in each direction. Johnston (1964) reports that 'In essentially normal posturing, there is an equal sense of freedom in both directions'.

If resistance is noted in one direction and not the other (or in both directions), the test is 'positive'.

The test is repeated several times (even if the first assessment results in equal degrees of freedom) in order to evaluate the persistence of the findings and also to ensure that the patient has a chance to relax, since the first effort may meet a voluntary tension which confuses the result.

In an acute setting, if (for example) there is free motion to the right and some restriction when moving toward the left, a postural shift of the pelvis toward the right should be evident.

Johnston reports that in a series of 1140 consecutive patients with musculoskeletal symptoms, 392 demonstrated a positive hip shift. Of these, 264 had low back problems, with 52 demonstrating objective hip shift distortion.

'Low back problems are not necessarily synonymous with lateral hip shift: 191 patients with low back pain had no hip shift, and 128 patients with hip shift had no presenting low back complaint.'

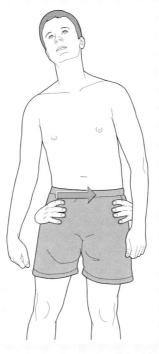

Fig. 9.15 Translation of the hips for assessment of gross motion.

continues

EXERCISE 9.35C   (*Continued*)

Reflections on possible learning outcomes

Were you able to sense any asymmetry when performing the test – either in range or in the quality of the end-feel when a barrier was reached?

If so, record what the difference was and what you think the implications might be.

If there was asymmetry, where do you believe the restriction was located?

Were you able to judge that you were using the least possible effort to induce a smooth and comfortable shift from one side to the other?

EXERCISE 9.35D: LATERAL LEG SWING TEST (JOHNSTON 1964)

Time suggested: 3–5 minutes

This test involves a totally passive side bending of the lumbar spine.

Your partner lies supine, arms elevated above shoulder level for stability and to allow easier observation of the waist area. The feet and ankles should extend slightly beyond the end of the table. You stand at the end and hold the legs just proximal to the ankles.

Apply light traction, just sufficient to take out soft tissue slack, and move the legs toward one side, say the left, until a sense of resistance is noted (see Fig. 9.16).

The legs are taken back to the midline and are then swung slowly to the right, to the first sign of resistance.

By repeating this action several times it should be possible to, first, evaluate whether the movement is symmetrical and, second, try to evaluate where any restriction is situated – hip or low back?

If resistance is noted in one direction and not the other (or in both directions), the test is 'positive'.

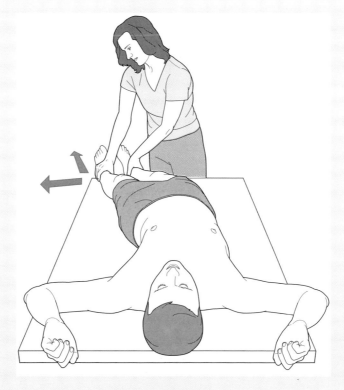

Fig. 9.16   Lateral swing of the legs to assess gross motion.

continues

Repeat the leg swing test, with the patient's arms lying at the sides and reevaluate the range and nature of the movement.

Reflections on possible learning outcomes

Were you able to sense any asymmetry when performing the test – either in range or in the quality of the end-feel when a barrier was reached?
If so, record what the difference was and what you think the implications might be.
If there was asymmetry, where do you believe the restriction was located?
Did you ensure that you were using the least possible effort to induce smooth and comfortable movements during the test?

Now reflect on which of the many ways of making sense of the body, as experimented with in this chapter, offer you the best methods for your way of working. If any of the tests in this exercise were positive, what would you do next to discover the nature of the dysfunction?

Conclusion

This chapter has attempted to involve you in discovering ways of extracting information, by means of palpation assessment. If you have worked through the exercises you should now see the need for both 'gross' and detailed observation, palpation and assessment of structure and function, in order to feel confident in your decision making as to treatment choices.

The next chapter offers a brief glimpse of the vast topic of visceral palpation.

REFERENCES

Cailliet R 1962 Low back pain syndrome. Blackwells, Oxford
Chaitow L 1999 Cranial manipulation: theory and practice. Churchill Livingstone, Edinburgh
Chaitow L 2001 Muscle energy techniques, 2nd edn. Churchill Livingstone, Edinburgh
De Jarnette B 1935 Spinal distortions. De Jarnette, Nebraska City
Denslow J 1960 Palpation of the musculoskeletal system. Journal of the American Osteopathic Association 60:
Fryett H 1954 Principles of osteopathic technic. National Printing Company, Kirksville, MI
Greenman P 1989 Principles of manual medicine. Williams and Wilkins, Baltimore
Jacob A, McKenzie R 1996 Spinal therapeutics based on responses to loading. In: Liebenson C (ed) Rehabilitation of the spine. Williams and Wilkins, Baltimore
Grieve G 1984 Mobilisation of the spine. Churchill Livingstone, London
Johnston W 1964 Hip shift: testing a basic postural dysfunction. Journal of the American Osteopathic Association 63(5): 35–42
Johnston W 1982 Passive gross motion testing (part 1): its role in physical examination. Journal of the American Osteopathic Association 81(5): 59–64
Lee D 1999 The pelvic girdle. Churchill Livingstone, Edinburgh
Lee D 2002 The palpation reliability debate. Journal of Bodywork and Movement Therapies 6(1): 18–37
Lewit K 1985 Manipulative therapy in rehabilitation of the locomotor system. Butterworths, London
Lewit K 1992 Manipulation in rehabilitation of the locomotor system, 2nd edn. Butterworths, London
Lewit K 1999 Manipulation in rehabilitation of the locomotor system, 3rd edn. Butterworths, London
Mitchell F, Moran P, Pruzzo N 1979 An evaluation of osteopathic muscle energy procedures. Valley Park, Missouri
Petty N, Moore A 1998 Neuromusculoskeletal examination and assessment. Churchill Livingstone, Edinburgh
Sutton S 1977 An osteopathic method of history taking and physical examination. Yearbook of Academy of Applied Osteopathy, Colorado Springs
Vleeming A, Snijders C, Stoeckart R, Mens J 1997 The role of the sacroiliac joints in coupling between spine, pelvis, legs and arms. In: Vleeming A, Mooney V, Dorman T, Snijders C, Stoeckart R (eds) Movement, stability and low back pain. Churchill Livingstone, Edinburgh
Walton W 1971 Palpatory diagnosis of the osteopathic lesion. Journal of the American Osteopathic Association 71:
Zink G, Lawson W 1979 Osteopathic structural examination and functional interpretation of the soma. Osteopathic Annals 7(12): 433–440

SPECIAL TOPIC 10
Percussion palpation

Percussion has been used as a means of manual treatment and diagnosis for many years.

The first major definitive study of the topic was that of Albert Abrams (of 'Black Box' fame) whose vast text *Spondylotherapy* was first published in 1910 (Abrams 1910). The preface to that book tells us that:

> In spondylotherapy the employment of mechanical vibration fills one of the most useful roles in therapeutics. It is easily controlled and is practical and effective of application in the hands of those familiar with the methods for employing spinal percussion.

Abrams described how he applied the percussive force.

> For simple concussion [I] employ a piece of soft rubber or linoleum about 6 inches [15 cm] long, 1.5 inches [4 cm] wide and about a quarter of an inch [0.5 cm] in thickness, as a pleximeter for receiving the stroke, and a plexor with a large rubber head for delivering the blow. In the absence of the latter a mallet or even an ordinary tack-hammer will suffice. One may also strike the spinous process with the knuckles, or better still the fingers may be used as a pleximeter and the clenched fist as a plexor . . . [Ideally] the strip of linoleum is applied to the spinous process or processes to be concussed, and with hammer a series of sharp and vigorous blows are allowed to fall on the pleximeter. Naturally the blows jar the patient somewhat, but beyond this no inconvenience is suffered.

Caution: Neither the degree of effort or the instruments suggested by Abrams are recommended – they are reported in this book as being of historical interest.

Some years later Johnson (1939) described the use of the hand or a mechanical instrument to apply percussive vibrations, 'which are only effective when applied with sufficient rapidity'.

What percussive sounds 'mean'

Percussion as a means of defining the position, and to some extent the status of organs, has a long history, with major variations in its use in Western and Oriental traditions of medicine.

A wide range of sounds may be heard when percussion is employed and their interpretation has been described in numerous medical texts, but in few more thoroughly than in that of Sir Robert Hutchinson (1897), published over a century ago and still in print. He described in detail the ways in which percussion examination can determine organ boundaries as well as the normal and abnormal variations in resonance of individual organs.

For example, in discussing thoracic percussion he describes both quantitative (ranging from hyperresonance to absolute dullness) and qualitative sound differences (various tympanic pitches, skodaic, boxy, cracked-pot, bell-sound/coin percussion, amphoric, etc.). Each of the qualitative variations is of potential diagnostic and prognostic value as it is interpreted in relation to other information available to the examiner.

Variations in sound will depend upon the relative solidity or hollowness, as well as the shape of the palpated organ, the nature and degree of intervening tissues, whether these are of bone, muscle, fat or other soft tissues, and the amount of air in the tissues being evaluated, as well as the manner in which percussion is applied (see Special Topic Figs 10A and 10B).

Method

Hutchinson suggests that the middle finger of the left hand be used as a pleximeter. This is laid firmly on the tissues to be percussed so that no air intervenes between finger and skin. The middle finger of the right hand then strikes this. The pleximeter finger can also be useful as a source of information regarding tissue resistance during percussion.

> The back of the middle phalanx (of the left middle finger) is struck with the tip of the middle finger of the right hand. The stroke should be delivered from the wrist and finger-joints and not the elbow, and the percussing finger should be so bent that when the blow is delivered its terminal phalanx is at right angles to the metacarpal bones, and strikes the pleximeter perpendicularly. As soon as the blow has been given, the striking finger must be raised, lest it should impair the vibrations it has excited, just as the hammers of a piano fall back from the wires as

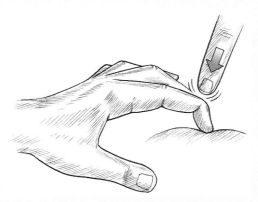

Special Topic Fig. 10A Distal phalanx position held as vertical to the palpated surface as possible, as described by Abrams, for percussion ('orthopercussion') assessment.

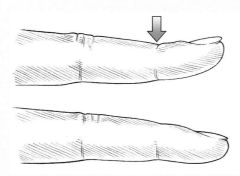

Special Topic Fig. 10B A finger which is to be used as a pleximeter should have the distal phalanx slightly raised (upper finger) and not resting along its length on the palpated surface (lower finger) (after Abrams). The arrow represents the ideal point which should be struck for optimal percussion efficiency.

soon as these have been struck. In cases where percussion requires to be firmer, several fingers may be used; but it is better, whenever possible to employ only one percussing finger . . . It is seldom necessary to deliver more than two or three strokes at any one situation. The points to be noted on percussion are the volume and *pitch* of the resonance elicited, and the sense of *resistance* experienced by the finger.

There are three cardinal percussion rules, states Hutchinson:

The first is that in defining the boundaries between contiguous organs the percussion should invariably be performed from the resonant [more hollow] towards the less resonant [more solid]. The second is that the longer axis of the pleximeter [finger] should be parallel to the edge of the organ whose delimitation is being attempted, and the line of percussion should be at right angles to that edge. The third is that the pleximeter finger must be kept in firm contact with the tissues [being evaluated].

In abdominal percussion, Hutchinson tells us that the pitch we hear depends upon the depth of the air space and the tension of the containing wall of the organ and that these two important elements vary greatly in the same viscus at different times. For example, the presence of free gas in the peritoneal cavity causes the normal dullness elicited in liver or spleen percussion to disappear. If abnormal dullness is detected we need to find out whether this is constant in all positions or whether it shifts when the position of the patient is altered, something of particular importance if an unnatural degree of fluid presence is suspected, as in ascites. He gives the example of an unusual distension of the abdomen which could result from gas, ascites or a new growth. Both a tumour and fluid would produce a dull percussion sound but the fluid would move (and the sound would therefore change) if the patient's position were altered, while the tumour would not.

Trigger point percussion technique or spondylotherapy

Trigger points can effectively be treated using a series of percussive strokes, according to Travell & Simons (1992). They state:

1. the muscle is lengthened to the point of onset of passive resistance
2. the clinician or patient uses a hard rubber mallet or reflex hammer to hit the trigger point at precisely the same place approximately 10 times
3. this should be done at a slow rate of no more than one impact per second but at least one impact every 5 seconds; the slower rates are likely to be more effective.

Travell & Simons suggest that this enhances, or substitutes for, intermittent cold with stretch ('spray and stretch') methods. The muscles which they list as benefiting most from percussion techniques include quadratus, brachioradialis, long finger extensors and peroneus longus and brevis.

Caution: It is specifically suggested that the anterior and posterior compartment of the leg muscle should not be treated by percussion, due to the risk of compartment syndrome, should bleeding occur in the muscle.

TCM percussion

Contraindications:

- acute disease
- severe heart disease
- TB

- malignant tumours
- haemorrhagic disease
- skin disease in area to be treated
- poor constitutional states such as malnutrition or asthenia.

In recent years, Chinese research involving percussion has dramatically added to our knowledge of the potential of these methods (Zhao-Pu 1991). In Traditional Chinese Medicine (TCM), percussion methods are incorporated into a broad heading of 'acupressure'.

Zhao-Pu states:

> Acupressure is based on the same theory as acupuncture and uses the same points and meridians. The therapeutic effect of acupressure technique lies in the way in which it regulates and normalizes blocked functions.

Included in these functions (as well as hypothesised energy transmission) are 'stimulating circulation of blood . . . and improving conductivity of nerves'.

In TCM, percussion techniques involve one of three variations.

1. One-finger percussion using the middle finger braced by the thumb and index finger.
2. Three-finger percussion using the thumb, index and middle fingers.
3. Five-finger percussion using the thumb and all fingers.

The degree of force applied during TCM percussion is also divided into three.

1. Light, which involves a movement of the hand from the wrist joint.
2. Medium, which involves a movement from the elbow joint with wrist fairly rigid.
3. Strong, which involves a movement of the upper arm, from the shoulder, with a rigid wrist.

Treatment is offered daily, on alternate days or once in 3 days and a course would involve 20 sessions. Patients often receive three courses or more. Zhao-Pu describes remarkable clinical results in patients with paralysis and cerebral birth injuries. He states:

> Research was carried out on the cerebral haemodynamics of patients with cerebral birth injury before and after acupressure (percussion and pressure techniques) therapy. Scanning techniques were used in monitoring the short half-life radioactive materials through the cerebral circulation; in almost one-third of the patients the regional cerebral blood flow was increased after acupressure therapy ranging from 28 to 60 sessions.

This approach does not produce instant results but attempts to influence and gradually harness the potential for recovery and improvement latent in the tissues of the patient. For more information on Oriental bodywork approaches, a complete manual of Chinese therapeutic massage (with many aspects which echo NMT methodology) edited by Sun Chengnan is highly recommended (Chengnan 1990).

Western percussion

Contraindications:

- osteoporosis
- malignancy
- inflammation in the area to be treated
- recent trauma in the area to be treated
- pain during application of percussive treatment.

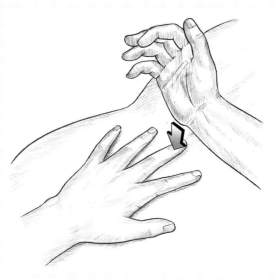

Special Topic Fig. 10C   Percussion for reflexive effects
on trigger points or spondylotherapy.

In order to stimulate organs via the spinal pathways, direct percussion techniques have long been employed by osteopathic and chiropractic practitioners. Over the past century in the USA a number of mechanical methods of percussion have evolved (Abrams 1910), as have effective manual systems in which the middle finger is placed on the appropriate spinous process(es), whilst the other hand concusses the finger with a series of rapidly rebounding blows. This approach is known as spondylotherapy (Johnson 1939) (see Special Topic Fig. 10C). One or two percussive repetitions are applied per second. Spondylotherapy percussion is usually applied to a series of three or four (or more) adjacent vertebrae.

An example of this is the treatment, as above, of the fifth thoracic spinous process, proceeding downwards to the ninth, in the case of liver dysfunction. Treatment would only be applied if the area was painful to palpating pressure. Similarly concussion over the 10th, 11th and 12th thoracic spinous processes would stimulate kidney function.

In order to stimulate the organ or tissues using the spinal reflexes, percussion would involve only a short amount of time: 15–30 second applications repeated three or four times, over approximately 4–5 minutes. A mild 'flare-up' of symptoms and increased sensitivity in the area treated would normally indicate that the desired degree of stimulation had been achieved. In order to inhibit function or to produce dilation of local blood vessels, Johnson (1939) suggests that percussive repetitions would be repeated for prolonged periods in order to fatigue the reflex.

SPECIAL TOPIC EXERCISE 10.1: PRACTISING PERCUSSION TO DEFINE THE UPPER AND LOWER BORDERS OF THE LIVER

Time suggested: 10–12 minutes

To perceive liver dullness, it is suggested that the person being palpated/percussed should be supine for anterior percussion and seated or standing for posterior percussion.

Percuss from the second rib downwards, to get a good lung note.

Percuss down from rib to rib till a duller sound is detected. Then repeat the process, going from space to space instead of from rib to rib. Percuss in this way down the mammary, midaxillary and scapular lines.

The upper limit of liver dullness in the middle line cannot be distinguished from heart dullness.

To map it out, draw a straight line from the apex beat to the angle where the right edge of the heart and the deep liver dullness meet.

The upper limit of liver dullness forms an almost horizontal line around the chest.

In defining the lower border of the liver, use very light percussion and pass upwards.

The exact position of the lower edge of the liver is extremely variable. Usually it coincides with the costal margin in the mammary line. It may be considerably above or below this without there being any pathological change in the organ. In percussing the surface of the liver where it is not covered by the lung, it should be observed that the organ has a certain degree of resistance or resilience. The normal amount of this can only be learned by practice.

If the organ is enlarged or congested, its resistance to percussion is increased owing to its being more firmly pressed against the chest wall.

Percuss the liver as suggested – can you define its borders?

Percussion is a form of palpation which deserves to be more widely used and the use of percussion therapeutically is a natural extension of the acquisition of this skill.

REFERENCES

Abrams A 1910 Spondylotherapy. Philopolis Press, San Francisco, CA

Chengnan S 1990 Chinese bodywork. Pacific View Press, Berkeley, CA

Hutchinson R 1897 Clinical methods. Cassel and Company, London

Johnson A 1939 Principles and practice of drugless therapeutics. Chiropractic Educational Extension Bureau, Los Angeles, CA

Travell J, Simons D 1992 Myofascial pain and dysfunction, vol 2. Williams and Wilkins, Baltimore

Zhao-Pu W 1991 Acupressure therapy. Churchill Livingstone, Edinburgh

10

Visceral palpation and respiratory function assessment

Accurate visceral palpation requires a high degree of palpatory literacy and that can only be accomplished by practice, practice, practice. And there is much to practise on. Goldthwaite and his colleagues (1945), in their classic text, described the changes which were commonly found in association with a slumped posture leading to loss of diaphragmatic efficiency and abdominal ptosis (see Chapter 5).

- Breathing dysfunction and restrictions develop.
- There is drag on the fascia supporting the heart, displacing this organ and resulting in traction on the aorta. Nerve structures supplying the heart are similarly stressed mechanically.
- The cervical fascia is stretched (recall that this can lead to distortion anywhere from the cranium to the feet, as the fascia is continuous throughout the body).
- Venous stasis develops below the diaphragm (pelvic organs and so on) as its pumping action is inhibited and diminished, leading to varicose veins and haemorrhoids.
- The stomach becomes depressed and tilted, affecting its efficiency mechanically.
- The oesophagus becomes stretched, as does the coeliac artery. Symptoms ranging from hiatus hernia to dyspepsia and constipation become more likely.
- The pancreas is mechanically affected, interfering with its circulation.
- The liver is tilted backwards, there is inversion of the bladder, the support of the kidneys is altered and the colon and intestines generally become mechanically crowded and depressed (as does the bladder). None of these can therefore function well.
- The prostate becomes affected due to circulatory dysfunction and increased pressure, making hypertrophy more likely. Similarly, menstrual irregularities become more likely.
- Increased muscular tension becomes a drain on energy, leading to fatigue which is aggravated by inefficient oxygen intake and poor elimination of wastes.
- Spinal and rib restrictions become chronic, making this problem worse.
- Postural joints become stressed, leading to spinal, hip, knee and foot dysfunction, increasing wear and tear.

All these changes are palpable and all are correctable, if caught early enough. A more precise examination of the biomechanical aspects of visceral dysfunction is now available through texts such as the highly recommended *Visceral manipulation* (Barral & Mercier 1988) which gives a host of directions, instructions and useful hints for anyone interested in this area of palpation and treatment. These British-trained French osteopaths have developed the art of visceral palpation and manipulation to a very high level of expertise. Additional exploration of this topic is to be found in *The science and art of osteopathy* (Stone 1999).

In their opening chapter Barral & Mercier (1988) outline what we need to know about visceral motility and mobility.

> There is an inherent axis of rotation in each of these motions (mobility and motility). In healthy organs, the axes of mobility and motility are generally the same. With disease, they are often at variance with one another, as certain restrictions affect one motion more than another. What a surprise it was for us to discover that the axes of motion reproduce exactly those of embryological development! Neither preconceived ideas nor hypotheses directed this research. The discovery of this phenomenon was purely empirical, and tends to confirm the idea that 'cells do not forget'.

Additionally visceral motion is influenced by:

1. the somatic nervous system (body movement, muscular tone and activity, posture). An example mentioned by Barral & Mercier is the motion of the liver during flexion, as it slides forwards over the duodenum and the hepatic flexure of the colon below. Similar motions occur in all viscera, determined by the particular support they have and their anatomical relationships

2. autonomic nervous system. This includes diaphragmatic motion, cardiac pulsation and motion as well as peristaltic activity. Clearly these automatic motions influence other closely associated organs, as well as some at a distance (for example, diaphragmatic motion, 24 000 times daily, influences and to some extent moves or vibrates all organs)

3. craniosacral rhythm. As we have seen in earlier chapters, this involves palpable movement throughout the body, including the viscera.

Embryological influences

These three influences produce visceral mobility and there is also inherent organ motility which Barral & Mercier have indicated relates very much to the embryological development phases. As an example, they describe how, during the development of the fetus, the stomach rotates to the right in the transverse plane and clockwise in the frontal plane. The transverse rotation therefore orients the anterior lesser curve of the stomach to the right and the greater posterior curvature to the left. The pylorus is therefore rotated superiorly and the cardia inferiorly.

Barral & Mercier found that these directions 'remain inscribed in the visceral tissues' with motion occurring around an axis, a point of balance, as it moves further into the direction of embryological motion and then returns to neutral (very similar to what takes place in the craniosacral mechanisms during flexion and extension of the structures of the skull).

Inspir and expir

The motility cycle is divided by Barral & Mercier (1988) into two phases which are termed *inspir* and *expir*. These are unrelated to the breathing cycle, being similar to the descriptions used in cranial osteopathy for cranial motion, flexion and extension.

Inspir describes the inherent motion and expir the return to neutral afterwards (7–8 cycles per minute). An example of this is that the liver's inherent inspir phase involves rotation posterosuperiorly (its mobility, as influenced by inhalation's diaphragmatic movement, is almost exactly opposite, anteroinferior).

In palpation, it is often easier to feel the expir phase (although inspir is more 'active' as there is less resistance to it), being a return to neutral.

Chronobiology

An additional vital, yet potentially confusing element is chronobiological influence. The 'energy clock' was initially described in Traditional Chinese Medicine (TCM) but is now universally recognised as delineating very pertinent changes in physiological function through the 24-hour period. The peak times for energy circulation through the meridians in TCM are as follows.

- Lungs 3.00–5.00 am
- Large intestines 5.00–7.00 am
- Stomach 7.00–9.00 am
- Spleen 9.00–11.00 am
- Heart 11.00 am–1.00 pm
- Small Intestine 1.00–3.00 pm
- Bladder 3.00–5.00 pm
- Kidney 5.00–7.00 pm
- Pericardium 7.00–9.00 pm
- Triple Burner 9.00–11.00 pm
- Gall Bladder 11.00 pm–1.00 am
- Liver 1.00–3.00 am

Other monthly, seasonal and annual cycles may also require consideration in visceral palpation/manipulation.

Visceral articulation

Just as joints have articulations, so do viscera. These are made of sliding surfaces (meninges in the CNS, pleura in the lungs, peritoneum in the abdominal cavity and pericardium in the heart) as well as a system of attachments (including ligaments, intercavity pressure, various folds of peritoneal structures forming containment and supportive elements). Unlike most joints, few muscular forces directly move organs.

Stone (1999) describes the movement of organs:

> Visceral biomechanics relate to the movements that the organs make against each other, and against the walls of the body cavities that contain them. The viscera 'articulate' by utilizing sliding surfaces formed by the peritoneal (and pleural or pericardial) membranes that surround the organs and line the body cavities. [Due to normal body movement including bending and locomotion, as well as body process such as micturition] . . . as the body cavities distort and change their shape, so the individual organs must adapt to those changes, and they do so by slightly sliding over each other, given the constraints of their attachments and surrounds.

By moving in these ways organs adapt to mechanical pressures and as they do so, they impart 'internal massage' and assist in fluid motion. Restrictions to normal visceral motion can derive from externally applied changes (restrictions, shortened soft tissue structures, etc.) involving the musculoskeletal system while conversely, local visceral scarring or adhesions can impact on the musculoskeletal system, via adverse tensions involving the suspensory ligaments which attach to, for example, the spine (see Fig. 10.1).

Figure 10.1 shows the way in which mesenteric attachments to the thoracic and lumbar spine support intestinal structures. Spinal changes (restrictions, positional modifications, increased or decreased spinal curves, etc.) could affect organ position and function and internal changes to the mesenteric ligaments (in a case of visceroptosis, for example) could affect the spinal structures to which they attach.

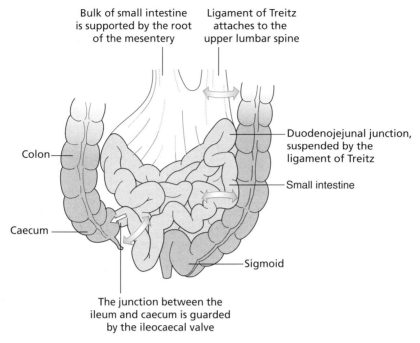

Fig. 10.1 Suspensory mesenteric ligaments supporting the small intestine attach to the spine (after Stone 1999).

Three visceral palpation elements

Barral & Mercier (1988) suggest that there are three elements involved in evaluation of visceral function and these are the traditional ones of:

- palpation (which informs as to tone of the walls of the visceral cavity)
- percussion (which informs about the position and size of the organ in question)
- auscultation (which informs as to factors such as circulation of air, blood and secretions such as bile).

Muscular influences

Barral & Mercier stress the importance of the influence on visceral function of muscular activity and urge mobility tests to identify dysfunction in the musculoskeletal system. However, they state that: 'We believe that visceral restrictions are the causative lesions much more frequently than are musculoskeletal restrictions'.

Mobility and motility

Mobility describes the potential for movement at an articulation or interface. The movement associated with mobility would be produced by external forces, such as active muscular contractions or passive movements.

Motility, on the other hand, describes the inherent movement, such as pulsation, of an area, organ or specific tissues: for example, the rhythmic motions palpated in the cranium, as described in Chapter 3.

How do you palpate an organ for mobility?

By precise movements, say Barral & Mercier. In order to do this, though, you need to know the normal movements of the organ in question. They give an example of the liver which 'you literally lift up to appreciate the elasticity of its supporting structures and the extent of its movement'.

Mobility assessment (which provides information as to elasticity, laxity/ptosis, spasm and structural injury of muscular or ligamentous supports) requires less skill than does finer evaluation of inherent motility and variations in it from the norm.

How do you palpate organs for motility?

The most effective method for evaluating motility, say Barral & Mercier, is that described by Rollin Becker (see Chapter 6) in which the hand 'listens' for information. This is how the French osteopaths describe application of Becker's work to this task.

> Place your hand over the organ to be tested, with a pressure of 20–100 g, depending on the depth of the organ. In some cases the hand can adapt itself to the form of the organ. The hand is totally passive, but there is an extension of the sense of touch used during this examination. Let the hand passively follow what it feels – a slow movement of feeble amplitude which will show itself, stop and then begin again (7–8 per minute in health).
> This is visceral motility.

It is then desirable, after a few cycles, to estimate elements such as frequency, amplitude and direction of the motility. The advice is very much as given by Becker, Upledger, Smith and others (see Chapter 6). Do not have preconceived ideas as to what will be felt. Trust what you feel. Empty the mind and let the hand listen. (Both organs of a pair should be assessed and compared.)

One visceral palpation exercise for motility (based on the work of Barral & Mercier) is suggested below. Those exercises relating to Becker's work, as outlined in Chapter 6, should have been performed satisfactorily before performing this exercise. Study of visceral manipulation and attendance at seminars and workshops covering this subject is suggested for those keen to explore this subtle and rewarding field.

EXERCISE 10.1: PALPATION FOR LIVER MOTILITY

Time suggested: 10 minutes

The person to be palpated should be supine. You should be seated or standing on the right of the patient, facing her.

Place your right hand over the lower ribs, moulding to their curve, covering the outer aspect of the liver. Your left hand should be laid over the right hand. Your mind should be stilled as you visualise the liver.

You are trying to assess the return to neutral (the expir phase of the motility cycle), which means that the direction of active motion would be the opposite to that palpated during this phase.

Barral & Mercier (1988) suggest that the expir phase is the easiest for the beginner to palpate. During this phase, three simultaneous motions may be noted.

● In the frontal plane, a counter-clockwise motion, from right to left, around the sagittal axis (of your hand and therefore the liver). This takes the palm of the hand towards the umbilicus (Fig. 10.2).

continues

EXERCISE 10.1 *(Continued)*

- In the sagittal plane the superior part of the hand should rotate anteroinferiorly around a transverse axis through the middle of your hand.

- In the transverse plane, the hand rotates to the left around a vertical axis, bringing the palm off the body as the fingers seem to press more closely.

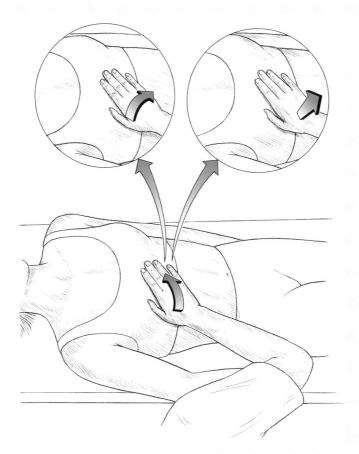

Fig. 10.2 Palpation of the liver (after Barral & Mercier) in which frontal, sagittal and transverse planes of motion are sequentially assessed.

Each of these planes of movement can be assessed separately before they are assessed simultaneously, providing a clear picture of liver motility in the expir phase of the cycle (inspir is the exact opposite).

This palpation exercise should be performed with eyes closed.

Periodically the patient should be asked to hold the breath for a 20-second period, to see whether this provides a less confused feeling of motion.

It may be useful to recall Becker's method of assessment (Chapter 6), in which elbows or forearm are used as a fulcrum to enhance palpatory sensitivity and perception.

Palpation for respiratory dysfunction

Lewit (1999) has synthesised much of the current knowledge about respiratory influence on body mechanics and describes useful methods for assessing its efficiency and coordination.

> Thinking of breathing, one naturally has in mind the respiratory system. Yet it is the locomotor system that makes the lungs work, and the locomotor system that has to coordinate the specific respiratory movements with the rest of the body's locomotor activity. This task is so complex that it would be a miracle if disturbances did not occur.

It is important to distinguish between respiratory problems which relate to habitual use patterns and those which derive from pathology. Breathing pattern disorders (such as tendency toward hyperventilation) are extremely common and are often remediable through a combination of breathing retraining and bodywork (Chaitow et al 2002). Respiratory disease (such as emphysema) is also common and usually requires expert medical attention (Pryor & Prasad 2001). Palpation exercises are described later in this chapter which can help to make this distinction.

Structural considerations

Garland (1994) has summarised the structural modifications which are likely to inhibit successful breathing retraining as well as psychological intervention, until they are at least in part normalised. He describes a series of changes including:

> Visceral stasis/pelvic floor weakness, abdominal and erector spinae muscle imbalance, fascial restrictions from the central tendon via the pericardial fascia to the basi-occiput, upper rib elevation with increased costal cartilage tension, thoracic spine dysfunction and possible sympathetic disturbance, accessory breathing muscle hypertonia and fibrosis, promotion of rigidity in the cervical spine with promotion of fixed lordosis, reduction in mobility of 2nd cervical segment and disturbance of vagal outflow . . . and more.

These changes, he states:

> Run physically and physiologically against biologically sustainable patterns, and in a vicious circle, promote abnormal function which alters structure which then disallows a return to normal function.

In simple terms, until there is some degree of normalisation of the breathing mechanism, it cannot be used normally, whatever instructions the individual gives it. However:

> If assistance can be given to an individual who hyperventilates, by minimising the effect of somatic changes, and if these structural changes can be provided with an ability to modify, therapeutic interventions via breath retraining and counselling will be more effective.

Garland concludes:

> In hyperventilation, where psychology overwhelms physiology the role of the osteopath can be very beneficial.

Lewit (1980) has given due attention to structure and function as it relates to respiration, and states that:

> The most important disturbance of breathing is overstrain of the upper auxiliary muscles by lifting of the thorax during quiet respiration.

The implications of this have been described by Garland, as detailed above. Other researchers have examined the relationship between respiration and the function of the musculoskeletal system. For example, Cummings & Howell

(1990) have looked at the influence of respiration on myofascial tension and have clearly demonstrated that there is a mechanical effect of respiration on resting myofascial tissue (using the elbow flexors as the tissue being evaluated).

They also quote the work of Kisselkova & Georgiev (1976), who reported that resting EMG activity of the biceps brachii, quadriceps femoris and gastrocnemius muscles 'cycled with respiration following bicycle ergonometer exercise, thus demonstrating that nonrespiratory muscles receive input from the respiratory centres'.

The conclusion was that:

These studies document both a mechanically and a neurologically mediated influence on the tension produced by myofascial tissues, which gives objective verification of the clinically observed influence of respiration on the musculoskeletal system and validation of its potential role in manipulative therapy.

Breathing and muscle pain

Dr Mark Pellegrino (1993/1994) of Ohio State University has studied fibromyalgia syndrome and its link with chest pain. He notes that 'FMS patients are more prone to getting anxiety or panic attacks, especially when placed in a stressful situation'.

Breathing irregularities often have a connection with the symptoms of anxiety. Hyperventilation and anxiety also have an intimate link with poor stress-coping abilities.

At its simplest, the connections can look as follows (Timmons & Ley 1994).

- A person responds habitually to what they find to be a stressful situation by breathing shallowly, using the upper chest and not the diaphragm.
- This breathing pattern becomes a habit, so that it continues even when whatever they see as stress is not present (even when sleeping), although it tends to be much more obvious when they are stressed.
- With such a pattern of breathing the accessory breathing muscles become overactive and tense and often develop painful local areas.
- Headaches due to irritation of local nerve structures in these muscles and/or interference with circulation to, and drainage from, the head can occur – with lightheadedness, dizziness and possibly headaches resulting.
- The overbreathing pattern leads to excess carbon dioxide being exhaled, causing carbonic acid levels in the blood to be lowered, leading to the bloodstream becoming too alkaline.
- Alkalisation leads automatically to a feeling of apprehension/anxiety and the abnormal breathing pattern becoming worse. Panic attacks and even phobic behaviour are not uncommon following this.
- Alkalisation also leads to nerve endings becoming increasingly sensitive so that the individual is more likely to report pain when previously only discomfort would have been reported.
- Alkalisation results also in vasoconstriction of the blood vessels in the head, further reducing oxygenation of the region.
- Along with heightened arousal/anxiety and cerebral oxygen lack there is also a tendency for what oxygen there is in the bloodstream to become more tightly bound to its haemoglobin carrier molecule, leading to decreased oxygenation of tissues and easy fatiguability.
- Inadequate oxygenation and retention of acid wastes in overused muscles takes place and these become painful and stiff.
- The muscles being overused in the inappropriate breathing pattern are mainly postural stabilising muscles (scalenes, SCS, trapezius, pectoral, levator

scapulae) and will, with the repetitive stress involved in the overbreathing, become short, tight and painful and will develop trigger points. Remember that the most common sites for tender points of FMS – and trigger points – lie in just these muscles of the neck, shoulder and chest.

● The increased tension in these muscles adds to feelings of fatigue since the muscles are constantly using energy in a non-productive way even during sleep.

● The poor breathing pattern leads to a restriction of the spinal joints which attach to the ribs which, because they are not moving much due to shallow breathing, are deprived of regular (each breath) movement, leading to stiffness and discomfort.

● The rib attachments to the sternum are also restricted, leading to pain.

● A similar lack of movement of the diaphragm leads to digestive organs missing out on a regular (each breath) rhythmic 'massage' as the diaphragm rises and falls.

● Shallow breathing restricts the pumping mechanism between the chest and the abdomen, which normally assists in the return of blood from the legs to the heart. Cold feet and legs could be caused, or at least aggravated, by this.

● The intercostal muscles become tense and tight with the likelihood of chest pain and a feeling of inability to get a full and deep breath.

The consequences of respiratory dysfunction which falls short of actual hyperventilation should not be underestimated since, although the impact on health may well be less dramatic than the sequence indicated above, the same tendencies will be apparent (see Special Topic 12 on hyperventilation).

Breathing and muscle and joint activity

In general, muscular activity is enhanced by inspiration and inhibited by expiration. There are exceptions to this, such as the abdominal muscles, which are facilitated by forced exhalation (Lewit 1999).

Flexion of the cervical and lumbar spines is enhanced by maximum exhalation whereas flexion of the thoracic spine is enhanced by maximum inspiration and these phases of respiration can be usefully employed in mobilisation (and assessment, including palpation) of this region.

A further influence on spinal mechanics of respiration is described by Lewit (1999).

> The most surprising effect of inspiration and expiration is the alternating facilitation and inhibition of individual segments of the spinal column during sidebending, discovered by Gaymans (1980). It can be regularly shown that during sidebending, resistance increases in the cervical as well as the thoracic regions, in the even segments (occiput-atlas, C2 etc. and again T2, T4, etc.) during inspiration; during expiration we gain the mobilising effect in these segments. Conversely, resistance increases in the odd segments during expiration (C1, C3, etc., T3, T5, etc.). There is a neutral zone between C7 and T1.

Inspiration increases resistance to movement in the atlas-occiput region in all directions, while expiration eases its motion in all directions, a most useful piece of information, of value during manipulation or assessment/palpation of motion. Where maximum muscular effort is required we tend to neither inhale nor exhale, but to hold the inhaled breath (Valsalva manoeuvre). This achieves postural stability (no facilitation of spinal motion in any segments) at the cost of momentary loss of respiratory function. The diaphragm has therefore been described (according to Lewit (1999)) as 'a respiratory muscle with postural function', while the abdominal muscles are 'postural muscles with respiratory function'.

These comments highlight the role of the diaphragm in supporting the spine. As Lewit explains, the abdominal cavity is a fluid-filled space which is not compressible as long as the abdominal muscles and the perineum are contracted (the shout of the judo wrestler, ski jumper and weight lifter all attest to this enhanced stability being used).

A further stabilising feature is the fact that, as we rise on our toes, the diaphragm contracts (at the start of a race or when jumping, for example), this being interpreted as a postural reaction. Lewit sees inspiration as largely dependent on contraction of the diaphragm which lifts the lower ribs as long as the central tendon is supported by counterpressure from sound abdominal muscles. This, he says, is the only explanation for the widening of the thorax from below (see also Latey's assessments of this function in Chapter 12).

The thorax must be widened from below to achieve postural stability during respiration, never raised from above. Therefore the shoulders, clavicles and upper ribs are not lifted but rotate slightly to accommodate the movement from below as the thorax widens. This does not happen when supine or on all-fours, where no postural stabilising effect is needed and pure abdominal respiration becomes physiologically normal, with the abdomen bulging while its wall remains relaxed.

Assessing breathing function

These preliminary explanations are necessary to understand what we should look for in the presence of respiratory dysfunction. What then should we observe and palpate?

Inactive abdominal muscles are clearly undesirable for respiratory and postural normality, for the spine then loses its diaphragmatic support. The abdominal tone can be assessed with the patient seated and relaxed. There should be no flabbiness on palpation. On stooping from the standing position the abdominals should be felt to contract. Recall that Janda has shown (Chapter 5) that tight erector spinae muscles will effectively reciprocally inhibit the abdominal musculature and that no amount of toning exercise can restore normality until the erector spinae group is stretched and normalised.

The test for abdominal muscle efficiency involves having the patient sit up from the supine position while knees and hips are flexed. In order to have coordinated action from the glutei (maximus) in this action, the heels may press backwards against a firm cushion or support. If this is difficult, then lying backwards from a seated position will train the abdominals. The spine is flexed first and one segment at a time is laid on the table/floor without raising the feet from the floor. If the feet start to leave the floor, stop the move backwards at this point and slowly return to the upright seated position. Keep repeating the lay back, trying to increase the distance travelled before the feet start to rise.

The thorax must be seen to widen from below on inhalation. Also, when sitting flexed or lying prone, there must be a visible ability to breathe 'into' the posterior thoracic wall. This is evidenced by the respiratory 'wave' described previously (see Chapter 9). Where this wave is limited, failing to start in the low lumbars and progressing throughout inhalation up to the cervicodorsal junction, there will be palpable restrictions in the thoracic spine due to the absence of the mobilising effect of the breathing function.

The most obvious evidence of poor respiratory function is the raising of the upper chest structures by means of contraction of the upper fixators of the shoulder and the auxiliary cervical muscles (upper trapezius, levator scapulae, scalenes, sternomastoid). This is both inefficient as a means of breathing and the cause of stress and overuse to the cervical structures. It is clearly evident (see below) when severe but may require a deep inhalation to show itself if only slight.

EXERCISE 10.2: ASSESSING RESPIRATORY FUNCTION

Time suggested: 20 minutes

The person to be evaluated should be seated. You stand behind and place your hands, fingers facing forwards, over the lower ribs, thumbs touching on the midline posteriorly (see Fig. 10.3).

The person exhales to her comfortable limit (i.e. not a forced exhalation) and then inhales slowly and fully.

Is there a lateral widening and if so, to what degree? Pryor & Prasad (2001) report that normal total excursion is between 3 and 5 cm (1.5–2 inches).

Or do your hands seem to be raised upwards? The hands should move apart but they will rise if inappropriate breathing is being performed involving the accessory breathing muscles and upper fixators of the shoulders.

Does one side seem to move more than the other? If so, local restrictions or muscle tensions are probably involved.

Is there evidence of paradoxical breathing? Pryor & Prasad (2001) report:

> Paradoxical breathing is where some or all of the chest wall moves inward on inspiration and outward on expiration . . . localized paradox occurs when the integrity of the chest wall is disrupted.

Causes can range from rib fracture to diaphragmatic paralysis and cases involving chronic airflow limitation.

While the person being tested continues to breathe slowly and deeply you should try to evaluate 'continuity of motion' in the inhalation/exhalation phases. Observe any starting and stopping, asymmetry or apparent malcoordination and any unexpected departures from smooth mobility.

Rest the hands over the upper shoulder area, fingers facing forwards. On inhalation, do the hands rise? Does either clavicle rise on inhalation? Neither the clavicles nor your hands should rise, except on maximal inhalation.

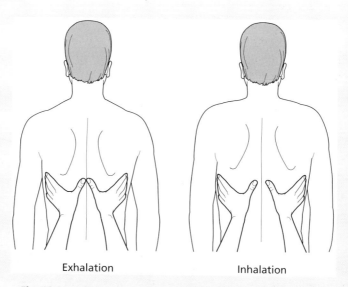

Exhalation   Inhalation

Fig. 10.3   Palpation of thoracic expansion on inhalation (after Pryor & Prasad 2001).

continues

While in this position, assess whether one side moves more than the other. If so, local restrictions or muscle tensions may be implicated.

Observe the upper trapezius muscles as they curve towards the neck. Are they convex (bowing outwards)? If so, these so-called 'gothic' shoulders are very taut and probably accompany inappropriate breathing, lifting the upper ribs (along with scalenes, sternomastoid and levator scapulae). Palpate these muscles and test them for shortness (see Chapter 5).

Palpate the abdomen, still with the person seated, as she inhales deeply. Does the abdomen (slightly) bulge on inhalation? This is normal. In some instances, breathing is so faulty that the abdomen is drawn in on inhalation and pushed outwards on exhalation – further evidence of a paradoxical pattern.

Now return to the first position, with your hands on the sides of the lower ribs. Feel the degree of contraction on exhalation. Does this seem to be a complete exhalation? Or does the person not quite get the end of the breath exhaled before commencing the next inhalation? If so, this leads to retention of excessive levels of tidal air, preventing a full inhalation. Inhalation efficiency can be said to depend on the completeness of the exhalation.

Now ask the person to take as long as possible to breathe in completely. How long did it take? If less than 5 seconds, there is probably dysfunction. Next, after a complete inhalation, ask the person to take as long as possible to exhale, breathing out slowly all the time. This should also take not less than 5 seconds, although people with dysfunctional breathing status or who hyperventilate, and those in states of anxiety, often fail to take even as long as 3 seconds to inhale or exhale.

Now time the complete cycle of breathing (inhalation plus exhalation). This should take not less than 10 seconds in good function.

The person should now lie supine, knees flexed. Rest a hand, lightly, just above the umbilicus and have the patient inhale deeply. Does your hand move towards the ceiling (ideally 'yes')? Are the abdominal muscles relaxed (ideally 'yes')? Or did your hand actually move toward the floor on inhalation (ideally 'no')? If the abdomen rises, was this the first part of the respiratory mechanism to move or did it inappropriately follow an initial movement of the upper or lower chest? Paradoxical breathing such as this involves the mechanism being used in just such an uncoordinated manner.

Then ask your palpation partner to lie prone. Observe the wave as inhalation occurs, moving upwards in a fan-like manner from the lumbars to the base of the neck. This wave can be observed by watching the spinous processes or the paraspinal musculature or palpated by a featherlight touch on the spine or paraspinal structures.

Cross-referral to other palpatory findings

Whatever restrictions or uncoordinated movements you observe or palpate during this exercise can now usefully be related to findings of spinal joint and rib restrictions (see Chapter 9), respiratory and postural muscular shortening as well as trigger point activity – especially in the intercostal muscles (Chapter 5), postural imbalance, pelvic dysfunction and short leg anomalies (Chapter 9), emotional involvement (Chapter 12).

Integrating the various components of palpation, as described throughout this book, enhances clinical thinking, as evidence from one source is supported or contradicted by additional (palpation and other) findings.

Charting results

Boxes 10.1 and 10.2 offer examples of the kind of forms you can create to record breathing dysfunction in individual cases.

Observation

Bradley (Chaitow et al 2002) describes those features which should be observed when breathing function is being evaluated, whether in the presence of pathology or a habitual breathing pattern disorder.

- Resting respiratory rate? (Normal adult range 10–14 per minute; West 2000)
- Nose or mouth breather?
- Resting breathing pattern:
  - effortless upper chest/hyperinflation
  - accessory muscle use
  - frequent sighs/yawns
  - breath-holding ('statue breathing')
  - abdominal splinting
- Combinations of the above
- Repeated throat clearing/air gulping

Observe:
- Jaw, facial and general postural tension, tremor, tics, twitches, bitten nails
- Chest wall abnormalities, for example:
  - pectus carinatum (anterior sternal protrusion)
  - pectus excavatum (depression or hollowing of the sternum)
- Kyphosis (abnormal forward anteroposterior spinal curvature)
- Scoliosis (lateral spinal curvature)
- Kyphoscoliosis, a combination of the former two
- Adaptive upper thoracic and shoulder girdle muscle changes, e.g. raised shoulders, protracted scapulae (see Chapter 5)

Assessing for pathology

This book cannot cover detailed palpation for pathology but several evaluations involving palpation can be usefully practised to enhance clinical skills.

Box 10.1 Primary and accessory respiratory muscle assessment for shortness (see previous chapters for guidance on individual muscle assessments)

E = Equal (circle if both are short)
L and R (circle if left or right is short)

1. Psoas	E	L	R
2. Quadratus lumborum	E	L	R
3. Pectoralis major	E	L	R
4. Latissimus dorsi	E	L	R
5. Upper trapezius	E	L	R
6. Scalenes	E	L	R
7. Sternocleidomastoid	E	L	R
8. Levator scapulae	E	L	R
9. Spinal flattening: seated, legs flexed	LowL MidT	LD UpperT	LowT
10. Cervical spine extensors short?	Yes	No	

Box 10.2 Palpation assessment and evaluation

Seated

a. Is lateral rib expansion symmetrical? Specify	YES	NO
b. Measure range of unforced expansion*: From:............... cm to .... cm	EXHALED	INHALED
c. Measure range of full expansion*: From: .... cm to .... cm	EXHALED	INHALED
d. Does inhalation start before exhalation complete?	YES	NO
e. Does clavicle rise on inhalation?	YES	NO
f. If there is movement, is it symmetrical? Specify	YES	NO
g. Does abdomen draw inwards paradoxically on inhalation?	YES	NO
h. Time breathing elements		
Does inhalation last at least 5 seconds?	YES	NO
Record inhalation secs		
Does exhalation last at least 5 seconds?	YES	NO
Record exhalation secs		
Does full cycle last at least 10 seconds?	YES	NO
Record cycle: secs		
i. Evaluate thoracic spinal restrictions.		
j. List and chart findings.		

Prone

k. Observe 'breathing wave' of prone patient as they take full breath. Is there a wave-like movement from the base of the sacrum to the base of the neck?	YES	NO

   Where does the wave start and stop?
       LowL   LDJ   LowT   MidT   UpperT

Supine

l. Evaluate for elevated or depressed rib restrictions.
m. Note any asymmetry in breathing function (e.g. lateral expansion).

*To measure the amount of expansion taking place, sit or stand facing your patient/model and place your thumbs, with their tips touching, on the anterior or posterior midline, with the index fingers resting along the shafts of a pair of ribs. As your palpation partner inhales, either fully or normally, your thumbs will separate. Judging the degree and equality of expansion by this means is rapid and accurate.

   Alternatively, use a flexible tape measure to record the unexpanded circumference and the expanded circumference in order to measure the range of expansion.

Palpation of vocal fremitus

When speaking, vibrations pass through the entire thoracic cavity and these can be palpated on the chest wall by placing the flat hands bilaterally and comparing the sensation as the person being evaluated repetitively speaks the words 'ninety nine'.

Pryor & Prasad note:

> The hands are moved from the apices to bases, anteriorly and posteriorly, comparing the vibration felt. Vocal fremitus is increased when the lung underneath is relatively solid (consolidated), as this transmits sound better. As sound transmission is decreased through any interface between lung and air or fluid, vocal fremitus is decreased in patients with pneumothorax or pleural effusion.

Percussion

See Special Topic 10 on the subject of percussion. Percussion of the chest is a useful means of evaluating areas of consolidation. Pryor & Prasad explain:

> Resonance is generated by the chest wall vibrating over the underlying tissues. Normal resonance is heard over aerated lungs, while consolidated lung sounds dull, and a pleural effusion sounds 'stony dull'. Increased resonance is heard when the chest wall is free to vibrate over an air-filled space, such as pneumothorax or bulla. In . . . obese patients the percussion note may sound dull even if the underlying lung is normal.

EXERCISE 10.3: PERCUSSION AND VOCAL FREMITUS PALPATION

Time suggested: 3–4 minutes

Perform the vocal fremitus and the percussion evaluation as described above and relate this to the body type of the person. If possible perform these exercises on a variety of different body types.

Conclusion

If all the exercises in this chapter have been successfully attempted, ideally more than once, you should have gained an appreciation of the importance and subtlety of these methods. While not everyone will be drawn to or feel comfortable regarding visceral palpation as such, the evaluation of breathing function is one of the skills which simply 'have to' be acquired, if a comprehensive understanding of the patient/client is to be gained. Awareness of breathing pattern disorders leads naturally to a need to uncover structural modifications (short tight muscles, restricted ribs, etc.) which might be impacting on this vital function. Reviewing the notes in Special Topic 12 (hyperventilation) and the chapters which cover muscle and joint evaluation will provide a solid foundation for clinical interventions.

REFERENCES

Barral J-P, Mercier P 1988 Visceral manipulation. Eastland Press, Seattle

Chaitow L, Bradley D, Gilbert C 2002 Multidisciplinary approaches to breathing pattern disorders. Churchill Livingstone, Edinburgh

Cummings J, Howell J 1990 The role of respiration in the tension production of myofascial tissues. Journal of the American Osteopathic Association 90 (9): 842

Garland W 1994 Somatic changes in hyperventilating subject – an osteopathic perspective. Presentation to Paris Symposium

Goldthwaite J et al 1945 Bodymechanics. JB Lippincott, Philadelphia

Kisselkova, Georgiev J 1976 Applied Physiology 46: 1093–1095

Lewit K 1980 Relation of faulty respiration to posture. Journal of the American Osteopathic Association 79(8): 525–529

Lewit K 1999 Manipulation in rehabilitation of the motor system, 3rd edn. Butterworths, London

Pellegrino M 1933/1994 Fibromyalgia Network Newsletters. Tucson, AZ

Pryor J, Prasad S 2001 Physiotherapy for respiratory and cardiac problems. Churchill Livingstone, Edinburgh

Stone C 1999 The science and art of osteopathy. Stanley Thornes, Cheltenham

Timmons B, Ley R 1994 Behavioral and psychological approaches to breathing disorders. Plenum Press, New York

West J 2000 Respiratory physiology. Williams and Wilkins, Philadelphia

SPECIAL TOPIC 11
Palpating the traditional Chinese pulses

A method of diagnosis which has existed and been refined over a period of 5000 years deserves to be taken seriously, even if its precepts and conclusions seem to fly in the face of current medical thinking.

Not surprisingly, there are different versions and interpretations of pulse diagnosis. However, the basic methodology is similar in all schools.

As an exercise in palpation the methods of pulse diagnosis have much to commend them, even if the interpretations of what is being palpated are not generally accepted by Western medicine or if the way these findings are expressed is difficult to follow in relation to Western terminology.

Precisely the same can be said for cranial palpation, in which there is little dispute that 'something' is being felt when 'cranial impulses' are being assessed, although there is a great deal of debate as to what 'it' is and what 'it' may mean in health terms.

It should be remembered that the TCM practitioner who is utilising pulse diagnosis incorporates the impressions gained in this way with other methods of assessment, including the presenting signs and symptoms and history as well as methods such as tongue diagnosis (where descriptors such as 'pale', 'fat', 'moist', 'dry', 'yellow', and so on, are used to discriminate one pathophysiological state of the tongue from another, each indicating an imbalance of one sort or another) (Ryan & Shattuck 1994).

History

Austin (1974) points out that in Western medicine, taking the pulse is an important part of the diagnostic process.

> How many beats to each breath, strong or weak, even or irregular? and the blood flow, when it is felt where a blood vessel is conveniently near the surface, is the flow full or thin, strong or weak, hard or soft, regular or intermittent, etc.?

TCM pulses

The Chinese pulse is, however, quite a different story.

> The truly great discovery made by the Chinese, as regards the pulse, was that through the pulse it is possible to read not merely the health of the organism as a whole, but that of each inner organ separately – whether it had much or little energy, whether it was congested, over-full, or escaping, deficient; whether it was hyper or hypo active; whether the polarity predominance and polarity changes were in proper order, and so on (Austin 1974).

The Chinese identified 12 (some say 14) positions on the radial pulse which could be used to indicate the status of specific organs and functions. How is this possible?

Austin explains:

> If you have fluid flowing through a resilient tube, a rubber or plastic tube attached to a water tap, and very lightly touch the tube with a finger, the flow of water can be felt. The tube need hardly be compressed at all for us to feel the flow quite distinctly. Let the finger tip linger a while, so that the kind of sensation of flow registers in you; now steadily compress the tube by increasing the pressure until you have stopped the flow, then lift ever so slightly – maintain this pressure and note what you are feeling. The kind of sensation you now experience in your finger tip is different from that of the first light touch. You may, for example, be more aware of the resilience of the tube itself, at one pressure level rather than another; or of volume, water pressure, speed of flow etc. Continue your experiment by varying the surface on which the tube rests. A tube resting on a hard surface will feel different from when it is resting upon a soft surface (folded towel, for example). This will apply to both levels of palpation. There will also be a difference if one places a layer of material between finger and tube.

If, instead of the tube described by Austin, we think of an artery, and of the hard surface as an underlying bone, and of the gauze as soft tissues, we can see that it may indeed be quite possible for palpation to detect variations in flow depending upon what lies between your finger and the vein and what lies below the vein.

Some of the many descriptors used in TCM to describe the different sensations imparted by the various pulses include, 'wiry', 'bounding', 'full', 'rapid', 'empty', 'thin', 'thready'. Each of these represent the current state of energy balance, relative to the organ and its functions which are being assessed in this way. When you attempt this exercise (see Exercise 11.2 below) see how many different descriptors you can contrive (Ryan & Shattuck 1994).

SPECIAL TOPIC EXERCISE 11.1: PALPATING WATER FLOW THROUGH A TUBE

Time suggested: 2–3 minutes

Connect a plastic or rubber tube to a bath or kitchen tap and conduct the experiment as described by Austin.

Can you sense differences depending upon the surface the tube rests on and materials between your finger and the tube?

SPECIAL TOPIC EXERCISE 11.2: PULSE PALPATION ON SELF AND OTHERS

Time suggested: 3–5 minutes

Learn to assess your own pulses and those of patients, friends or volunteers. George Oshawa (1973) states that:

> The extreme end of the finger, the pulp, which is the most sensitive part, should be used to evaluate the pulses. The last phalanges should be perpendicular to the plane of the wrist. The nails must be cut short.

> The superficial yin pulse corresponds to the hollow organs; the deep yang pulse corresponds to the full yang organs.

> You judge the superficial pulse by feeling the position lightly and then gradually increasing the pressure of the finger. To determine the deep pulse, one compresses the artery completely at the beginning and then releases it little by little.

SPECIAL TOPIC EXERCISE 11.2 *(Continued)*

The deep pulse corresponds to the blood pressure, to the fundamental composition of blood; the superficial pulse to the variable blood pressure.

Method

Sit in a relaxed manner and with your right hand feel the (TCM) pulses of the left wrist.

Resting the back of your, or your patient's, left hand on the palm of your right hand, curl your fingers so that they rest on the radial artery. Place the middle finger at the level of the styloid prominence, just below the wrist crease. Your forefinger will then rest naturally on the crease, near the thenar eminence, and the ring finger will fall naturally onto the third pulse position.

Position 1 is where your index finger rests, position 2 is where the middle finger rests and position 3 is where the ring finger rests.

Adopt the palpation position as described, right hand palpating the left radial pulse.

Left wrist: TCM interpretations

Position 1 light pressure (superficial) is said to relate to the Small Intestine meridian and deep pressure detects the Heart meridian status.

Position 2 light pressure (superficial) relates to Gall Bladder and deep pressure detects Liver meridian status.

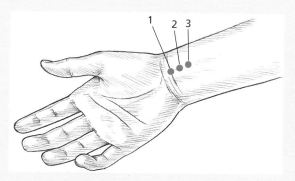

Special Topic Fig. 11A Location of pulses (right hand only illustrated) for assessment in Traditional Chinese Medicine.

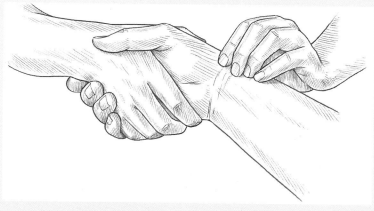

Special Topic Fig. 11B Taking the pulse in TCM. One finger at a time would apply suitable degrees of pressure to make an assessment, superficially or at depth.

continues

SPECIAL TOPIC EXERCISE 11.2 (Continued)

Position 3 light pressure (superficial) relates to Bladder meridian and deep detects the Kidney meridian.

Right wrist: TCM interpretations

Position 1 light pressure (superficial) is for Large Intestine and deep is for Lungs.

Position 2 light pressure (superficial) is for Stomach and deep is for Spleen.

Position 3 light pressure (superficial) is Triple Heater and deep is Circulation.

Note: Oshawa states that the allocation of organs to pulses on the right and left hand as described above relates to men only. The pulse allocations are said by him to be reversed in women. This sort of controversial statement helps to explain why so many Western-trained therapists find difficulty in accepting the conclusions drawn from TCM pulse diagnosis.

A simpler view

Stiefvater (1956) gives the following simplified breakdown of what pulse readings may indicate.

- Small, thin, fine indicates insufficiency.
- Full and hard indicates hypertension and hyperfunction.
- Soft and strong indicates inflammation.
- Small, hard and pointed indicates spasticity, contracture and the associated organ will usually be painful.
- Overflowing and large indicates excess, usually with inflammation and pain.
- Very weak, scarcely perceptible indicates energy depletion.

Giving a numerical value to the palpated pulse

As you palpate, try to gain a sense of normal (score of 4), excess (score of 5–8) or deficiency (score of 0–3).

Lawson-Wood (1965) states that a score of 0 is applicable to someone who is 'almost dead' and a score of 8 represents a patient '*in extremis*'.

When feeling the pulses the practitioner 'listens' to them much as one listens to an orchestra – each pulse representing one of the instrumentalists. Taken together the 'melody' should be a happy and harmonious one. If the melody is not joyous and harmonious at least one of the players is out of tune. You need to locate which is the discordant player. You must be relaxed and receptive and when you palpate each level quite deliberately say to yourself, 'I am now listening to the pulse of (name of meridian) to hear and understand what it has to say to me'.

The exercises in this segment should help you to sense the difference in what you feel in the various indicated pulse positions. You are not meant to make a diagnosis on this basis or to necessarily accept the interpretations of TCM offered above, merely to gain an awareness of what is being suggested by TCM.

REFERENCES

Austin M 1974 Acupuncture therapy. Turnstone Books, London

Lawson-Wood D 1965 Five elements of acupuncture and Chinese massage. Health Science Press, Rustington, Sussex

Oshawa G 1973 Acupuncture and the philosophy of the Far East. Tao Publications, Boston, MA

Ryan M, Shattuck A 1994 Treating AIDS with Chinese medicine. Pacific View Press, Berkeley, CA

Stiefvater A 1956 Akupunktur als Neuraltherapie. Hang, Heidelberg

11 Palpation without touch

The field of the 'laying on of hands', 'bioenergy', 'spiritual healing', intercessory prayer, 'absent healing', Qigong, Reiki, 'chakra balancing' and various other methods of non-touch treatment have been researched scientifically for many years.

Most recently, an investigation of these phenomena by Oschman (2000) has clarified what was until recently largely anecdotal. To be sure, anecdotal evidence itself can have weight, if there is enough of it, as demonstrated by the data collected, collated and discussed by Benor (1992).

Benor has shown that the results (in many clinical studies) of non-touch healing are impressive in their extent and implications, ranging as they do from beneficial changes in patients with anxiety, pain and chronic headaches; improvements in haemoglobin and haematocrit levels; the healing of dermal wounds; improved blood pressure levels; significantly reduced complications in patients in a coronary care unit; prevention of stroke in hypertensive patients, to improved myopia.

The fact that such methods are also shown to help recovery of damaged and dysfunctional enzymes, single-celled organisms, fungi, bacteria, plants and animals – as well as humans – should remove most of the 'it's all in the mind' suggestion as to their efficacy.

Clearly, anyone holding their hands above the surface of the body is not really palpating or manipulating the physical tissues themselves. However, the boundary between what we take to be the physical and something distinctly palpable above the surface requires investigation. As we can see from Fritz Smith's work (and that of other 'energy' workers, discussed in Chapter 6), it helps if we can 'visualise' an energy field/body when working in this as yet ill-defined area. It is Oschman (2000) who has taken our understanding forward, explaining the mechanisms which may be operating when non-touch (and a good deal of hands-on) healing is performed.

Some of the evidence is summarised in Box 11.1.

Therapeutic touch

Therapeutic touch, as developed by Dolores Krieger, is a modern derivative of the laying on of hands, which involves barely touching the patient's body, or the holding of hands away from the body surface, with an intent to help or heal. This method is now taught to many members of the nursing profession worldwide and recent research has validated its therapeutic value.

A fascinating, if somewhat inexplicable benefit, under controlled conditions, has been reported by Keller & Bzdek (1989).

Sixty volunteers with tension headaches were divided randomly into two groups. In one group patients were treated with therapeutic touch – in which

Box 11.1   Oschman's evidence

These notes are an abbreviated version of an article by James Oschman which appeared in the *Journal of Bodywork and Movement Therapies*, April 2002.

Research at Yale Medical School between 1932 and 1956 offered evidence that early stages of pathology, including cancer, can be diagnosed as disturbances in the body's electrical field and that reestablishing a normal field will halt the progress of disease (Burr 1957).

The heart's magnetic field was first measured in the laboratory in 1963 at the electrical engineering department of Syracuse University in New York (Baule & McFee 1963).

In 1964 Josephson developed the concept of quantum tunnelling for which he eventually received a Nobel Prize (Josephson 1964, 1973). This led to the development of a magnetometer of unprecedented sensitivity (Zimmerman et al 1970) known as the SQUID (Superconducting Quantum Interference Device). By 1967, workers at MIT had perfected the SQUID to the point that it could produce recordings of the heart's biomagnetic field with great clarity and sensitivity (Cohen 1967). By 1972, further refinements of the SQUID enabled the recording of the biomagnetic field of the brain (magnetoencephalogram) (Cohen 1972, Cohen et al 1970).

Bassett and colleagues, at Columbia University College of Physicians and Surgeons, developed a pulsing electromagnetic field therapy (PEMF) that stimulates repair of fracture non-unions. This was approved as 'safe and effective' in 1979. PEMF therapy was used on hundreds of thousands of non-unions, worldwide, between 1979 and 1995 (Bassett 1995).

The PEMF method has since been modified for treating soft tissues, such as nerves, ligaments, skin and capillaries. Each tissue requires a different frequency of stimulation. Nerves respond to 2 Hz, bone to 7 Hz, ligaments to 10 Hz and skin and capillaries to 15, 20 and 72 Hz (Sisken & Walker 1995).

The mechanisms involved include a cascade of reactions which enables a single molecular event at the cell surface to initiate, accelerate or inhibit biological processes. A tiny field, far too weak to power any cellular activity, seems to trigger a change at the regulatory level which then leads to a substantial physiological response that is carried out using the energy of cell metabolism (Pilla et al 1987).

Various components of the regulatory cascade, including receptors, calcium channels and enzymatic processes within the cell, are sensitive to magnetic fields. New research is revealing how free radicals, including nitric oxide, are involved in the coupling of electromagnetic fields to chemical events in the signal cascade. Again, the medical importance of this research was recognised by a Nobel Prize in 1998 (Furchgott et al 1998).

Several groups of researchers have now documented energy exchanges taking place when people touch or are in proximity. Specifically, it has been demonstrated that one's electrocardiogram (ECG) signal can be registered in another person's electroencephalogram (EEG) and elsewhere on the other person's body (Russek & Schwartz 1996).

The fact that the heart's biomagnetic field is hundreds of times stronger than that of the brain provides a simple physical explanation for the apparent entrainment of one person's electroencephalogram (EEG) by another person's electrocardiogram (ECG). Physicists use the term 'entrainment' to describe a situation in which two rhythms that have nearly the same frequency become coupled to each other. Technically, entrainment means the mutual phase locking of two or more oscillators.

In essence, a regular periodic signal can entrain ambient noise to boost the signal to a level above the threshold value, enabling it to generate measurable effects. Stochastic resonance has been firmly established as a valid phenomenon in a wide range of sensory and neural systems and is being exploited in electronic equipment (Bulsara & Gammaitoni 1996, Wiesenfeld & Moss 1995).

Given what we now know about these phenomena, it is conceivable that we will be able to document a scheme for beneficial energy field interactions that can take place between individuals. Such a scheme may

continues

Box 11.1 (*continued*)

involve brain waves and, possibly, effects on the autonomic nervous system, neuropeptide release, and the immune system. We now have logical and testable hypotheses to begin to explain the clinical effects of a wide variety of approaches such as Reiki, Therapeutic Touch, Polarity Therapy, Massage, and Acupuncture (Oschman 2002).

If a healthy, well-balanced practitioner/therapist, in a state which is calm, centred and focused (a series of conditions which implies a good degree of sympathetic/parasympathetic balance), applies manual (or non-touching) treatment with a positive therapeutic intent, this interaction might influence the patient's dysfunctional state towards a more balanced and healthy one. Another key piece of evidence for non-touch healing was the demonstration by Zimmerman (using SQUID technology, see above) that electromagnetic fields could be measured emanating from the hands of various healing professionals and practitioners of martial arts. Biomagnetic waves which pulsed from 0.3 Hz to 30 Hz were measured, with most activity being in the range of 7–8 Hz, precisely that shown to produce healing effects when PEMF technology is used to treat damaged tissues (see Fig. 11.1).

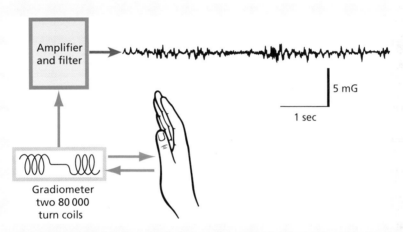

Fig. 11.1 Biomagnetic measurement of 'energy' (chi) emission from the hand of a Japanese female healer (redrawn after Oschman 1997, Fig. 4).

5 minutes of non-touching energy balancing with healing intent was applied – while in the other group patients received 5 minutes of apparently identical methodology (hand position the same and so on) but with the therapist deliberately concentrating on mental arithmetic during the treatment. Both groups were asked to sit quietly and breathe deeply during the real and placebo sessions and no physical contact was used on either group. Standard McGill– Melzack pain assessment questionnaires were used before, immediately after and 4 hours after each treatment or placebo treatment. Ninety percent of those exposed to therapeutic touch experienced sustained reduction in intensity in headache pain with an average of 70% pain reduction, twice the average achieved immediately after therapeutic touch.

Dummy therapeutic touch (placebo) reduced pain in 80% of patients but only by a level of 37% for a shorter duration, since half the placebo group resorted to medication in the 4-hour period after, as compared with only five of the therapeutic touch group.

So what do the therapists actually do?

Keller & Bzdek:

> The intervention began with the researcher centering herself into a meditative quiet and making conscious intent to help the subject. She then passed her hands 6 to 12 inches [15–30 cm] from the subject without physical contact to assess the energy field . . . and to redirect areas of accumulated tensions out of the field. She then let her hands rest around (not on) the head or solar plexus in areas of energy imbalance or deficit and directed life energy to the subject.

Those who do not, thus far, use such methods might care to think more about just what happens under these conditions and to learn how to 'feel' the fluctuations in energy, something which is apparently palpable with practice.

As part of an attempt to achieve this and to understand the mechanics of such interventions, we will now assess the methods recommended by a number of experts in this field for palpating and treating, using 'energy'.

Dr Dolores Krieger

During the 1960s, a series of experiments was conducted involving enzymes, plants and animals, in which the 'laying on of hands' was demonstrated to have profoundly protective effects in the face of a variety of negative influences, ranging from a deficiency diet to irradiation. Anyone who wishes to read a succinct account of these should study *Vibrational medicine* by Richard Gerber (1988).

It was following the publication of such research – specifically research by Dr Bernard Grad, of McGill University, indicating an increase in chlorophyll in plants nourished by water which had been 'treated' by healers – that Dolores Krieger, a professor of nursing at New York University, began to investigate the human potential of these methods. It was reasoned that since chlorophyll was chemically identical to haemoglobin, except that in the former a magnesium atom exists instead of iron, it should be possible to improve haemoglobin levels in humans by similar means.

A healer who had been involved in the plant experiments 'magnetically charged' rolls of cotton batting for a group of sick people to keep with them, as well as conducting a laying on of hands. A year later these patients were compared with a control group who had received no such 'treatment' and were found by Dr Krieger to have significantly raised haemoglobin levels. This was confirmed in later experiments and led Dr Krieger to begin teaching her method, dubbed 'therapeutic touch', to senior nurses. By this time Krieger had become convinced that what was being manipulated was *prana* (subtle energy) as described in Hindu and yogic tradition.

In its simplest terms, the method was conceived as the balancing of the energy field of someone in whom it had become disrupted or weakened, either as a result of ill health or as a predisposing factor to that ill health. Individuals who are basically healthy have an abundance of energy and seem able to use this to help those in whom it is disturbed, with profoundly beneficial effects, both physically and emotionally (see Box 11.1).

The potential to apply this form of healing resides in us all, says Krieger (her book *The therapeutic touch* is highly recommended; Krieger 1979) and its use can be developed by simple exercises. Krieger states that its two most noticeable effects are the eliciting of a profound, generalised relaxation as well as relieving pain. What is called for, before practicing or performing therapeutic touch, is a 'centering' process in which you learn to find within yourself an inner reference of stability.

Krieger says:

Centering . . . can be thought of as a place of inner being, a place of quietude within oneself where one can be truly integrated, unified and focused. This place is well known to those who practise meditation and deep relaxation. It cannot be found by effort or strain: it is a conscious direction of attention inwards, an 'effortless effort' that is conceptual but that can be experiential.

It is not within the scope of this text to teach the reader to find that quiet state; numerous texts and tapes exist, as well as opportunities for individual or group instruction which can all lead to this state of 'balance, of equipoise, and of quietude that marks the experience of centering'.

Once you have achieved this, Krieger provides clear guidelines as to how we should begin palpating energy variables.

EXERCISE 11.1: LEARNING TO PALPATE ENERGY

Time suggested: 5–10 minutes

Centre yourself and sit comfortably with both feet on the floor and place your hands so that the palms face each other. Your elbows should be held away from your trunk, the lower arms unsupported by anything.

Bring the palms as close together as you can without actually allowing them to touch (perhaps as close as under 0.5 cm – just under a quarter of an inch). Slowly separate your hands to a gap of around 5 cm (2 inches) and then return them to the first position (0.5 cm gap). Next take them 10 cm (4 inches) apart and then slowly return them to the first position. Now go to a 15 cm (6 inches) gap (always very slowly) and come again to the first position (Fig. 11.2).

Do you feel anything as the hands come close together? A build-up of 'pressure' in that small space, perhaps? Or do you feel any other sensation, such as a tingling or vibration?

Now take your palms 20 cm (8 inches) apart and this time do not bring them together again immediately but rather do so in 5 cm (2 inch) increments; first to 15 cm (6 inches) apart, then 10 cm (4 inches), 5 cm (2 inches) and finally, the starting position.

At each position stop and sense and 'test' what you can feel between your hands (Fig. 11.3).

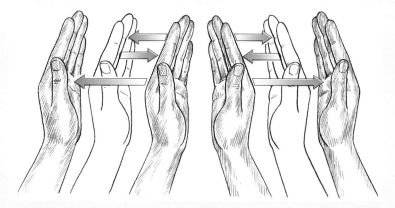

Fig. 11.2 Bring hands as close together as you can without the palms touching each other. Then bring hands apart about 5 cm. Return hands slowly to original position. Repeat and on each repetition, separate the palms by an additional 5 cm, until they are finally 20 cm apart.

continues

Do you sense a 'compression' of something between your hands? A 'bouncy' feeling? If so, at what distance did this become apparent?

Take a minute or more each time to practise this exercise over and over again. Try to experience what you are feeling and note the characteristics of the elastic, bouncy, energy field you are holding between your hands.

Do you feel heat, cold, tingling, pulsation or something else altogether?

Try to put into words the sensations you feel.

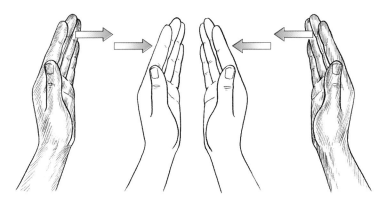

Fig. 11.3 When the hands are about 20 cm (8 inches) apart, slowly bring them together. Every 5 cm, (2 inches) test the field between your hands for a sense of bounciness or elasticity.

This exercise can be practised whenever you have a spare moment until you are confident that what you feel is real and its characteristics become familiar. Do it with your eyes closed or open and see which is best for you.

As Krieger says, 'You do not stop at your skin' and this exercise proves this to you and allows you to develop the sensitivity for application of therapeutic touch.

Krieger provides a series of exercises which incrementally help you to become more aware of your own potential in this field and her book is suggested as a working tool for those attracted to these methods.

EXERCISE 11.2: SCANNING SOMEONE'S ENERGY FIELD

Time suggested: 10–15 minutes

Having developed your skills in energy palpation with the first exercise and having centred yourself (a calm, rested state of mind and body), practise the following assessment of someone else's energy field.

Have a 'model', or a real patient, who is sitting or lying. Place your hands 5–8 cm (2–3 inches) from their skin surface, perhaps starting at the head.

'Test' the area to the left of the head for any sensations similar to those noted when doing Exercise 11.1 and compare this with the right side.

Scan from the top of the head over the face to the chin, taking about 10 seconds to cover that area.

Be aware of whatever you feel, changes in sensation, temperature and so on, but do not dwell on questions such as 'Did I or did I not feel something?'. Simply sense what comes through your hands.

Gradually move over the entire front of the body and then move to the back. Speed of movement is slow but steady.

continues

EXERCISE 11.2 *(Continued)*

When the complete scan is finished, recheck any areas which seemed unusual (especially those which seemed 'hot' or 'cold' or 'dense') and recheck your first impressions.

It may be that where there are significant variations in the energy field you will note temperature fluctuations through your hands. Or you may feel pressure changes, tingling, vibration, minute electric shock type sensations or pulsations instead.

All may be significant. Note and record what you sense.

EXERCISE 11.3: BEGINNING TO SCAN THE CHAKRAS

Time suggested: 3–5 minutes per person

Relax and centre yourself and then scan the body of a partner or patient to see whether you feel any variations or changes in the texture and nature of the energy field in the regions of the chakras, as described in Chapter 5, by Upledger (Fig. 11.4).

Try to formulate a sense of normality and abnormality, balanced and disturbed energy regions.

When the opportunity arises compare what you feel/sense in the various chakra positions when assessing/scanning 'normal' healthy energetic individuals and those who are unwell or fatigued.

See whether particular forms of ill health relate to particular patterns of energy fluctuation.

Note and record your findings.

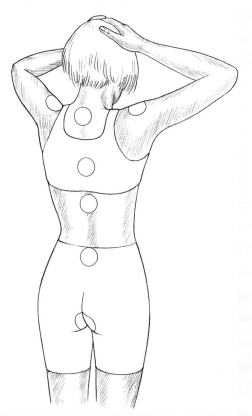

Fig. 11.4   Map of 'energy (or chakra) fields' of spinal region.

The concepts of Brugh Joy

Along with Dr Krieger's book, a thoughtful and delightful introduction to energy medicine will be found in *Joy's way* by Dr Brugh Joy (1979). There is much which is similar to Krieger but a good deal which is unique, with abundant material to help the reader in developing the ability to feel radiating energy fields as well as guidance in methods for 'transfer of energy to others'.

Joy describes what he teaches as 'transformational therapy' and stresses that one set of exercises should be mastered before the next is attempted, describing them under the headings of:

1. resonation circle
2. exploration of greatly amplified musical sounds
3. modified spiral meditation
4. dyadic exercises
5. triadic exercises
6. hand scanning
7. energy transfer.

It can be seen from this list alone that before getting to the place where Krieger starts (scanning), Joy suggests a good deal of work. Joy's book is one of the best ways of obtaining detailed directions in the first five of the above requirements. His description of hand scanning of chakras is also worth studying as it gives a clear outline of his approach:

> During the hand-scanning phase of body-energy work the consciousness of the scanner must become totally receptive and his/her awareness must be centred entirely in the hand or hands. The witness state of consciousness is activated. One must be careful not to project what one thinks should be there into the space surrounding the person to be scanned. Instead the task is to explore that space in order to find out what is actually there. The hand that is acting as the detector is relaxed. The fingers should be slightly apart and may be bent, as in the classical ballet pose. A rigid flat hand, with the fingers held tightly together, is not nearly so effective a detector.

Joy suggests that you roll up long sleeves, exposing the skin of your forearm, as this is often a more sensitive detector than the hand. He also suggests that beginners should start with the right hand (if they are right handed) as it is hard to be efficient with both hands at first; both will eventually become suitably sensitive.

Speed of movement is important during scanning, as going too quickly prevents the mind from registering sensory input and going too slowly allows the scanner's own energy to be reflected back from the body surface, so that all surfaces feel the same. Covering approximately 30 cm (12 inches) every 2 seconds is about the right speed (faster than Krieger's suggested speed of 10 seconds for the face alone).

Joy suggests that a common sensation for the beginner is to feel 'over-charged', characterised by a tingle or pulsation or even an ache or pain. This prevents awareness of incoming stimuli. Joy suggests flicking the hands to relieve the sensation or patting them on your own thigh. This may result from too much trying, which is not what is called for as you palpate the energy fields. The feeling has to be allowed to 'come through', not chased after.

Joy likens the process of learning this subtle palpation to what happens to medical students as they learn to detect heart murmurs.

> First they must learn where to centre their hearing awareness, because their ordinary hearing mechanism simply does not listen to the ranges where these murmurs can be heard. The same is true with the subtle sense of touch, at least at the beginning stages.

The distance from the body of the scanning hand should be 20–30 cm (8–12 inches), says Joy, with the person to be scanned lying face upwards on a wooden bed or table (metal apparently interferes with the energy field). All jewellery should be removed, as should metal buckles and watches. The person being scanned should feel relaxed and free to move (to scratch, for example, or stretch) if they wish. Talking, however, should be discouraged.

Joy suggests a start be made by taking the pulse of the 'patient' in order to attune the scanner's consciousness to that of the patient. With the other hand, scanning can then begin over the chest and upper body and lower abdomen, as here the energy fields are strong and relatively easy to assess. He suggests the scanning hand starts off from the side of the body, beyond its edge, moving into the area above the body and then out again, for a contrast to be noted. As one becomes familiar with the 'feel' of an energy field this is less necessary. He recommends the eyes be closed when working in this way (just as in skin or muscle palpation, for better focusing of the mind).

He gives a most important pointer when he says:

> The fields are not felt when the hand is held over them but as the hand moves through them. This principle is fundamental. During a scan the hand must be in perpetual motion. It must pass in and out of the fields.

Thus, by 'slicing' through the energy field at different levels, its shape can be determined, as well as its distance from the surface, its density and its degree of 'health'.

Joy notes that after years of experience he can detect a field two or three times further from the body surface than can a beginner. At first, simply registering the fact that an energy vortex exists over a chakra is a major step forward. The ones over the groin and the top of the head are relatively easy to detect. The variations in intensity should be registered as the scanning hand passes from chakra to chakra.

The region over the throat chakra requires that the patient hold their breath for a short while, so that it does not confuse the scanning process. Practise in a group, if possible, so that the differences one from another are available to reinforce the learning process.

After scanning the front of the body, the patient turns over and the back is assessed in much the same manner.

EXERCISE 11.4: CHAKRA SCANNING WITHOUT A MAP

Time suggested: 4–7 minutes

Try scanning the back of the body, from the head to the base of the spine, without having first referred to a chakra 'map' of where the fields are most dense, and compare your findings with such a map later.

EXERCISE 11.5: SCANNING THROUGH ANOTHER MEDIUM

Time suggested: 5–8 minutes

With your partner lying face down, palpate the energy fields on the front of the body by scanning under the table.

Compare your findings with what you assessed when they were face upward. The energy field is said to pass through the material of the table readily and should be easily palpable at the same distance from the body as previously.

Before attempting to transfer energy (as in therapeutic touch), Joy suggests, it is essential to be able to scan in this way. He urges you to practise until all the chakras can be readily detected.

Following the guidelines of Krieger and Joy (as well as those given below) will open this area of palpation and those interested in carrying their knowledge further will find excellent help in the books referred to in this chapter.

Brennan's methods

Barbara Ann Brennan, in her fine explanation of her approach to healing through the human energy fields (Brennan 1987), explains what is known via scientific enquiry, and much that is still speculated upon, as she leads the reader through a series of training processes towards an ability to work in this area with confidence.

She describes a series of exercises which can help you to visualise the human aura (energy field) which she says is the manifestation of universal energy intimately involved in your (human) life. This is divided into various 'layers' or 'bodies' which interpenetrate each other, each succeeding one being of finer vibrational quality than the body which it surrounds and interpenetrates.

EXERCISE 11.6: GROUP WORK

Time suggested: 10–15 minutes

In a group, make a circle in which you all hold hands. Sense a pulsating flow of energy if you can. In which direction is it travelling (almost always from left to right around the circle)? Ask your neighbour whether they feel the same thing.

Without moving anything or altering the hand contact, Brennan asks you to 'stop the flow of energy'. Everyone in the circle should simultaneously hold this energy still for a short while before allowing it to flow again.

This should be repeated several times as you feel the difference between energy flow and stillness.

EXERCISE 11.7: TRANSFERRING ENERGY

Time suggested: 10 minutes

Sit opposite a partner with your palms facing theirs.

Let any energy flow occur naturally. Then direct energy out of your left palm to the other person's hand. Then stop this and bring energy into your right palm from the other person's hand.

Reverse and vary these flows and then stop it altogether.

continues

EXERCISE 11.7 *(Continued)*

Then attempt to 'push' energy out of both hands at the same time and finally 'suck' energy into both simultaneously.

A feeling of tickling, 'tingling or pressure', something like static electricity, indicates that the energy fields are touching the skin or that the fields are touching each other.

'Push, pull and stop are the three basic ways of manipulating energy in healing,' says Brennan.

EXERCISE 11.8: FEELING YOUR OWN ENERGY

Time suggested: 10 minutes

Brennan then suggests you practise the scanning exercise (11.1 above) given by Krieger as a first step in assessing the field between your hands, as you take them to varying distances apart and then slowly bring them together again until you feel the compressed energy in the space between your hands:

> If your hands are one and a quarter inches [3 cm] apart (when you feel the compression forces) you have touched your etheric body edges together (first layer of the aura). If your hands are three to four inches [7–10 cm] apart, you have touched the outside edges of your emotional body together (second layer of the aura).

Brennan suggests you hold the hands about 18 cm (a fraction over 7 inches) apart and point your right index finger at the palm of the left hand and slowly draw circles with it. See whether you can feel this (eyes closed, centred and relaxed) as a tickling sensation.

EXERCISE 11.9: VISUALISING ENERGY

Time suggested: 10–15 minutes

Dim the room lights and hold your hands with fingertips pointing towards each other. The hands should be held in front of your face, about 60 cm (24 inches) away from your eyes.

Have a plain white wall behind your hands. Relax your gaze and softly look at the space between your fingertips which should be about 4–5 cm (around 2 inches) apart.

As you move the fingers towards and away from each other slightly, or take one hand slightly upwards and the other down slightly, Brennan asks that you note what you might be seeing between your fingers or around the hand.

She suggests that for approximately 95% of people what is noted will be as follows:

> Most people see a haze around the fingers and hands . . . it looks somewhat like the heat haze over a radiator. It is sometimes seen in various colours, such as a blue tint . . . The energy bodies pull like toffee between the fingers as the haze from each fingertip connects to the haze at the fingertip of the opposite hand.

Energy blocks

Brennan takes her reader through a host of gradually more complex exercises towards a full ability to palpate and manipulate the subtle energies around us all.

Of practical value to those working in bodywork are her instructions regarding identification and interpretation of 'energy blocks', which she divides into six types. The way these are formed will depend largely, she believes, on variations of tactics we all adopt in our 'energetic defence systems', which we use to defend ourselves aggressively or passively, to repel incoming threatening forces. The end results of such defensive/protective strategies are palpable in the space just away from the body's 'energy blocks' which she categorises as follows.

1. The 'blah' block. The result of 'depressing one's feelings', causing a stagnation of energy, with accumulation of fluid in the region involved. The physical body will be bloated at this region, the energy having a low intensity rather than 'high energy'. The related emotions often have a despairing quality or are associated with anger (in a blaming manner). Colitis and angina pectoris are examples of an end result. The 'feeling' of such a block is sticky, like mucus.

2. Compaction blocks are related to suppressed feelings, containing accumulated rage (volcanic, ready to explode). An 'ominous' feeling is associated with palpation or observation of such a block. Body fat or muscle accumulates in the regions affected. Diseases such as pelvic inflammatory disease may occur. The individual is usually aware of the suppressed rage, with a feeling of being trapped. Sexuality and a sense of humiliation may also be involved.

3. 'Mesh armour' is another pattern of block, used to help the individual avoid feelings, especially fear. The blocks are therefore shifted around when there is a challenge. Thus, if therapy releases associated tensions, they reappear elsewhere very rapidly. This type of block may not result in disease, the individual often appearing a 'perfect wife and mother', but with a vague sense of something lacking in life. Deep feelings are usually only tolerated for brief periods with intermittent crises occurring (sudden illness, affair, accident) as a pattern of life.

4. Emotions in the person with 'plate armour' are frozen. There is a palpable high-tension quality in the energy fields around the body. This allows the person to apparently build an effective, well-structured life. Physically they seem to be firm, well-built, with good muscular tone. The individual is, however, often unfulfilled due to a low level of sensitivity. Cardiac or ulcerative conditions may develop, as well as musculoskeletal problems such as tendonitis. While appearing to have a well-ordered life, the lack of feeling often leads to a life crisis, such as a coronary attack, which may prove a watershed for restructuring their life.

5. In some people an 'energy depletion' block exists, in which the flow of energy to the ends of the limbs is drastically reduced (making it obvious during scanning) and resulting in weakness or even physical problems related to the limbs. The energy and physical alterations may be a metaphor for an inability to 'stand on their own two feet' in life or as a representation of a feeling of failure.

6. Finally, there is the 'energy leak' where, instead of a smooth flow onwards from particular joints, energy seems to 'leak' from them. This may relate to an unconscious inability to respond to the environment or circumstances (based perhaps on a belief gained in childhood that response is dangerous or 'improper'). Physically, it will relate to malcoordination or other physical joint abnormalities or problems. The limbs will be cold and may feel vulnerable. The leaking energy is palpable close to the joints in such limbs.

Brennan asks you to ask yourself which blocks you have used in your life as a result of early experience or conditioning.

Fritz Smith again

Let us briefly return to the work of Fritz Smith (1986), who gives this view of the energy body which Krieger, Joy and Brennan have shown us how to palpate in their respective ways.

> The working energy model of the human body is composed of three functional units: first, the non-organised background field of energy; second, the vertical movement of current conducted through the body which orients us to our environment; and third, the internal flows of the body which are produced because of the body's unique and individualised presence and which organise us into discrete functioning units. The last pattern – energy flow within the body – is further divided into three levels: the deep current through the bone and skeletal system; the middle currents through the soft tissues of the body; and the superficial level of vibration beneath the skin surface.

It is Smith's aim to make direct contact with these vibrational fields and he uses his unique 'bridging' methods (pressure, traction, bending, twisting or a non-moving fulcrum), as described earlier (see Chapter 5), to achieve this end. Via these means, he assesses the clarity, density, pliability and other characteristics of energy, as well as the speed with which it responds (as evidenced by changes in rapid eye movement or breathing pattern, for example) to such contact (or to needles in acupuncture).

Particular areas of energy dysfunction relate, he believes, to specific forms of mento-emotional discord. Thus sexual problems relate to the sacral area, security/insecurity to the pelvic bowl, power to the lumbar area, anger and frustration to the hips and jaw, compassion to the heart, sadness to the chest, creativity to the throat and intuition to the brow. He uses these generalisations (his word) to help assess the physical-emotional (or energetic) nature of the patient.

Pavek's physioemotional release

Richard Pavek (1987) has developed a system of 'physioemotional release therapy' called SHEN, which uses methods similar to those described in this chapter to release, or normalise, energy dysfunction (SHEN calls this biophysical dysfunction) resulting from emotional stress. He states that it is not difficult to feel the 'physioemotional' field, in the same ways described by Krieger, Joy and Brennan, in the palm of the scanning hand(s) as 'changes in temperature, tingles, prickles, pressure, "electricity" or "magnetism" '.

He amplifies these views as follows.

> The sensations [felt by the scanning hand] are usually different when the hand is over an area of physical pain, inflammation, tension and/or when release of emotion occurs when the hand is over an emotion region. The sensations picked up over an area of pain do not feel the same as the ones over a centre that is releasing emotion.

A series of exercises are given, some of which are the same as those already described in this (and previous) chapter(s), but with some useful variations.

EXERCISE 11.10: PLAYING WITH ENERGY

Time suggested: 5–7 minutes

Perform Exercise 11.1 again (feeling the 'bounce' of the energy field between the palms of your hands as you vary the distance between them).

After sensing the energy as a pressure, hold this and then begin to rotate your palms in small circles as though you were holding a ball between the palms, the hands travelling in a series of circular motions away from and then towards yourself, one hand travelling forward as the other travels back, all the while keeping the palms facing each other, as far apart as you noted the sense of 'pressure'. The circles described should be about 25 cm (10 inches) in diameter. Does the field change?

Pavek suggests that this process should alter the feel, as it 'energises' the field, much as a nail stroked across a magnet will become energised. This, he suggests, is a useful way of enhancing sensitivity prior to performing energy balancing or diagnosis.

SHEN, as a system, demands a great deal of practice, as do all the clinical applications of the methods touched on above. These few examples are by no means a complete representation of the depth of the work described by Krieger, Joy, Brennan, Smith or Pavek, being merely introductory concepts and exercises, which can be carried further if they trigger an interest. The reading of Oschman's text (2001), as discussed earlier in this chapter, might well be the key which opens that door!

Further exploration . . . the work of Eeman and others

Those who would like to explore this apparently uncharted area of healing even further should also read the research work of LE Eeman (1947). Eeman was a pioneer in his studies of human energy patterns who finally concluded:

Do not the experiments described recall the aura so frequently described by occultists, mystics and clairvoyants?
  Do they not combine to suggest that there may, in fact, be, for right handers:
a. a flow of electro-magnetic(?) force down the left and up the right side of the body (clockwise), and also
b. clockwise inner vortices, and
c. the reverse for left-handers?

He appeals for research to continue in this field, since physical medicine has no evidence to offer on the subject. Useful study should also be made of other areas such as:

● the Japanese system of Aikido, explained in two books (Japan Publications 1978a, b)
● the Chinese system of Qigong (China Sports Magazine 1985)
● polarity therapy, on which numerous books exist (e.g. Seidman 1986, Stone 1954).

As mentioned at the start of this chapter, a compilation of research evidence into the effects of non-touch therapeutic measures (such as therapeutic touch) has been made by Dr Daniel Benor (1992), and this is highly recommended.

REFERENCES

Bassett CAL 1995 Bioelectromagnetics in the service of medicine. In: Blank M (ed) Electromagnetic fields: biological interactions and mechanisms. Advances in Chemistry Series 250. American Chemical Society, Washington DC, pp 261–275

Baule GM, McFee R 1963 Detection of the magnetic field of the heart. American Heart Journal 66: 95–96

Benor D 1992 Healing research – holistic energy medicine and spirituality, vol 1. Helix, Munich

Brennan B 1987 Hands of light. Bantam New Age, Toronto

Bulsara AR, Gammaitoni L 1996 Tuning into noise. Physics Today (March): 39–45

Burr HS 1957 Harold Saxton Burr. A biography and bibliography of his publications. Yale Journal of Biology and Medicine 30(3): 161–167

China Sports Magazine 1985 The wonders of Qigong. Wayfarer Publications, Los Angeles, CA

Cohen D 1967 Magnetic fields around the torso: production by electrical activity of the human heart. Science 156: 652–654

Cohen D 1972 Magnetoencephalography: detection of the brain's electrical activity with a superconducting magnetometer. Science 175: 664–666

Cohen D, Edelsack EA, Zimmerman JE 1970 Magnetocardiograms taken inside a shielded room with a superconducting point-contact magnetometer. Applied Physics Letters 16: 278–280

Eeman LE 1947 Cooperative healing. Frederick Muller, London, p 351

Furchgott RF, Ignarro KH, Murad F 1998 Nitric oxide as a signaling molecule in the cardiovascular system. Nobel Prize in Physiology or Medicine, Karolinska Institutet

Gerber R 1988 Vibrational medicine. Bear & Co

Japan Publications 1978a Ki in daily life. Tokyo

Japan Publications 1978b Book of Ki: coordinating mind and body in daily life. Tokyo

Josephson BD 1964 Supercurrents through barriers. Advances in Physics 14: 419–451

Josephson BD 1973 Theoretical predictions of the properties of supercurrent through a tunnel barrier. Nobel Prize in Physics, Karolinska Institutet

Joy B 1979 Joy's way. JP Turner Inc

Keller E, Bzdek M 1989 Effects of therapeutic touch on tension headache pain. Cooperative Connection X(2):

Krieger D 1979 The therapeutic touch. Prentice Hall, New York

Oschman J 2000 Energy medicine. Churchill Livingstone, Edinburgh

Oschman J 2002 Clinical aspects of biological fields. Journal of Bodywork and Movement Therapies 6(2): 117–125

Pavek R 1987 Handbook of SHEN: physioemotional release therapy. Shen Institute, California

Pilla AA, Kaufman JJ, Ryaby JT 1987 Electrochemical kinetics at the cell membrane: a physicochemical link for electromagnetic bioeffects. In: Blank M, Findl E (eds) Mechanistic approaches to interactions of electric and electromagnetic fields with living systems. Plenum Press, New York, pp 39–62

Russek L, Schwartz G 1996 Energy cardiology: a dynamical energy systems approach for integrating conventional and alternative medicine. Advances 12(4): 4–24

Seidman M 1986 A guide to polarity therapy. Newcastle Publishing, North Hollywood

Sisken BF, Walker J 1995 Therapeutic aspects of electromagnetic fields for soft-tissue healing. In: Blank M (ed) Electromagnetic fields: biological interactions and mechanisms. Advances in Chemistry Series 250. American Chemical Society, Washington DC, pp 277–285

Smith F 1986 Inner bridges – a guide to energy movement and body structures. Humanics New Age, New York

Stone R 1954 Polarity therapy. Published by the author

Wiesenfeld K, Moss F 1995 Stochastic resonance and the benefits of noise: from ice ages to crayfish and SQUIDs. Nature 373: 33–36

Zimmerman JE, Thien P, Harding JT 1970 Design and operation of stable rf-biased superconducting point-contact quantum devices, and a note on the properties of perfectly clean metal contacts. Journal of Applied Physics 41(4): 1572–1580

SPECIAL TOPIC 12
About hyperventilation

The effect of overbreathing is to rapidly reduce the levels of carbon dioxide in the blood, altering the acid–alkaline balance (increasing alkalinity), increasing nociceptor sensitivity and a sense of apprehension and anxiety, resulting in a variety of unpleasant symptoms.

Many studies have concentrated on the widespread problem of overbreathing and much of this has related to its connection with anxiety states, panic attacks of an incapacitating nature and, all too often, phobic behaviour (Chaitow et al 2002, Timmons 1994).

The symptoms most often associated with hyperventilation include: giddiness, dizziness, faintness, numbness in the upper limbs, face or trunk, loss of consciousness (fainting), visual disturbances in which blurring or even temporary loss of vision is experienced, headaches of a general nature often accompanied by nausea and frequently diagnosed as migraine, inability to walk properly (ataxia) as well as trembling and noises in the head.

A number of symptoms often associated with cardiac function can become apparent during or after hyperventilation, including: palpitation, chest discomfort, difficulty in taking a deep breath, feelings of pressure in the throat, insomnia, fatigue, weakness in the limbs and much more.

Of patients diagnosed with hyperventilation, more than half are found to be undergoing stress, related to marriage, work or finance. Hyperventilation is not, however, always associated with psychiatric stress and this is made clear in correspondence in the *Journal of the Royal Society of Medicine* (1987) in which it is stated that: 'The underlying disorder (of hyperventilation) may be psychiatric, organic, a habit disorder or a combination of these'.

Indeed, one of the leading researchers into this topic, Dr L Lum (1984), states:

> Neurological considerations can leave little doubt that the habitually unstable breathing is the prime cause of symptoms. Why they breathe in this way must be a matter for speculation, but manifestly the salient characteristics are pure habit.

Lum has summarised some of the confusion surrounding the phenomenon:

> Although Kerr et al (1937) had pointed out that the clinical manifestations of anxiety were produced by hyperventilation, it was Rice (1950) who turned this concept upside down by stating that the anxiety was produced by the symptoms and, furthermore, that patients could be cured by eliminating faulty breathing habits. Lewis identified the role of anxiety as a trigger, rather than the prime cause. Given habitual hyperventilation, a variety of triggers, psychic or somatic, can initiate the vicious cycle of increased breathing, symptoms, anxiety arising from symptoms exacerbating hyperventilation and thus generating more symptoms and more anxiety.

Despite the literature providing evidence of various symptom patterns being linked to hyperventilation, the concept of selecting patients for treatment and breathing retraining on the basis of symptoms alone might be flawed according to some.

Bass (Bass & Gardner 1985) points out:

Diagnostic criteria for the hyperventilation syndrome [HVS] are imprecise. The practice of basing diagnosis on symptom checklists is unreliable and equivalent to diagnosing diabetes on the basis of symptoms without measuring blood glucose concentrations.

When Bass & Gardner examined 21 patients with unequivocal hyperventilation and a host of unexplained symptoms they found that all but one complained of 'inability to take a satisfying breath' but that there was enormous variety when a host of different physical and psychological markers and signs were evaluated. They concluded: 'Severe hyperventilation can occur in the absence of formal psychiatric or detectable respiratory or other organic abnormalities'.

Not everyone agrees with Bass's view that symptoms cannot provide a clue as to whether HVS exists. A symptom questionnaire (Nijmegen Questionnaire) was evaluated by Van Dixhoorn & Duivenvoorden (1985). They compared the results of the questionnaire when completed by 75 confirmed HVS patients and 80 non-HVS individuals (health workers!). Three dimensions were measured in the questionnaire:

- shortness of breath (HVS1)
- peripheral tetany (HVS2)
- central tetany (HVS3).

All three components had an unequivocally high ability to differentiate between HVS and non-HVS individuals. Together they provided a 93% correct classification. Statistical double cross validation resulted in 90–94% correct classifications. The sensitivity of the Nijmegen Questionnaire in relation to diagnosis was 91% and the specificity 95%.

How to deal with hyperventilation

In most instances of hyperventilation a combination exists of a learned pattern of breathing coming into operation in response to real or assumed stressful situations. This is usually found to coexist alongside severely contracted muscles relating to the rib cage, spinal regions and the diaphragm area. These are readily palpable or observable. Such changes are a common feature amongst people who are chronically fatigued, since the combination of energy wastage, through long-held tension, and reduced oxygenation due to impaired respiratory function can produce profound fatigue.

Muscles which are chronically hypertonic, shortened or contracted cannot function normally and this is usually the case in people who hyperventilate who, it seems, have learned to overbreathe excessively in response to both stressful events and non-stressful ones. (See Chapter 10 for more detail on structural changes associated with breathing dysfunction.)

It is perfectly normal to hyperventilate when excessive demands are required of the body, for example on physical exertion. If, however, this response occurs inappropriately, in the face of a perceived but unreal crisis, such as exists when we are abnormally anxious about something, then the sequence of overbreathing would lead to imbalanced blood gas levels, changes in acidity/alkalinity and the whole sequence of hyperventilation symptoms previously listed.

This may become a habitual method of responding to all minor stress situations, leading to the complete misery of phobic states compounded by panic attacks and virtual incapacity and inability to function.

People affected in this way often respond well to breathing retraining. By recognising that it is possible to learn to use more appropriate patterns of breathing in the face of a stressful (real or imagined) situation, they can stop the symptoms, because they simply will not hyperventilate.

Ample research evidence exists to indicate that arousal levels (how rapidly and severely an individual responds to stressful situations) can be markedly reduced via the habitual use of specific patterns of calming breathing.

Bonn et al (1984), Cappo & Holmes (1984) and Grossman et al (1985), among many others, have shown that breathing retraining is a valid and highly successful approach; however, none of them incorporated physical therapy into their protocols which, it is suggested, would have allowed for even better results.

Pranayama breathing

Cappo & Holmes in particular have incorporated into their methodology a form of traditional yoga breathing which produces specific benefits which have gone largely unrecognised in the protocols of most other workers.

The pattern calls for a ratio of inhalation to exhalation of 1:4 if possible, but in any case, for exhalation to take appreciably longer than inhalation. Research indicates that this pattern markedly lowers arousal.

Conclusion

There is a clear link between abnormal breathing patterns, excessive use of the accessory breathing muscles, upper chest breathing, etc. and increased muscle tone, which is itself a major cause of fatigue, over and above the impact on the economy of the body of reduced oxygenation and the unbalanced, malcoordinated patterns of use which stem from the structural and functional changes, as detailed by Garland (Chapter 10).

These patients will be fatigued, plagued by head, neck, shoulder and chest discomfort and a host of minor musculoskeletal problems as well as feeling apprehensive or frankly anxious. Many will have digestive symptoms (bloating, belching and possibly hiatal hernia symptoms, etc.) associated with aerophagia which commonly accompanies this pattern of breathing, as well as a catalogue of symptoms.

And yet none of the major medical researchers into hyperventilation seem to have examined the structural machinery of respiration! There is scant attention in the quoted literature to the status of the muscles which perform the task of breathing.

And none of them seem to have considered that modifying the structural component (muscles, rib cage, spinal attachments, etc.) could encourage more normal function, despite evidence from manual medicine that this is possible (Lewit 1991).

Nor is there any seeming concern for those many patients whose condition does not fit the strict criteria for a diagnosis of hyperventilation, those whose breathing is demonstrably out of balance but who fail to display evidence of arterial hypocapnia.

There is always a spectrum in such cases, with some being patent and obvious, others being borderline and many being somewhere on their way towards a point where they will indeed show evidence of arterial hypocapnia and thus achieve the status of 'real' hyperventilators.

The fact that before someone displays frank symptoms they are possibly progressing towards that state should be our concern in breathing dysfunction, to recognise people who are borderline hyperventilators and to prevent that progression, as well of course as trying to help those already entrenched in this pattern of dysfunction.

REFERENCES

Bass C, Gardner W 1985 Respiratory and psychiatric abnormalities in chronic symptomatic hyperventilation. British Medical Journal 11 May: 1387–1390

Bonn J, Readhead C, Timmons B 1984 Enhanced adaptive behavioural response in agoraphobic patients pretreated with breathing retraining. Lancet ii: 665–669

Cappo B, Holmes D 1984 Utility of prolonged respiratory exhalation for reducing physiological and psychological arousal in non-threatening and threatening situations. Journal of Psychosomatic Research 28(4): 265–273

Chaitow L, Bradley D, Gilbert C 2002 Multidisciplinary approaches to breathing pattern disorders. Churchill Livingstone, Edinburgh

Grossman P, DeSwart, Defares 1985 A controlled study of breathing therapy for treatment of hyperventilation syndrome. Journal of Psychosomatic Research 29(1): 49–58

Journal of the Royal Society of Medicine 1987 Correspondence. November

Kerr W et al 1937 Annals of Internal Medicine 11: 962

Lewit K 1991 Manipulative therapy in rehabilitation of the locomotor system. Butterworths, London

Lum L 1984 Hyperventilation and anxiety state. Journal of the Royal Society of Medicine January: 1–4

Timmons B 1994 Behavioral and psychological approaches to breathing disorders. Plenum Press, New York

Van Dixhoorn J, Duivenvoorden H 1985 Efficacy of Nijmegen questionnaire in recognition of hyperventilation syndrome. Journal of Psychosomatic Research 29(2): 199–206

12 Palpation and emotional states

Sherrington (1937) asked:

> Can we stress too much that . . . any path we trace in the brain leads directly or indirectly to muscle?

Wilfred Barlow (1959) stated:

> There is an intimate relationship between states of anxiety and observable (and therefore palpable) states of muscular tension.

Use of electromyographic techniques has shown a statistical correlation between unconscious hostility and arm tension as well as leg muscle tension and sexual themes (Malmo 1949).

Sainsbury (1954) showed that when 'neurotic' patients complained of feeling tension in the scalp muscles, there was electromyographic evidence of scalp muscle tension.

Wolff (1948), in his famous book *Headache and other head pains*, proved that the majority of patients with headache showed:

> Marked contraction in the muscles of the neck . . . most commonly due to sustained contractions associated with emotional strain, dissatisfaction, apprehension and anxiety.

Even thinking about activity produces muscular changes. Jacobson (1930) demonstrated that:

> It is impossible to conceive an activity without causing fine contractions in all those muscles which produce the activity in reality.

Barlow sums up his views on the emotion/muscle connection thus.

> Muscle is not only the vehicle of speech and expressive gesture, but has at least a finger in a number of other emotional pies – for example, breathing regulation, control of excretion, sexual functioning and above all an influence on the body schema through proprioception. Not only are emotional attitudes, say, of fear, and aggression mirrored immediately in the muscle, but also such moods as depression, excitement and evasion have their characteristic muscular patterns and postures.

Ford (1989), in his book *Where healing waters meet*, summarises the early, less controversial work of Wilhelm Reich, who rejected the exclusivity of the concepts that underlying physical conditions created the environment in which psychological dysfunction would occur or that physical dysfunction was necessarily the result of psychological forces. Rather, he synthesised the two positions, stating that:

> Muscular attitudes and character attitudes have the same function . . . They can replace one another and be influenced by one another. Basically they cannot be separated.

As Ford puts it:

> When he encountered difficult psychological resistance (character armouring) in a patient, he moved to the corresponding areas of physical tension (muscular armouring) in the body, and used various forms of somatic therapy to correct the underlying physical distortions . . . Similarly if he was unable to affect a change in the tension of the patient's body through somatic therapy, he resorted to working with the psychological issues beneath the tension.

Palpation, insofar as it relates to emotional states, therefore requires the ability to observe (patterns of use, posture, attitudes, tics and habits) and feel for changes in the soft tissues which relate to emotionally charged states, acute or chronic. One of the key elements in this relates to breathing function which is intimately connected with emotion (see Chapter 10 and Special Topic 11).

British osteopath Philip Latey (1980) has described patterns of distortion which coincide with particular clinical problems. He uses an analogy of 'three fists' because, he says, the unclenching of a fist correlates with physiological relaxation while the clenched fist indicates fixity, rigidity, overcontracted muscles, emotional turmoil, withdrawal from communication and so on:

> The lower fist is centred entirely on pelvic function. When I describe the upper fist I will include the head, neck, shoulders and arms with the upper chest throat and jaw. The middle fist will be focused mainly on the lower chest and upper abdomen.

Evidence of selective muscle contraction due to emotion

Is there evidence for these observations, apart from clinical experiences and opinion?

Waersted et al (1992, 1993) have shown that selective motor unit involvement results from psychogenic influences on muscles. Researchers at the National Institute of Occupational Health in Oslo, Norway, have demonstrated that a small number of motor units, in particular muscles, may display almost constant, or repeated, activity when influenced psychogenically. The implications of this information are profound since it suggests that emotional stress can selectively involve postural fibres of muscles, which shorten over time when stressed (Janda 1983). The possible 'metabolic crisis' suggested by this research has strong parallels with the evolution of myofascial trigger points as suggested by Simons et al (1999).

If emotional states can create specific and predictable musculoskeletal changes, at least aspects of this should be palpable and sometimes observable.

Postural interpretation

Latey describes the patient who enters the consulting room as showing an 'image posture', which is the impression the patient subconsciously wishes you to see of him. If instructed to relax as far as possible, the next image we see is that of 'slump posture', in which gravity acts on the body and it responds according to its unique attributes, tensions and weakness. Here it is common to observe overactive muscle groups coming into operation; hands, feet, jaw and facial muscles may writhe and clench or twitch.

Finally, when the patient lies down and relaxes, we come to the deeper image we wish to examine, the 'residual posture'. Here we find the tensions the patient cannot release. It is palpable and, says Latey, leaving aside sweat, skin and circulation, the deepest 'layer of the onion' available to examination.

Contraction patterns

What can be seen when someone is looked at from these perspectives varies from person to person, depending on the state of mind, degree of adaptation to life events and activities, as well as the current level of well-being of the individual. Apparent is a record, or psychophysical pattern, of the patient's responses, actions, transactions and interactions with his environment, historically and currently. The patterns of contraction which are found seem to bear a direct relationship with the patient's unconscious (see Waersted's research discussed above), and provide a reliable avenue for discovery and treatment. They are providing sensory input to the patient and this is of considerable importance.

One of Latey's concepts involves a mechanism which leads to muscular contraction as a means of disguising a sensory barrage resulting from an emotional state. Thus he describes:

- a sensation which might arise from the pit of the stomach being hidden by contraction of the muscles attached to the lower ribs, upper abdomen and the junction between the chest and lower spine
- genital and anal sensations which might be drowned out by contraction of hip, leg and low back musculature
- throat sensations which might be concealed with contraction of the shoulder girdle, neck, arms and hands.

Emotional contractions

A restrained expression of emotion itself results in suppression of activity and, ultimately, chronic contraction of the muscles which would be used were these emotions expressed, be they rage, fear, anger, joy, frustration, sorrow or anything else.

Latey points out that all areas of the body producing sensations which arouse emotional excitement may have their blood supply reduced by muscular contraction. Also, sphincters and hollow organs can be held tight until numb. He gives as examples the muscles which surround the genitals and anus as well as the mouth, nose, throat, lungs, stomach and bowel.

Three fists

In assessing these and other patterns of muscular tension in relation to emotional states, Latey divides the body into three regions which he describes as:

- 'lower fist' – (metaphor for a clenched fist) which centres entirely on pelvic function
- 'upper fist' – which includes head, neck, shoulders, arms, upper chest, throat and jaw
- 'middle fist' – which focuses mainly on the lower chest and upper abdomen.

Why are Latey's concepts so important? Because he comes close to an explanation of the mechanisms at work in the body – mind problems which are familiar to all who work on the human body with their hands. He avoids more conjectural explanations involving electromagnetic energy, chakras, auras or energy fields or flows; not that such explanations are necessarily any less valid than Latey's, but he provides another way of seeing the problem.

The lower fist

The lower fist describes the muscular function of the pelvis, low back, lower abdomen, hips, legs and feet, with their mechanical, medical and psychosomatic significance.

Latey identifies the central component of this region as the pelvic diaphragm, stretching as it does across the pelvic outlet, forming the floor of the abdominal cavity. The perineum allows egress for the bowel, vagina and urinary tract as well as the blood vessels and nerve supply for the genitalia, each opening being controlled by powerful muscular sphincters which can be compressed by contraction of the muscular sheet.

When our emotions or feelings demand that we need to contract the pelvic outlet, a further group of muscular units comes into play which increases the pressure on the area from the outside. These are the muscles which adduct the thighs and which tilt the pelvis forwards and rotate the legs inwards, dramatically increasing compressive forces on the perineum, especially if the legs are crossed.

The impression this creates is one of 'closing in around the genitals' and is observed easily in babies and young children when anxious or in danger of wetting themselves. You can reproduce these contractions experimentally as follows.

EXERCISE 12.1: SENSING YOUR OWN TENSIONS

Time suggested: 2 minutes

Stand upright, legs apart a little, and exert maximum pressure and weight through the arches of the feet, trying to flatten them to the floor.

Sustain this effort for at least 2 minutes and sense the changes in your overall posture – feel the details of what is happening in the feet, knees, legs, hips, pelvis and spine.

Feel the tensions begin to build around the pelvis and upper body parts. Note where discomfort begins.

Comment

If this sort of contraction is short-lived no damage occurs. If it is prolonged and repetitive, however (weeks rather than days), compensatory (adaptation stage) changes appear, involving those muscles which abduct the legs, rotate them outwards and which pull the pelvis upright (Selye 1956).

If this compensatory correction is incomplete the pelvis remains tilted forwards, requiring additional contraction of low back muscles in order to maintain an erect posture.

Buttock muscle tension

Another pattern which is sometimes observed is of tension in the muscles of the buttocks which act to reinforce the perineal tension from behind. This tends to compress the anus more than the genitals and produces a different postural picture.

EXERCISE 12.2: SELF-EVALUATION OF POSTURAL EFFECTS OF CLENCHED BUTTOCKS

Time suggested: 2–3 minutes

Demonstrate on yourself the effects of maintaining clenched buttocks for several minutes, by standing and squeezing your anus tight, contracting the buttocks really hard, and holding this for 2 or 3 minutes.

Focus on the changes of posture and feelings of tension, strength and weakness in different parts of your body as time passes.

What is happening to your low back, your upper back, your hips, knees and feet?

What happens to your breathing after a minute or so of this clenching?

Then note the postural and other changes which take place as you stand still for a minute after releasing the clenching action.

Lower fist problems

Problems of a mechanical nature which stem from the lower fist contraction include:

- internally rotated legs and 'knock-knees'
- unstable knee joints
- 'pigeon-toed' stance, resulting in flattened arches.

Here then may lie the onset of symptoms in 'knock-kneed, flat-footed children' and here also may reside the answer.

The main mechanical damage is, however, to the hip joints, due to compression and overcontraction of mutually opposed muscles. The hip is forced into its socket, muscles shorten and as there is loss of rotation and the ability to separate the legs, backward movement becomes limited. Uneven wear commences with obvious long-term end results. If this starts in childhood, damage may include deformity of the ball and socket joint of the hip.

Low back muscles are also involved and this may represent the beginning of chronic backache, pelvic dysfunction, coccygeal problems and disc damage. The abdominal muscles are also affected since they are connected to changes in breathing function which result from the inability of the lower diaphragm to relax and allow proper motion to take place.

Medical complications which can result from these muscular changes involve mainly circulatory function, since the circulation to the pelvis is vulnerable to stasis. Haemorrhoids, varicose veins and urethral constriction all become more likely, as do chances of urethritis and prostatic problems. All forms of gynaecological problems are more common and childbirth becomes more difficult.

EXERCISE 12.3: ASSESSING PELVIC MOTION WHILE PATIENT IS BREATHING

Time suggested: 5–7 minutes

12.3A
Have your palpation partner seated. You place a hand to cover the sacrum and feel for a gentle motion of the sacrum (pelvis) tipping forwards on inhalation and backwards on exhalation.

12.3B
Your palpation partner should be side-lying, knees bent together. You place a hand over the sacrum, allowing pelvic breathing motion to be assessed.

Where there is good function there should be a sense of a slight lengthening of the lower body (a flattening of the lumbar lordosis) on inhalation and a shortening on exhalation.

12.3C
Your palpation partner lies on her back, knees flexed and head supported about 5–10 cm (2–4 inches) from the surface. You sit at the side and rest your caudad arm across the front of the pelvic bones, your hand resting on the far ASIS, and feel for a slight rocking motion during respiration.

Do the ASIS contacts ease slightly cephalad on inhalation and slightly caudad on exhalation?

Now try resting your free (cephalad) hand just above the sacrum, under the patient's lower back, at the same time. This helps the patient to become aware of the subtle respiratory motion of the sacrum and pelvis.

EXERCISE 12.4: SELF-TREATMENT FOR RESTRICTED PELVIC MOTION

Time suggested: 3–5 minutes

If no such rhythmic motion (as described in Exercise 12.3) is palpable (and this is often the case), have the person lie face down (or do this on yourself), taking one arm back and down to cup their (your) own perineum.

Practise feeling, at the perineum, for the difference between normal motion of the phases of breathing when relaxed and the restricted pattern when the buttocks are clenched.

By breathing deeply while in this position, with buttocks unclenched, the abdomen is compressed against the floor or table and perineal motion is forced to occur.

The person/patient (and you) can learn to increase the excursion by consciously relaxing the muscles of the region. This improves further if the tense/shortened muscles of the region are released by treatment.

A profound weakness of the legs is often felt as relaxation of these muscles begins and this may last for hours. As tension goes, so vulnerability increases and reassurance is required.

This is only a part of the restoration of normal function, but it is a beginning.

While this is clearly a therapeutic/educational exercise, it has palpation overtones, since normal movements which were previously restricted should improve after performing the relaxation of the perineal area.

The middle fist

When considering the area he designates as the middle fist, Latey concentrates his attention on respiratory and diaphragmatic function and the many emotional inputs which affect this region. He discounts the popular misconception which states that breathing is produced by contraction of the diaphragm and the muscles which raise the rib cage, with exhalation being but a relaxation of these muscles.

Instead he asserts:

> This is quite untrue. Breathing is produced by an active balance between the muscles mentioned above [the diaphragm and the muscles which raise the rib cage] and the expiratory muscles that draw the rib-cage downwards and pull the ribs together. The even flow of easy breathing should be produced by dynamic interaction of these two sets of muscles.

The muscles which 'draw the rib cage downward' and so help to produce the active exhalation phase of breathing include the following.

1. Transversus thoracis which lies inside the front of the chest, attaching to the back of the sternum and fanning out inside the rib cage and then continuing to the lower ribs where they separate. This is the inverted 'V' below the chest (it is known as transversus abdominis in this region). He calls this 'probably the most remarkable muscle in the body'. It has, he says, direct intrinsic abilities to generate all manner of uniquely powerful sensations, with even light contact sometimes producing reflex contractions of the whole body, or of the abdomen or chest, and feelings of nausea and choking, all types of anxiety, fear, anger, laughter, sadness, weeping and so on.

The most common sensations described by patients when it is touched include 'nausea, weakness, vulnerability and emptiness'. He discounts the idea that its sensitivity is related to the 'solar plexus', maintaining that its closeness to the internal thoracic artery is probably more significant, since when it is contracted it can exert direct pressure on it.

Latey believes that physiological breathing has as its central event a rhythmical relaxation and contraction of this muscle. Rigidity is often seen in the patient with 'middle fist' problems, where 'control' dampens the emotions which relate to it.

2. The other main exhalation muscle is serratus posterior inferior which runs from the upper lumbar spine, fanning upwards and outwards over the lower ribs which it grasps from behind, pulling them down and inwards on exhalation.

These two muscles mirror each other, working together.

Latey comments on the remarkable changes in tone in serratus relating to speech.

> The tone of this muscle varies with the emotional content of the patient's speech, especially when the emotions are highly labile and thinly veiled near the surface. With the patients lying on their front the whole dorsolumbar region may be seen to ripple in ridge-shaped patterns as they talk. As their words become progressively more 'loaded' the patterns become more emphatic. However, it is more usual to find a static overcontracture of this muscle, with the underlying back muscles in a state of fibrous shortening and degeneration, reflecting the fixity of the transversus, and the extent of the emotional blockage.

Middle fist functions

Laughing, weeping and vomiting are three 'safety valve' functions of middle fist function which Latey is interested in. These are used by the body to help resolve internal imbalance. Anything stored internally, which cannot be contained, emerges explosively via this route. In all three functions transversus alternates between full contraction and relaxation. In laughing and weeping there is a definite rhythm of contraction/relaxation of transversus, whereas in vomiting it remains in total contraction throughout each eliminative wave. Between waves of vomiting the breathing remains in the inspiratory phase, with upper chest panting. Transversus is slack in this phase.

Latey suggests that often it is only muscle fatigue which breaks cycles of laughter/weeping/vomiting and he reminds us of phrases such as: 'I wept/laughed until my sides ached'.

Nausea and vomiting are often associated with feelings such as 'I swallowed my pride' and 'stomaching an insult'. He suggests seeking early feelings of hunger, need, fullness, emptiness, overfulness, nausea, rejection, expulsion and so on when working in this area, if we wish to uncover basic emotional links.

While Latey delves into areas which are clearly within the realm of psychotherapy, the form of bodywork he espouses, which seeks to understand and, where appropriate, to modify the adaptive changes in the soft tissues can be seen to be potentially important in this field.

EXERCISE 12.5: EXPLORING THE 'MIDDLE FIST'

Time suggested: 5–10 minutes

Latey suggests that:

> With the patient balanced, sitting upright or lying sideways with knees up – the practitioner can easily learn the movements he is trying to encourage. The feelings of the middle fist disturbance surface most readily with the patient lying on their back. With one hand resting below the sternum (assessing transversus movement) the practitioner's other hand can feel the upper or lower fist movement. Nausea is often felt strongly in this position.

What might you notice in the person as you hold this muscle?

If they are feeling nauseous you might see a sudden pallor, sweat and protrusion of the chin followed by retching and gagging. A receptacle should be on hand and you should ask 'do you want to be sick?'. After that you could ask 'what was stopping you?', for insights into underlying emotions.

If laughter is going to emerge this may be preceded by a squirming movement, a sideways look of 'naughtiness', superficial guilt, shame or embarrassment. A slight snort, snigger or grunt can lead to the main explosive laughter release. A comment such as 'It's ridiculous, isn't it?' can help.

Before weeping starts the eyes become moist, the mouth quivers, a catch is heard in the voice. There is an expectation of encouragement and of comfort being offered. These emotions are interchangeable and one may lead into another since these safety valves may be releasing feelings from quite different sources at the same time.

If panic starts it is characterised by a fluttering of the transversus and is unmistakable. This can build into a shaking of the whole body, with breathing and chest movements becoming jerky and tremulous. Limbs twitch and eyes open wide. This sort of emotional explosion can have roots in very early experiences.

Latey pays great attention to the transversus muscle during this exploration of the middle fist. He says:

continues

EXERCISE 12.5 *(Continued)*

A feeling of tightness behind or below the breastbone marks the beginning of a cycle of emotion linked to this muscle (recrimination, pity, disgust, etc.). Is heartache an overtightness of the transverses muscle!

As outlined above, he encourages movement of the middle fist components (via breathing and bodywork) and while doing so registers feelings of unease in the patient:

Panic starts as a very definite fluttering of the transversus muscle itself and is quite unmistakable. Given full play it rapidly builds into a shaking of the whole body. The chest movements and breathing are jerky and tremulous: the limbs are twitchy: the eyes wide and staring in alarm. I have to look elsewhere for the meaning of panic: the chains of investigation are tortuous and difficult – invariably when fully exposed they lead back to earliest feelings.

This is an exercise in which you are palpating tissues which are intimately connected to basic emotions, while at the same time you are trying to become aware of subtle changes (breathing pattern, facial expression, voice pitch, muscular tone, etc.) all or any of which may be precursors to an emotional release. See the notes immediately below for further exploration of this theme.

Middle fist problems

The clinical problems associated with middle fist dysfunction relate to resulting distortions of blood vessels, internal organs, autonomic nervous system involvement and alteration in the neuroendocrine balance. Diarrhoea, constipation or colitis may be involved but more direct results relate to lung and stomach problems. Thus bronchial asthma is an obvious example of middle fist fixation.

There is a typical associated posture, with the shoulder girdle raised and expanded as if any letting go would precipitate a crisis. Compensatory changes usually include very taut deep neck and shoulder muscles. In treating such a problem Latey starts by encouraging function of the middle fist itself then extending into the neck and shoulder muscles, encouraging them to relax and drop. He then goes back to the middle fist.

Dramatic expressions of alarm, unease and panic may be seen. The patient, on discussing what they feel, might report sensations of being smothered, drowned, choked, engulfed, crushed, obliterated. They relate to early life panic sensations and may go to the person's very core.

Asthma is not easy to treat. Some merely require to mourn the loss (or lack) of motherly tenderness, soothing and comfort. Most have a great deal more work to do.

When middle fist dysfunction involves digestive function this can be associated with postural alterations and emotional conflicts common in adolescents, says Latey:

The lower end of the oesophagus passes through the muscular part of the diaphragm before joining the stomach. There is an intriguing mechanism which allows for the passage of food, or regurgitation of vomit, between the chest and the abdomen. When the diaphragm is contracted the muscular opening is constricted. In order to allow free flow it must be relaxed (full expiration) with the lower ribs pulled slightly together (transversus contraction). This device frequently fails when there is a chronic disturbance of the middle fist – the 'lower end of swallowing' is not happening properly. This may merely lead to wind, burping or fullness. However, when the neuroendocrine/smooth muscle activity is also disturbed the consequences may be more severe. Peptic ulcers, heartburn, reflux oesophagitis, hiatus hernia and so on are all medical conditions associated with middle fist problems. Here the filling and emptying of the stomach and duodenum, with their internal secretions, have become chronically disordered.

We discussed briefly (Exercise 12.5) Latey's methods for the holding and releasing of the middle fist and he suggests that this can lead to total or partial resolution of such dysfunction:

> However, most patients only achieve partial resolution: when the middle fist disturbance begins to resolve the conflict is transferred to the mouth, neck and throat. Even though severe gastrointestinal symptoms may have dissipated, we may still be left with a more complex problem involving the upper fist (the first part of swallowing).

If patients begin to weep, stopping and starting this process of release, Latey suggests the safety valve is only slightly open. He sees the pelvic and middle fist rhythms as coordinated but the head, neck and shoulders may seem rigid, fighting the movement. In such cases he has found that the situation can change dramatically by laying one's hands across the front of the patient's throat, a very light but firm touch which seems to affect sensitivity in the sternocleidomastoid muscles.

In such cases weeping may become full-bodied, giving a total expression of grief with an orgasmic rhythm. Wailing and high-pitched crying may follow with expressions of complete misery and dejection, even leading to screams of terror. Unfettered rage, snapping and even biting are possible as the upper fist releases its pent-up tensions and expresses itself for the first time in years. Patently this is an area where many may not wish to venture. It is powerful and requires nerves of steel on the part of the practitioner; however, it is in such catharsis that healing of pains and hurts buried for decades may occur.

The upper fist

The metaphor of the clenched fist, which is used to describe regions of the body associated with chronic, often emotionally based contractions, is a powerful image. We have looked at the middle fist (diaphragm, respiratory muscles, abdomen) and also the lower fist which, not unnaturally, focused on the pelvic region (as well as low back and lower abdomen, hips, legs and feet).

The upper fist involves muscles which extend from the thorax to the back of the head, where the skull and spine join, extending sideways to include the muscles of the shoulder girdle. These muscles therefore set the relative positions of the head, neck, jaw, shoulders and upper chest, and to a large extent the rest of the body follows this lead (it was FM Alexander (1931) who showed that the head–neck relationship is the primary postural control mechanism).

This region, says Latey, almost with relish, is 'the centre, par excellence, of anxieties, tensions and other amorphous expressions of unease'.

In chronic states of disturbed upper fist function, he asserts, the main physical impression is one of restrained, overcontrolled, damped-down expression. The feeling of the muscles is that they are controlling an 'explosion of affect'.

In contrast to the lower fist, which impresses us with its grip on sensual functions, the upper fist has contracted in response to, or to restrain response to, the outer world.

Just what it is that is being restrained is never obvious from the muscles themselves, but interpreting facial muscles may give a clue. Far more important, though, than the expressions on the face are those which have been withheld. Those experiences which are not allowed free play on the face are expressed in the muscles of the skull and the base of the skull. This is, Latey believes, of central importance in problems of headache, especially migraine.

Says Latey: 'I have never seen a migraine sufferer who has not lost complete ranges of facial expression, at least temporarily'.

Effects of upper fist patterns

The mechanical consequences of upper fist fixations are many and varied, ranging from stiff neck to compression factors leading to disc degeneration and facet wear. Swallowing and speech difficulties are common, as are shoulder dysfunctions including brachial neuritis, Reynaud's syndrome and carpal tunnel problems.

Latey states:

> The medical significance of upper fist contracture is mainly circulatory. Just as lower fist contraction contributes to circulatory stasis in the legs, pelvis, perineum and lower abdomen; so may upper fist contracture have an even more profound effect. The blood supply to the head, face, special sense, the mucosa of the nose, mouth, upper respiratory tract, the heart itself and the main blood vessels are controlled by the sympathetic nervous system and its main 'junction boxes' (ganglia) lie just to the front of the vertebrae at the base of the neck.

Thus headaches, eye pain, ear, nose and throat problems, as well as many cardiovascular troubles may contain strong mechanical elements relating to upper fist muscle contractions.

He reminds us that it is not uncommon for cardiovascular problems to manifest at the same time as chronic muscular shoulder pain (avascular necrosis of the rotator cuff tendons) and that the longus colli muscles are often centrally involved in such states.

He looks to the nose, mouth, lips, tongue, teeth, jaws and throat for evidence of functional change related to upper fist dysfunction, with relatively simple psychosomatic disturbances underlying these. Sniffing, sucking, biting, chewing, tearing, swallowing, gulping, spitting, dribbling, burping, vomiting, sound making and so on are all significant functions which might be disturbed acutely or chronically.

And as with middle and lower fist dysfunction these can all be approached via breathing function.

> When all the components of the upper fist are relaxed, the act of expiration produces a noticeable rhythmical movement. The neck lengthens, the jaw rises slightly (rocking the whole head), the face fills out, the upper chest drops. When the patient is in difficulty I may try to encourage these movements by manual work on the muscles and gentle direction to assist relaxed expiration. Again, by asking the patient to let go and let feelings happen, I encourage resolution. Specific elements often emerge quite readily, especially those mentioned with the middle fist, the need to vomit, cry, scream, etc.

In relation to headache Latey observes:

> We can often see the headache to be a more general avoidance mechanism. The way in which the generalised focus of pain occupies attention is significant. It clouds and limits concept formation and observation. There is always a deadening and coarsening of sensation and expressiveness. It seems as though the patient uses the headache to hold some perturbation at bay until it can be coped with more responsively, or disappears.
>
> With more severe migraines, with disturbances of vision and nausea, it is often necessary to work through feelings of disgust in considerable detail. Fear of poisoning may be a strong component of nausea, and usually dates back to earliest disturbances of feeling.

Latey also spends time analysing shock and withdrawal, possibly experienced in the early months of life, as life's realities are recoiled from. This leads, he believes, to our failing to learn from experience as we flinch from emotionally unpleasant episodes. Withdrawal characteristics determine many of Latey's clinical perspectives.

Superficially, at any rate, they are easy to recognise.

The dull lifeless tone of the flesh; lifeless flaccidity of larger surface muscle (or spastic rigidity); lifeless hard fibrous state of deep residual postural muscles (with the possible exception of the head and neck muscles); the over-investment of the person in his eyes and ears – hearing and seeing.

More profound pointers to withdrawal are more subtle.

The ritualised expression of any 'emotion' in a depersonalised and unspontaneous fashion; the use of language that denies the central presence and unity of self, wards off threats (from outside or inside temptation perhaps) and grasps hold of common insanities of our civilisation. These insanities are greatly worsened by social/family mystification.

EXERCISE 12.6: PALPATING EMOTIONAL EFFECTS

Time suggested: 10–15 minutes

Patiently and slowly examine someone with known emotional stress symptoms and see whether you can identify patterns of muscular change, as outlined above in the discussion of Latey's 'clenched fist' model, seeking tissues which correspond with descriptors such as 'dull lifeless', 'lifeless flaccidity', 'spastic rigidity', 'lifeless hard fibrous', and so on.

Also seek evidence of associated breathing pattern dysfunction, as described in Chapter 10.

Additionally look for:

● 'ritualised expression of emotion'
● 'use of language that denies central presence and unity of self, wards off threats'
● lack of facial expression (which ones are missing?)
● statements about bodily feelings that seem unusual.

Ford's variations on the same theme

Latey suggests that we consider these three 'fists', or regions, of abnormal tension, contraction and restriction as we try to look and feel for the physical manifestations of emotional turmoil. A variation on precisely this same theme is found in the methods grouped together as 'somatosynthesis'. This is described quite beautifully by Ford (1989).

There is a close relationship between the diagnostic and therapeutic uses of touch. When touch is involved (palpation), it is not uncommon to hear of the diagnosis turning into therapy without the awareness of the therapist or the patient.

Ford continues:

My approach to therapeutic touch has always been to keep it simple, getting maximal results from minimal number of techniques and procedures.

Which areas does Ford suggest working on in dealing with emotional problems?

I might begin by working with the four major areas of cross-restriction in the body; the base of the pelvis [Latey's lower fist], the base of the rib cage [Latey's middle fist], the base of the neck and the base of the skull [together these are Latey's upper fist]. (Fig. 12.1)

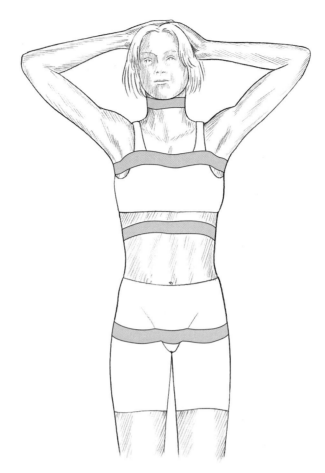

Fig. 12.1　Illustration of Ford's cross-restriction areas.

It is in these regions, Ford asserts, that the usual vertical orientation of soft tissues is different as they become horizontally directed:

> Usually the horizontal tissue cross-restricts the vertical tissue of the body, thereby hampering normal muscle movement, fluid flow and nerve transmission. *The practical result is that these areas turn out to be the places that most of us experience and retain stress, tension and pain in our bodies. And they are also the areas often related to the deeper psychological issues beneath our physical signs and symptoms. A simple straightforward approach to working with these cross-restrictions is to gently compress them from front to back.* [My italics]

How does he palpate and treat these (and other) dysfunctions?

Seasoned palpators have long known that the best hand is a light hand. The lighter the touch, the more information can be obtained.

Ford suggests that we 'remember that palpation and therapy are happening simultaneously'. This message should be one of our key considerations throughout palpation, particularly as it relates to emotional effects. It is by lightly palpating, projecting the sense of touch, and by being receptive to whatever information radiates into the hand that Ford identifies areas of maximal tension and dysfunction.

> Once I have palpated to determine where to touch (therapeutically), there are three things I take into account: depth, direction and duration. How deep does my touch need to be? Should it be at the level of the energy field where no physical contact is involved, at the skin surface . . . or pressing firmly into the (patient's) body.

He then decides in which direction this hand contact should move: straight down, right, left, pulling, pushing, steady or continuous movement or a

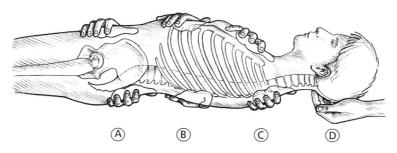

Fig. 12.2 The hand positions which would be used in Ford's treatment of horizontal cross-restrictions – (A) pelvic, (B) diaphragmatic, (C) thoracic outlet and (D) base of skull. By 'projecting' his sense of touch he palpates for 'depth, direction and duration' in order to treat these dysfunctions.

combination of these? And finally he allows the tissues themselves to determine how long the force should be held (Fig. 12.2).

We can now see that Latey and Ford approach these problems with slightly different methods, as does Marion Rosen whose work is considered next.

The Rosen method

Marion Rosen, a brilliant physical therapist, has evolved a method (Mayland 1980) which addresses the same physical manifestations of emotional turmoil as do the approaches of Latey and Ford.

The Rosen method is not a mechanical process. It is a journey taken together by client and practitioner towards self-discovery.

The practitioner observes the patient's back, as in the following exercises.

EXERCISE 12.7: OBSERVATION OF THE STRESSED INDIVIDUAL

Time suggested: 10–12 minutes

Have the person lie down prone (if possible the same person, with known emotional stress symptoms, used in Exercise 12.6). Sit silently and observe to see whether you can identify any of the following.

Are the muscles tense?

Where does breath move freely?

Where is it withheld?

What statement is the patient making with his body?

What has to happen so that he can relinquish that contracted space?

What is the direction in which the muscles are holding?

Does this holding bear down, hold him together, puff him up or separate the top from the bottom of the body by tightening in the middle (equivalent to Latey's middle fist)?

Compare these observations with the findings you made in Exercise 12.6.

EXERCISE 12.8: PALPATION OF THE (SAME) STRESSED INDIVIDUAL

Time suggested: 12–20 minutes

Lightly palpate the back muscles (ideally of the same person as in the previous exercise – someone with known emotional stress symptoms). Take your time to locate the most restricted muscular area of the back, where marked tension is palpated and where little or no movement is noted in response to breathing.

'Watch and feel for the place[s] on the back that is [are] most unmoving, held, or not included in his expression of himself. He is unaware that he is holding back.'

Hold a flat palpating hand against these tissues, meeting the tension, just taking out the slack.

Your other hand may be placed against another similarly tense area, as you patiently and silently wait for a change in the feel of the tissues or for breathing movement to begin to be noted where previously it was not evident.

After the same attention has been given to several tense areas, the hands should be run gently over the back muscles, seeking information, comparing what was initially observed and palpated with what is now being palpated.

How much has it changed?

Your task is to increase the person's awareness of areas of 'restriction and holding' in a non-judgemental manner.

You are also required to follow tense tissues as they release and relax, continuing until all the back is released and breathing function is freely observed in all the tissues.

Try to note:

- what happens to the very tense, unyielding tissues over a period of some minutes, and
- what changes, if any, take place in the breathing pattern itself.

Then attention turns to the diaphragm and the anterior aspect of the body. This major breathing muscle reveals tensions being held and changes in its function are readily palpated, at the same time as alterations in facial expression are commonly seen.

What may happen?

Compare the description given below, of what might be observed when the Rosen method is used, with the description given by Latey following Exercise 12.5.

Sometimes as the [Rosen therapy] practitioner works with the muscles that move the diaphragm, a flutter of the diaphragm itself can be seen. Movements in the abdomen might begin as they do when a person is sobbing or crying, although the expression on the face has not changed, leading her [the practitioner] to believe that the sadness that is being expressed in the body is not reaching the face and the consciousness of the client. (Mayland 1980)

What next?

With Rosen therapy, following on from the approach described in the previous exercise, after the back and diaphragm have received attention, other tensions, in the neck or chest perhaps, are then sought which are specifically palpated and worked on in the same manner, until releases occur. The work is accompanied by careful observation and skilled questioning.

As should be clear, the process of palpation is in fact the start of the treatment process (something which can also be said for Lief's neuromuscular technique).

The essence of this approach is the identification, via observation and palpation, of restricted areas in which the breathing function fails to manifest itself. Until this is addressed subsequent release is not easily achieved.

As Mayland says:

> All we want is for a person to get connected with what they are holding back. The degree to which they repress, that they will not allow themselves to experience, that they carry around with them . . . form a barrier to our living. They are like loads, like rocks in our being.

Pressure during Rosen work

It is perhaps helpful to note that the amount of pressure used on tense 'held' areas, when the Rosen method is applied, is very similar to that described by Fritz Smith and Stanley Lief in earlier chapters (Chapters 5 and 6).

The pressure 'meets' the muscle, not attempting to overwhelm it or make it do anything. Awareness is the key, with release occurring from the patient's side, not as a forced event.

Rosen's hierarchy of emotions

In the Rosen method, as in Latey's work, there is a hierarchy of emotions, linked to specific areas.

- Deep fear and deep love are associated with the region of the pelvis (or deep in the belly) and where the legs meet the pelvis.
- Repressed anger and sadness are often found in the upper torso or neck.
- Feelings towards others relate to the middle trunk and heart area.
- Fear and anxiety are repressed around the diaphragm.

Anger, sadness and fear are, according to Marion Rosen, easier to release than held emotions associated with love.

The goal of Rosen's method

The Rosen method is characterised by the gentleness of the approach. Emotions are reexperienced, not forced, as the client learns that feelings are just feelings and not the events which precipitated their being locked away. The method leads to self-acceptance and release from long-held tensions, identified by palpation and observation.

Upledger's contribution to emotional release and unwinding

Upledger's somatoemotional release (Upledger 1987) described in earlier chapters (Chapters 3, 6) is worthy of further mention at this point. Using gentle compressive or traction forces, such as:

- slight inferiorly directed compressive force upon the parietals of the seated patient
- compression of the cervical and thoracic vertebrae caudally
- gentle medial compression of the anterior ilia with the patient standing
- grasping of the ankles of the supine patient and introduction of slight compressive or traction force, etc.,

Upledger requires the therapist to follow the 'unwinding' process which the body may initiate when these (compressive, etc.) forces are applied.

Palpatory and proprioceptive skills of a high order are required to achieve this, since not only are the hands required to follow the slow unwinding process but also to register and prevent any tendency for the unwinding to follow a repetitive pathway.

While this method is used largely to release locked-in trauma-induced forces, 'repressed emotional components of the somatic injury are frequently and concurrently released'.

Panic or hysteria related to the trauma may be relived and adaptational energy released.

Upledger warns: 'Be alert. Do not inhibit your patient by dragging on their body movements. Try to follow where the patient's body leads you'. The patient may finally adopt the position in which the trauma occurred.

While somatoemotional release (as in the Rosen method) seems to describe therapy rather than palpation/assessment, the distinction is essentially blurred when these approaches are used as described by their developers.

Palpation skills determine the practitioner's ability to perform these therapeutic methods.

You will probably by now have noted the resemblance that these descriptions have with Smith's work (Chapter 6). Indeed, the overlap between the work of Latey, Rosen, Ford, Upledger and Smith (and indeed that of Lief and the Beckers) should not be surprising, since they are all looking at the physical somatic manifestations of emotional distress and are all attempting to both palpate, locate and initiate or assist in self-generated change in these altered soft tissues.

Cautions and questions

There is justifiably intense debate regarding the question of the induction by bodywork therapists of 'emotional release'.

If the most appropriate response an individual can make to the turmoil of their life is the 'locking away' of these in their musculoskeletal system, we need to ask if it is advisable to unlock the emotions that the tensions and contractions hold.

If there exists no current ability to psychologically process the pain that these somatic areas hold, are they not best left where they are until counselling or psychotherapy or self-awareness leads to the individual's ability to reflect, handle, deal with and eventually work through the issues and memories?

What is the advantage of triggering a release of emotions, manifested by crying, laughing, vomiting or whatever, as described by Latey and others, if neither the individual nor the manual therapist can then take the process further?

Answers?

The answers to these questions are not readily available although there are many opinions. However, it is suggested that each patient and each therapist/practitioner should reflect on these issues before removing (however gently and however temporarily) the defensive armouring that life may have obliged vulnerable individuals (all of us) to erect and maintain.

At the very least, all therapists and practitioners should learn skills which allow the safe handling of 'emotional releases', which may occur with or without deliberate efforts to induce them. Or we should have a referral process in place which leads to the patient having the ability to process, with suitably qualified practitioners, whatever is emerging from these therapeutic endeavours.

Conclusion

The exercises and discussions in this chapter have taken us to the end of this exploration of palpation potentials but certainly not to the end of the search for optimal palpation skills, which is a perpetual quest.

What should have become evident is the seamless way in which palpation becomes therapy and how manual therapy demands that palpation be continuous during its application.

Another thought is that while the therapist is touching the patient, the patient is also touching the therapist. The brief discussion of the entrainment process (see Chapter 11) might have alerted you to the chance that you are influencing the person you are touching (or perhaps not even touching) in profound ways and that this can be a two-way process.

The ultimate demand, then, is for the therapist to maintain optimal health, to be focused and centred when working, and to become so practised in palpation skills that the processes involved are performed with virtually intuitive direction.

I hope you have enjoyed this palpation journey and that this is the start of a never-ending process of exploration.

REFERENCES

Alexander FM 1931 The use of the self. Methuen, London
Barlow W 1959 Anxiety and muscle tension pain. British Journal of Clinical Practice 13(5)
Ford C 1989 Where healing waters meet. Station Hill Press, New York
Jacobson E 1930 American Journal of Physiology 91: 567
Janda V 1983 Muscle function testing. Butterworths, London
Latey P 1980 Muscular manifesto. Latey, London
Malmo R 1949 Psychosomatic Medicine 2: 9
Mayland E 1980 Rosen method. Mayland, Palo Alto, CA
Sainsbury P 1954 Journal of Neurology, Neurosurgery and Psychiatry 17: 3
Selye H 1956 The stress of life. McGraw-Hill, New York
Sherrington C 1937 Man on his nature.
Simons D, Travell J, Simons L 1999 Myofascial pain and dysfunction: the trigger point manual, vol 1, upper half of body, 2nd edn. Williams and Wilkins, Baltimore, MD
Upledger J 1987 Craniosacral therapy. Eastland Press, Seattle, WA
Waersted M, Eken T, Westgaard R 1992 Single motor unit activity in psychogenic trapezius muscle tension. Arbete och Halsa 17: 319–321
Waersted M, Eken T, Westgaard R 1993 Psychogenic motor unit activity – a possible muscle injury mechanism studied in a healthy subject. Journal of Musculoskeletal Pain 1(3/4): 185–190
Wolff H 1948 Headache and other head pains. Oxford University Press, Oxford

Appendix: location of Chapman's neurolymphatic reflexes

(See page 148 for Fig. 5.14–5.19)

No. Symptoms/area	Anterior	Fig.	Posterior	Fig.
1. Conjunctivitis and retinitis	Upper humerus	5.14	Occipital area	5.16
2. Nasal problems	Anterior aspect of first rib close to sternum	5.14	Posterior angle of the jaw on the tip of the transverse process of the first cervical vertebra	5.16
3. Arms (circulation)	Muscular attachments pectoralis minor to third, fourth and fifth ribs	5.14	Superior angle of scapula and superior third of the medial margin of the scapula	5.16
4. Tonsillitis	Between first and second ribs close to sternum	5.14	Midway between spinous process and tip of transverse process of first cervical vertebra	5.16
5. Thyroid	Second intercostal space close to sternum	5.14	Midway between spinous process and tip of transverse process of second thoracic vertebra	5.16
6. Bronchitis	Second intercostal space close to sternum	5.14	Midway between spinous process and tip of transverse process of second thoracic vertebra	5.18
7. Oesophagus	As No. 6	5.14	As No. 6	5.18
8. Myocarditis	As No. 6	5.14	Between the second and third thoracic transverse processes. Midway between the spinous process and the tip of the transverse process	5.17
9. Upper lung	Third intercostal space close to the sternum	5.14	As No. 8	5.17
10. Neuritis of upper limb	As No. 9	5.14	Between the third and fourth transverse processes, midway between the spinous process and the tip of the transverse process	5.17
11. Lower lung	Fourth intercostal space, close to sternum	5.14	Between fourth and fifth transverse processes. Midway between the spinous process and the tip of the transverse process	5.17
12. Small intestines	Eighth, ninth and tenth intercostal spaces close to cartilage	5.14	Eighth, ninth and tenth thoracic intertransverse spaces	5.16

No. Symptoms/area	Anterior	Fig.	Posterior	Fig.
13. Gastric hypercongestion	Sixth intercostal space to the left of the sternum	5.14	Sixth thoracic intertransverse space, left side	5.16
14. Gastric hyperacidity	Fifth intercostal space to the left of the sternum	5.14	Fifth thoracic intertransverse space, left side	5.19
15. Cystitis	Around the umbilicus and on the pubic symphysis close to the midline	5.14	Upper edge of the transverse processes of the second lumbar vertebra	5.19
16. Kidneys	Slightly superior to and lateral to the umbilicus	5.14	In the intertransverse space between the 12th thoracic and the first lumbar vertebrae	5.19
17. Atonic constipation	Between the anterior superior spine of the ilium and the trochanter	5.14	Eleventh costal vertebral junction	5.16
18. Abdominal tension	Superior border of the pubic bone	5.14	Tip of the transverse process of the second lumbar vertebra	5.17
19. Urethra	Inner edge of pubic ramus near superior aspect of symphysis	5.14	Superior aspect of transverse process of second lumbar vertebra	5.19
20. Dupuytren's contracture, and arm and shoulder pain	None		Anterior aspect of lateral margin of scapulae, inferior to the head of humerus	5.19
21. Cerebral congestion (related to paralysis or paresis)	(On the posterior aspect of the body) Lateral from the spines of the third, fourth and fifth cervical vertebrae	5.14	Between the transverse processes of the first and second cervical vertebrae	5.18
22. Clitoral imitation and vaginismus	Upper medial aspect of the thigh	5.14	Lateral to the junction of the sacrum and the coccyx	5.17
23. Prostate	Lateral aspect of the thigh from the trochanter to just above the knee. Also lateral to symphysis pubis as in uterine conditions (see No. 43)	5.14	Between the posterior superior spine of the ilium and the spinous process of the fifth lumbar vertebra	5.17
24. Spastic constipation or colitis	Within an area 1–2 inches wide extending from the trochanter to within an inch of the patella	5.14	From the transverse processes of the second, third and fourth lumbar vertebrae to the crest of the ilium	5.16
25. Leucorrhoea	Lower medial aspect of thigh, slightly posteriorly (on the posterior aspect of the body)	5.16	Between the posterior/superior spine of the ilium and the spinous process of the fifth lumbar vertebra	5.17
26. Sciatic neuritis	Anterior and posterior to the tibiofibular junction	5.14	1. On the sacroiliac synchondrosis 2. Between the ischial tuberosity and the acetabulum 3. Lateral and posterior aspects of the thigh	5.16
27. Torpid liver (nausea, fullness malaise)	Fifth intercostal space, from the mid-mammillary line to the sternum	5.15	Fifth thoracic intertransverse space on the right side	5.16

No. Symptoms/area	Anterior	Fig.	Posterior	Fig.
28. Cerebellar congestion (memory and concentration lapses)	Tip of coracoid process of scapula	5.15	Just inferior to the base of the skull on the first cervical vertebra	5.18
29. Otitis media	Upper edge of clavicle where it crosses the first rib	5.15	Superior aspect of first cervical transverse process (tip)	5.16
30. Pharyngitis	Anterior aspect of the first rib close to the sternum	5.15	Midway between the spinous process and the tip of the transverse process of the second cervical vertebra	5.18
31. Laryngitis	Upper surface of the second rib, 2 or 3 inches (5–8 cm) from the sternum	5.15	Midway between the spinous process and the tip of the second cervical vertebra	5.18
32. Sinusitis	Lateral to the sternum on the superior edge of the second rib in the first intercostal space	5.15	As No. 31	5.18
33. Pyloric stenosis	On the sternum	5.15	Tenth costovertebral junction on the right side	5.19
34. Neurasthenia (chronic fatigue)	All the muscular attachments of pectoralis major on the humerus, clavicle, sternum, ribs (especially fourth rib)	5.15	Below the superior medial edge of the scapula on the face of the fourth rib	5.17
35. Wry neck (torticollis)	Medial aspect of upper edge of the humerus	5.15	Transverse processes of the third, fourth, sixth and seventh cervical vertebrae	5.18
36. Splenitis	Seventh intercostal space close to the cartilaginous junction, on the left	5.15	Seventh intertransverse space on the left	5.16
37. Adrenals (allergies, exhaustion)	Superior and lateral to umbilicus	5.15	In the intertransverse space between the 11th and 12th thoracic vertebrae	5.19
38. Mesoappendix	Superior aspect of the 12th rib, close to the tip, on right	5.15	Lateral aspect of the 11th intercostal space on the right	5.16
39. Pancreas	Seventh intercostal space on the right, close to the cartilage	5.15	Seventh thoracic intertransverse space on the right	5.19
40. Liver and gall bladder congestion	Sixth intercostal space, from the mid-mammillary line to the sternum (right side)	5.14	Sixth thoracic intertransverse space, right side	5.19
41. Salpingitis or vesiculitis	Midway between the acetabulum and the sciatic notch (this is on the posterior aspect of the body)	5.19	Between the posterior superior spine of the ilium and the spinous process of the fifth lumbar vertebra	5.17
42. Ovaries	The round ligaments from the superior border of the pubic bone, inferiorly	5.15	Between the ninth and 10th intertransverse space and the 10th and 11th intertransverse space	5.17
43. Uterus	Anterior aspect of the junction of the ramus of the pubis and the ischium	5.15	Between the posterior superior spine of the ilium and the fifth lumbar spinous process	5.17

No. Symptoms/area	Anterior	Fig.	Posterior	Fig.
44. Uterine fibroma	Lateral to the symphysis, extending diagonally inferiorly	5.15	Between the tip of the transverse process of the fifth lumbar vertebra and the crest of the ilium	5.16
45. Rectum	Just inferior to the lesser trochanter	5.15	On the sacrum close to the ilium at the lower end of the iliosacral synchondrosis	5.19
46. Broad ligament (uterine involvement usual)	Lateral aspect of the thigh from the trochanter to just above the knee	5.15	Between the posterior superior spine of the ilium and the fifth lumbar spinous process	5.17
47. Groin glands (circulation and drainage of legs and pelvic organs)	Lower quarter of the sartorius muscle and its attachment to the tibia	5.15	On the sacrum close to the ilium at the lower end of the iliosacral synchondrosis	5.19
48. Haemorrhoids	Just superior to the ischial tuberosity. (These areas are on the posterior surface of the body)	5.17	On the sacrum close to the ilium, at the lower end of the iliosacral synchondrosis	5.17
49. Tongue	Anterior aspect of second rib at the cartilaginous junction with the sternum	5.14	Midway between the spinous process and the tip of the transverse process of the second cervical vertebra	5.18

Index

Page numbers in **bold** indicate figures and tables

Ford, Clyde (contd)
sense of touch, projection of, 52
somatosynthesis, 372–374
Where healing waters meet, 361–362
Forearm palpation
energy interface, 194, 195
for inherent motion, exercise, 61–62
layer palpation exercises, 68–71
Form closure, SI joint, 270, 271
Fractures, previous, and energy variation, 196
Fryett's short leg observations, 297–298
Frymann, Viola, 4–5, 47
bimanual inherent motion palpation, 62–63,
177–178
exercises, 55, 56, 58–59, 60, 61–62, 177–178
movement, evaluating, 177
off-body scanning for temperature differences,
88
palpatory pressure, 64
pulse taking, 63–64
Fulcrum
Becker's methods, 202–203, 205
Smith's `essential touch' palpation, 192, 198
Functional palpation, 235–254
atlantooccipital joint combined functional and
SCS palpation, 253–254
dynamic neutral, 235–236
Greenman's functional literacy, 247–248, 249
spinal palpation, 244–246, 248–249
Hoover's experiments, 241–243
clavicle palpation, 249–252
objectives, 236–241

G
General adaptation syndrome, Selye's, 110
Gibbons, Peter, palpation reliability debate, 24–25
Gillet test, 17–18, 267, 269–270
Glide or translation, joints, 255–256
Gluteal region and upper thigh, NMT
assessment, **131**
Goldthwaite et al, slumped posture, visceral
changes associated, 319
Goodridge, John
ease and bind palpation, 160
resistance palpation exercise, 159
Goossen, Shannon, palpation reliability debate,
25–28
Gothic shoulders, respiratory function, 330
Greenman, Philip
myofascial release techniques, 210–211
palpation
exercises, 68–71, 247, 248–249
objectives, 5
ribs, 288
spinal prescription, 167–169
three stages, 54
Grieve, referred pain, 231

H
Hair through paper, palpation exercises, 57
Half-moon vector, palpation using, exercise, 112,
193
Hamstrings
short and unstable SI joint, 13
shortness, palpation
lower fibres, 162
upper fibres, 161–162
shortness, palpation exercises for, 161–162
Hands
care of, 54
palmar surfaces, thermoreceptors, 86
as palpatory tools, 47, 51
Headache
therapeutic touch trial, 341, 343, 344
upper fist problems, 370, 371
Heat
and cold, sensations of, 48
transfer, rate of, 86

Heel lifts, short leg, objectives of correction,
299–300
High-velocity, low-amplitude thrust techniques,
palpatory proficiency for, 25
Hilton's law, 174
Hip joints
extension tests, 154, 270
F-AB-ER-E test, 16, **17**, 272
hip abduction test, 155–156
hip shift (translation) test, Johnston, 310–311
mechanical damage, lower fist problems, 365
rotation test, 309
Hoag, red reaction, 171
Hooke's Law, 191
Hoover, Harold
clavicle palpation, 249–252
ease, description of, 158
functional palpation exercises, 241–243
Horizontal cross restrictions, Ford, 373–374
Hruby, red reflex test, 174
Hutchinson, percussion, 313–315
Hyperalgesic skin zones, 82, 92–93
similarity to Varma's theories, 189
skin stretching, 93
Lewit, 93, 95, 96
and trigger points, 93
Hypermobile joints, 258
Hypertonicity, muscles
local irritation, 109–110, 111
postural muscle shortening, tests for, 158–169
tendon changes, 110
Hyperventilation, 357–360
and anxiety, 326–327
dealing with, 358–359
Hypotonicity, muscles, 153

I
Iliac outflare, 275
Iliosacral joint *see* Sacroiliac (SI) joint
Image posture, 362
Inanimate object discrimination, 57
Information, discrimination of, palpation
exercises, 64
Inhalation, complete, breathing function
assessment, 330
Inherent motion palpation, exercises, 60, 61–62,
62–63
Inspir and expir, 320
Intensity discrimination, physiology of touch, **49**
Intercostal
muscles, anterior, and abdominal palpation
assessment, 132–133
spaces
NMT assessment, 133
Interference arcing, Upledger, 189–190
Interference waves, Upledger, 206
Internal malleoli, palpation for, 273
Interneural fibrosis, 220
Interobserver reliability, palpation methods, 15,
26
Bullock-Saxton, Joanne, 21–22
Goossen, Shannon, 25–26
Lee, Diane, 28–29
Murphy, Donald, 34
Simons, David, 37
spinal levels, intertherapist ability to identify,
17
testing procedures, standardisation, 24
Interosseous changes and end-feel, 258
Interpretation of palpatory information, 54
Interpretive value, palpatory findings
Bullock-Saxton, Joanne, 24
Goossen, Shannon, 28
Lee, Diane, 30
Murphy, Donald, 36–37
Simons, David, 39
Intersegmental muscles, 119
Intervertebral joints, periosteal pain points, 147

Journals of related interest

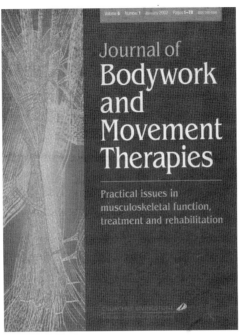
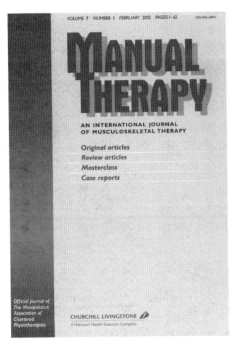
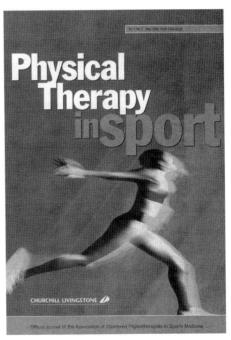
Subscribe online at
www.elsevierhealth.com

CHURCHILL LIVINGSTONE

Elsevier Limited
32 Jamestown Road, London NW1 7BY, UK
Tel: +44 (0) 208 308 5700   Fax: +44 (0) 207 424 4433
E-mail: journals@elsevierhealth.com
Call toll free in the US: 1-877-839-7126

ELSEVIER